Stroke

Stroke

Robert J. Wityk, MD, FAHA

Johns Hopkins University School of Medicine

Rafael H. Llinas, MD, FAHA

Johns Hopkins University School of Medicine

AMERICAN COLLEGE OF PHYSICIANS   PHILADELPHIA

Director, Editorial Production: Linda Drumheller
Associate Publisher and Manager, Books Publishing: Tom Hartman
Production Supervisor: Allan S. Kleinberg
Senior Production Editor: Karen C. Nolan
Publishing Coordinator: Angela Gabella
Design: Tom Hartman and Kate Nichols
Indexer: Nelle Garrecht

Printed in the United States of America
Printed by Versa Press
Composition by Scribe, Inc.

ISBN: 1-930513-70-4

The authors and publisher have exerted every effort to ensure that the drug selection and dosages set forth in this book are in accordance with current recommendations and practice at the time of publication. In view of ongoing research, occasional changes in government regulations, and the constant flow of information relating to drug therapy and drug reactions, the reader is urged to check the package insert for each drug for any change in indications and dosage and for additional warnings and precautions. This care is particularly important when the recommended agent is a new or infrequently used drug.

07 08 09 10 11 / 10 9 8 7 6 5 4 3 2 1

Contributors

Ishtiaq Ahmad, MD, PhD
Co-Director, Stroke Program
Department of Neurology
Saint Agnes Hospital
Baltimore, Maryland

Eric M. Aldrich, MD, PhD
Assistant Professor of Neurology
Johns Hopkins Hospital
Baltimore, Maryland

Anish Bhardwaj, MD, FAHA, FCCM
Professor of Neurology, Neuro-
   logical Surgery, Anesthesiology,
   and Peri-Operative Medicine
Director, Neurosciences Critical
   Care Program
Oregon Health & Science
   University
Portland, Oregon

Jaishri O. Blakeley, MD
Fellow, Department of Neurology
Johns Hopkins University School
   of Medicine
Baltimore, Maryland

Connie L. Chen, MD
Director, Stroke Unit
Neurology Consultants of Dallas
Dallas, Texas

Dorothy S. Chung, MD, PhD
Department of Neurology
Johns Hopkins University School
   of Medicine
Baltimore, Maryland

Irene Cortese, MD
Fellow, Department of Neurology
Johns Hopkins University School
   of Medicine
Baltimore, Maryland

Christopher Early, MD, PhD
Associate Professor, Department of
   Neurology
Johns Hopkins Bayview Medical
   Center
Baltimore, Maryland

Philippe Gailloud, MD
Associate Professor, Department
   of Radiology
Johns Hopkins University School
   of Medicine
Baltimore, Maryland

Romergryko Geocadin, MD
Assistant Professor
Departments of Neurology,
  Neurological Surgery &
  Anesthesiology, and Critical
  Care Medicine
Johns Hopkins University School
  of Medicine
Director, Neurosciences Critical
  Care Unit
Johns Hopkins Bayview Medical
  Center
Baltimore, Maryland

Adrian Goldszmidt, MD
Instructor, Department of
  Neurology
Johns Hopkins University School
  of Medicine
Director, Division of Neurology
Sinai Hospital of Baltimore
Baltimore, Maryland

Rebecca Gottesman, MD
Instructor, Department of
  Neurology
Johns Hopkins Hospital
Baltimore, Maryland

Argye Hillis, MD, MA
Professor of Neurology
Co-Director, Cerebrovascular
  Division
Johns Hopkins University School
  of Medicine
Baltimore, Maryland

Judy Huang, MD
Assistant Professor of Neurosurgery
Department of Neurosurgery
Johns Hopkins University School
  of Medicine
Baltimore, Maryland

Lori C. Jordan, MD
Cerebrovascular Fellow
Department of Neurology
Johns Hopkins University School
  of Medicine
Baltimore, Maryland

Matthew A. Koenig, MD
Post-Doctoral Fellow
Division of Neurocritical Care
Johns Hopkins Hospital
Baltimore, Maryland

Alan Levitt, MD
Director, Stroke Rehabilitation Unit,
  Kernan Hospital
Assistant Professor, Department
  of Medicine
University of Maryland School
  of Medicine
Baltimore, Maryland

Rafael H. Llinas, MD, FAHA
Assistant Professor of Neurology
Cerebrovascular Neurology
  Division
Johns Hopkins Bayview Medical
  Center
Baltimore, Maryland

Louise D. McCullough, MD, PhD
Assistant Professor of Neurology
  and Neuroscience
Director of Stroke Research
University of Connecticut Health
  Center
Farmington, Connecticut

Kieran Murphy, MD
Associate Professor
Department of Radiology
Director of Interventional
  Neuroradiology
Johns Hopkins Hospital
Baltimore, Maryland

Lucas Restrepo, MD
Molecular, Cellular and Integrative
  Physiology LR
Department of Physiological
  Science
University of California, Los
  Angeles
Los Angeles, California

Daniele Rigamonti, MD, FACS
Professor and Vice Chairman,
  Department of Neurosurgery
Director, Stereotactic Radiosurgery
Co-Director, Hydrocephalus
  Program
Johns Hopkins Medical Institutions
Baltimore, Maryland

Jason D. Rosenberg, MD
Assistant Professor, Department
  of Neurology
Johns Hopkins University School
  of Medicine
Baltimore, Maryland

Rafael J. Tamargo, MD, FACS
Professor, Department of
  Neurosurgery
Johns Hopkins University School
  of Medicine
Baltimore, Maryland

Quoc-Anh Thai, MD
Instructor and Assistant Chief of
  Service
Department of Neurosurgery
Johns Hopkins University School
  of Medicine
Baltimore, Maryland

George Thomas, MD, MPH
Resident, Department of Internal
  Medicine
Caritas St. Elizabeth's Medical
  Center
Boston, Massachusetts

Michel Torbey, MD, MPH, FAHA
Director, Stroke Critical Care
  Program
Director, Neurointensive Care Unit
Assistant Professor, Neurology and
  Neurosurgery
Medical College of Wisconsin
Milwaukee, Wisconsin

Robert J. Wityk, MD, FAHA
Associate Professor of Neurology
  and Medicine
Co-Director, Cerebrovascular
  Division
Johns Hopkins Hospital
Baltimore, Maryland

Foreword

When I was a medical student in the late 1960s, a "cerebrovascular accident" (CVA) was defined as the sudden or rapid onset of a neurological deficit, caused by a cerebrovascular disease, lasting longer than 24 hours. Transient ischemic attacks (TIAs) were the same except patients returned to their baseline in less than a day. It was felt that people with TIA had a much better prognosis than those with stroke. It was known that strokes could be either ischemic or hemorrhagic in nature and that carotid artery occlusion was an important cause of the former and hypertension the latter, but it was believed that atrial fibrillation was only an important contributor to strokes when there was associated significant rheumatic or congenital valvular disease.

The only available brain imaging was nuclear scanning, first with arsenic and then with technetium, methods which rarely could visualize the acutely damaged brain. When abnormalities *were* seen by these methods, they were only the largest catastrophes, usually seen days or weeks after the event. There was virtually no treatment. A few practitioners administered heparin, only to find that some strokes would become hemorrhagic, leading to a worsening of the patient's condition or even death. Neurological intensive care units did not yet exist, so most patients were nursed in the back of general medical wards where many died of aspiration pneumonia caused by the dysphagia seen in many stroke patients.

Rehabilitation was felt to be rather ineffective, and very little was known about preventing a stroke or recognizing its risk factors. Medical house officers and their mentors, even seasoned internists, were sophisticated about the care of myocardial infarction but suffered from severe therapeutic nihilism when it came to managing patients with strokes.

When one reflects on what was known about strokes in the late 1960s, it is truly remarkable how our understanding of this important group of diseases has grown in the past two generations. Yet one is still struck by the persistence of relative naivety regarding the causes, pathogenesis, and treatment of the family of illnesses that we now call stroke. By its very nature, stroke is at the interface of several fields of medicine, including neurology, internal medicine, cerebrovascular surgery, radiology, and emergency medicine. It is critical for patient care and future progress that all physicians and surgeons be conversant in the general principles of stroke prevention, treatment, and recovery. It is this challenge that is taken on in *Stroke*.

Aiming at the non-neurologist, Drs Wityk and Llinas have assembled an impressive group of experts, mostly from Johns Hopkins affiliated institutions, to create a clearly written modern manual of stroke diagnosis and treatment. Individual chapters are aimed at general approach and terminology, prevention, diagnostic testing, and treatment of the many disorders that are generally considered strokes, including carotid artery disease, cardioembolic stroke, lacunar stroke, intracerebral and subarachnoid hemorrhages, and vertebrobasilar disease. Special topics, such as stroke in the young, stroke caused by hypercoagulability, and stroke in women are given specific attention, and modern approaches to stroke rehabilitation are covered as well.

This book is very much needed. As the field of stroke has matured, it has become more and more specialized. Several large textbooks are devoted to stroke, and its own journal is sponsored by the American Heart Association, but most of this massive literature is inaccessible to non-neurologists who are intimately involved in the management of stroke patients in the real world. The fact that emergency physicians have found it so difficult to embrace the new thrombolytic therapies for acute ischemic stroke is a manifestation of the poor communication and support provided by stroke experts to those physicians on the front lines in emergency departments who must deliver immediate care. Without a clear understanding of a literature free from conflicts of interest, or the necessary neurological and neuro-imaging support that is required in real time in the emergency setting, one cannot expect emergency physicians to take on all the risk for the less-than-optimal outcomes to be expected as a new therapy evolves.

Stroke goes a long way towards closing the gap between what is known about these sudden attacks and what is actually done for patients (and for people who would like to avoid becoming patients) when they are seen in the internist's office, in the emergency department, on the wards of a general hospital, and in the rehabilitation setting. Stroke care has come a long way; this book should ensure that all relevant participants in the process know about it.

Martin A. Samuels, MD, DSc(Hon), FAAN, FACP
Chairman and Neurologist-in-Chief, Department of Neurology
Brigham and Women's Hospital
Boston, Massachusetts

Contents

Chapter 1

Overview of the Approach to the Stroke Patient

RAFAEL H. LLINAS, MD

Medical terminology will often vary depending on the specialty or subspecialty of the practitioner who is using it: practitioners in one specialty may use different terms than clinicians in another specialty to refer to the same disorders or to express the same concepts. The authors of the chapters in this text are neurologists and neurosurgeons, but the chapters are written with the needs of non-neurologists in mind. Therefore, this chapter introduces the terminology used throughout the rest of the text. Additionally, it reviews basic neuroanatomy and briefly introduces the clinical approach to patients with different types of stroke.

Definitions and Semantics in Stroke

"Stroke" is a general term used to describe a focal neurologic event that is acute in onset and may have a vascular cause, etiology, or relevance. Adjectives can be added to make this general term more specific; for example, hemorrhagic stroke, ischemic stroke, lacunar stroke, embolic stroke, young stroke, thrombotic stroke, spinal cord stroke, venous stroke, brainstem stroke, and cerebellar stroke. In general the adjective before the word stroke suggests etiology and is more specific than the term "cerebral vascular accident (CVA)," which is not used by many stroke neurologists. This is because strokes are, in fact, "not always cerebral, not necessarily primarily vascular, and *never* an accident."

Stroke can occur in the brainstem, cerebellum, or spinal cord and is therefore not always cerebral. While strokes are typically vascular-origin neurologic lesions, hypercoaguable states cause stroke and may be defined as rheumatologic or hematologic events. Finally, stroke is not an accident.

It is most often due to predictable causes such as a family history of stroke, atrial fibrillation, and carotid stenosis, and sometimes preventable causes such as smoking and elevated cholesterol levels. Furthermore, referring to them as accidents only adds to the mystery that many clinicians associate with stroke.

"Brain-attack" is a newer term for acute stroke. This term was coined primarily to add acuity to the concept of stroke and perhaps to try to move away from the CVA term. It is meant to be accessible to laypersons, utilizing the familiarity of the term "heart attack" and implying that "brain attack" has a similar etiology. Use of the term is also intended to change the perception of stroke as a horrible medical problem with no treatment that will cause death or permanent dependency: brain-attack sounds like a medical emergency for which there are emergency treatments. This is entirely acceptable; however, patients know what a stroke is and, ironically, sometimes struggle with the term "brain-attack."

Ischemic Stroke

Ischemic stroke accounts for 80% of stroke. Ischemic stroke is defined as an acute interruption of blood to the brain, cerebellum, brainstem, or spinal cord in a focal area leading to infarction. Generalized loss of blood flow to the brain due to profound hypotension or anoxia is typically referred to as hypoxic/ischemic injury but can produce focal ischemia and infarction, as in stroke, on imaging. Ischemic stroke results in bland (non-hemorrhagic) ischemia and infarction in a typically vascular distribution. The vascular distribution is often very helpful in differentiating stroke from tumor or demyelination. Ischemic stroke can be caused by emboli from the heart due to atrial fibrillation or emboli from large arteries such as the carotid artery stenosis. These are often referred to as embolic stroke when an embolic source is found. Thrombotic strokes are when there is an occlusion of a cerebral artery without a proximal embolic source, often from local atherosclerotic disease resulting in stenosis and occlusion. Thrombosis can also occur secondary to arterial dissection or from hypercoaguable states. Both are referred to as ischemic stroke, but "embolic" or "thrombotic" indicates specific stroke etiology.

Hemorrhagic Stroke

The term "hemorrhagic stroke" refers to events in the central nervous system that are caused by too much blood or bleeding into the brain instead of bland ischemic infarcts. Of note, ischemic stroke can undergo hemorrhagic conversion of a bland infarct, acutely becoming a hemorrhagic infarct due to reperfusion. The way to differentiate bland from hemorrhagic strokes is with imaging. Computed tomography (CT) or magnetic resonance imaging (MRI) can quickly differentiate between bland and hemorrhagic strokes. It is extremely difficult to differentiate one from another on purely clinical grounds. Severity of deficit, headaches, nausea, vomiting, and hypertension are signs classically found in hemorrhagic stroke but can be found in large ischemic strokes also. Causes of hemorrhagic stroke are most commonly hypertension, vascular malformations, abnormalities of cerebral blood vessels, venous occlusions, hemorrhagic transformation of ischemic strokes, and bleeding disorders. Treatment tends to be more supportive or surgical for expanding hemorrhages or hemorrhages from aneurysms. Subarachnoid hemorrhages refer to blood collection within the space below the arachnoid layer but above the pial layer where arteries run. Ruptured aneurysms, vascular malformations, and trauma lead to subarachnoid hemorrhages. See Chapters 15, 16, and 17 for more information.

Lacunar Stroke

Lacunar stroke is an ischemic stroke. "Lacune" comes from the French word for lake. It implies an etiology of small vessel atherosclerotic disease and arteriosclerosis (lipohyalinosis) and thrombosis. The arterioles that thrombose are the small penetrating arterioles in the brain. It implies a thrombotic etiology and not an embolic etiology, although small emboli can resemble lacunar strokes on imaging. Work-up for this type of stroke revolves around ruling out an embolic source. Lacunar strokes tend to be small, 1.5 cm or less, and involve the deep white matter and brainstem. The deficits can be dense initially, but the recovery is usually excellent. Stroke syndromes that are classically lacunar are discussed in Chapter 11.

Transient Ischemic Attack

Transient ischemic attack (TIA) is a neurologic deficit thought to be of vascular origin that lasts less than 24 hours. In fact, TIAs typically last less than 30 minutes. Most deficits that last longer are actually resolving stroke (cell death occurs). TIAs can be of embolic, hemorrhagic, or thrombotic origin and can occur due to local hypoperfusion of the brain. Hypoperfusion states, like systemic drops in blood pressure, can present with transient neurologic events when there is a high-grade stenosis of an intracerebral or extracerebral artery. TIAs don't tend to be hemorrhagic, with the exception of subdural hematoma and multiple micro-hemorrhages of amyloid antipathy, which can present like ischemic TIAs. Classically, TIAs are ischemic in origin with carotid artery stenosis and intracranial stenosis presenting with increasingly frequent TIAs. TIAs should be worked up quickly; they are the neurologic equivalent to unstable angina. Rates of stroke after TIA can be as high as 4%-8% in 30 days and 24%-29% in 5 years (1). TIAs are discussed in Chapter 3.

Epidemiology of Stroke

Ischemic stroke is similar in prevalence and epidemiology to ischemic heart disease. Often physicians and patients alike underestimate the rate and impact of stroke, especially in relation to cardiac disease or Alzheimer's disease.

Stroke is the third leading cause of death in the US in those 40 or more years old, ranking just below cancer and heart disease. Stroke, not Alzheimer's disease, is the most common cause of disability and long-term care. The monetary cost to society is upwards of $40 billion per year, of which only a relatively small amount goes to medical professionals and for medication (2.2 and 0.3 billion, respectively). Most of the money, $24.2 billion, goes to hospital costs and nursing home costs due to the high rate of long-term disability associated with the disease (2).

There are 700,000 new or recurrent strokes each year: one stroke every 45 seconds and 275,000 deaths per year. There are 4,700,000 stroke survivors alive today (2). Strokes are 80% ischemic and 20% hemorrhagic in origin. Approximately 8% to 12% of ischemic strokes and 37% to 38% of hemorrhagic strokes are fatal. According to a study looking at the number of hospital patients (3.2 million) admitted with various vascular diagnoses, 1,094,000 were diagnosed with coronary atherothrombosis, 1,010,000 with cerebrovascular disease, 783,000 with acute myocardial infarction, and 308,000 with other ischemic heart disease (4).

What the public knows about stroke is variable and dependent on local education efforts. Although a majority of patients polled know what a stroke is and how it presents, only 25% can name a single stroke symptom (Table 1-1). Sudden onset of these symptoms needs to be addressed immediately if the symptoms are felt to be of vascular origin. Education of patients and their physicians clearly is extremely important. With improved identification of the illness by the patient and the primary care provider, more patients can be treated acutely, and stroke can be prevented by correctly diagnosing and working up transient ischemic attacks.

The risk factors for stroke are similar to those of ischemic heart disease (Table 1-2). Fortunately medical professionals addressing cardiovascular risk factors are also addressing primary stroke prevention. Secondary prevention of stroke is an important issue and revolves primarily around finding the cause of the stroke and addressing the etiology to reduce

---

Table 1-1   Acute Stroke Symptoms

- Sudden onset of weakness or numbness
- Sudden onset of problems speaking
- Sudden onset of problems seeing
- Sudden onset of dizziness or problems walking
- Sudden onset of headache

Table 1-2   Major Risk Factors for Stroke

• Smoking	• Diabetes
• Hypertension	• Family history
• High cholesterol	• Coronary artery disease

recurrence. Chapter 2 deals in more detail with primary and secondary prevention of ischemic stroke.

The high rate of stroke, especially in relation to heart disease, puts into perspective the large numbers of stroke patients that we see. Clearly, in terms of primary prevention of stroke, every intervention is a significant reduction not only in death from stroke but also in the disability that can come with stroke. Education for patients and their health care professionals regarding stroke is of the utmost importance. It will increase the number of patients who present early and increase the amount of identification and control of modifiable stroke risk factors in at-risk populations.

Review of Basic Neuroanatomy

A review of basic neuroanatomy is necessary here. Understanding this subject is of the utmost importance in examining and determining localization and risk in stroke patients. In general, although exceptions exist, the larger the stroke, the more likely is a poor outcome and the more likely it is that swelling after the stroke will cause a worsening and life-threatening situation. Therefore, determining size and location of strokes is important. CT scanning will not show acute strokes for 6-24 hours, so clinical impression and diagnosis is important (Figure 1-1). MRI can detect stroke earlier, especially with diffusion-weighted imaging (DWI). This will be discussed in Chapter 4.

Vascular Anatomy

The anatomy of the vasculature of the brain, cerebellum, and brainstem can be boiled down to the distribution of four basic arteries (Figures 1-2, *A*, and 1-3). Blood enters the brain through a left and right carotid artery in the anterior neck and through right and left vertebral arteries in the posterior neck. Within the brain these arteries form a circle called the *circle of Willis*. The junction of the carotid arteries and anterior cerebral arteries forms the anterior portion of the circle of Willis. This circle is of great importance because it is the source of collateral flow. An intact circle of Willis can help compensate for a vertebral or even carotid occlusion. Posterior communicating arteries join the internal carotid arteries to the posterior cerebral arteries (PCAs), which arise from a joining of the two vertebral arteries, called the *basilar artery*.

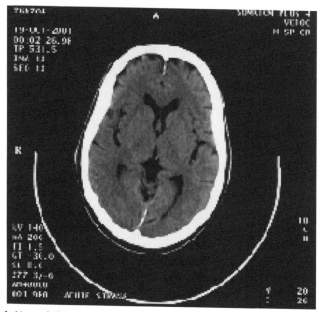

Figure 1-1 Normal CT scan in a patient with clinical evidence of a very large right-hemisphere stroke. CT scan done in the first 3–4 hours. Stroke visible on CT imaging 24 hours later.

Anterior Cerebral Artery

Anterior cerebral arteries (ACAs) are paired arteries coming off each carotid artery, running anteriorly. They supply blood to the anterior most portions of the brain and superiorly along the medial portion of the hemisphere of the brain. Occlusion of the ACA gives a typical appearance of frontal and medial cerebral infarction as seen in Figure 1-4. The anterior cerebral artery provides blood to the medial portion of the cerebral cortex. The ACA vascular territory serves the contralateral hip and leg area motor and sensory cortex, sparing other parts of the body. ACA stroke can present with unilateral leg weakness and numbness along with abulia (a decrease in cognitive spontaneity) and urinary incontinence (Table 1-3).

Middle Cerebral Artery

The middle cerebral artery (MCA) comes off the carotid artery and moves laterally and posteriorly. It supplies blood to the largest portion of the cortex. Branches of the MCA feed the frontal lobe, temporal lobe, and parietal lobe, as well as much of the deep white matter. Strokes of the entire MCA are devastating (Figure 1-5). Damage to left frontal lobe (in right-handed people) will cause frontal aphasias (expressive or Broca's aphasias). Right frontal strokes may have no aphasia at all. The frontal lobe of the brain also

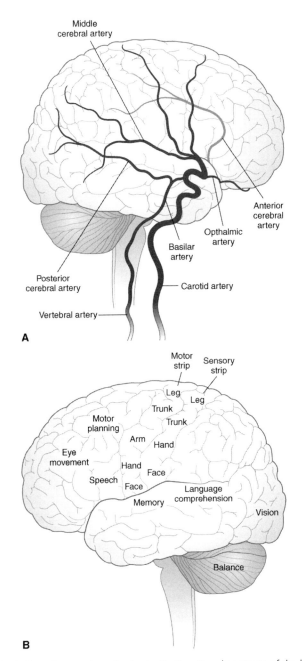

Figure 1-2. **A**, Vascular supply to the brain. **B**, Functional anatomy of the brain.

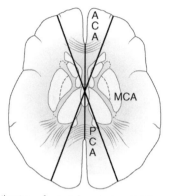

Figure 1-3 Vascular distribution of arterial occlusion (ACA = anterior cerebral artery territory; MCA = middle cerebral artery territory; PCA = posterior cerebral artery territory) as seen on CT or MRI. See Table 1-3.

Table 1-3 Cerebral Artery Stroke Syndromes

Artery	Area Affected	Clinical Deficits
ACA	Medial frontal lobe Medial parietal lobe	Weakness/numbness Contralateral leg Abulia Urinary incontinence
MCA	Frontal lobe Temporal lobe Parietal lobe	Aphasia Gaze deviation Hemiplegia (face/arm) Sensory loss Neglect
PCA	Medial temporal lobe Occipital lobe	Memory loss, confusion Loss of vision in one visual field

controls horizontal eye movements and when damaged in the acute setting will lead to forced gaze deviation away from the weak side of the body. Hemiplegia results from damage to the motor cortex with weakness and spasticity affecting contralateral face and arm, and leg to a lesser extent. Damage to parietal lobe causes sensory loss and neglects. Neglect is when patients with parietal lobe dysfunction lose the ability to attend to stimuli. Right hemisphere damage produces the densest neglect. These patients may ignore visual and sensory stimuli, including family and objects around them. Damage to temporal lobe causes posterior aphasias (receptive or Wernicke's aphasias), as well auditory neglect, the ignoring of auditory stimuli. The MCA has many branches; therefore, branch occlusions of the MCA can present with one or more of the above symptoms and signs without all being present.

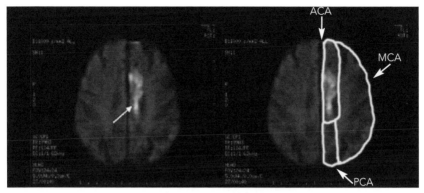

Figure 1-4 Diffusion weighted MRI of an anterior cerebral artery stroke (*left arrow*). Vascular distributions of ACA, MCA, and PCA are outlined by arrows at right.

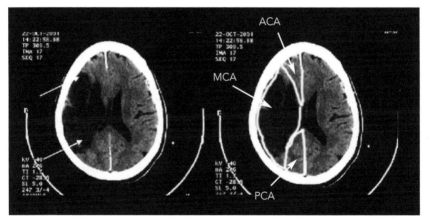

Figure 1-5 Middle cerebral artery stroke seen on head CT scan (*left arrows*). Vascular distributions of MCA, ACA, and PCA are outlined by arrows at right.

Posterior Cerebral Artery

Posterior cerebral arteries (PCAs) arise from the posterior circulation. The vertebral arteries join to form the basilar artery (Figure 1-2) and then divide again to form the PCAs. Each PCA feeds the occipital lobe of the brain as well as the medial temporal lobe and much of a deep structure called the *thalamus* (Figure 1-6). Classically, PCA stroke causes damage to visual fibers in the occipital lobe, leading to visual field cuts or a homonymous hemianopia. That is loss of vision in both eyes contralateral to the occipital stroke (Table 1-3).

Vertebral Artery

The vertebral arteries enter the skull after running in the transverse foramen in the cervical vertebral bodies. Before they join they give off a posterior

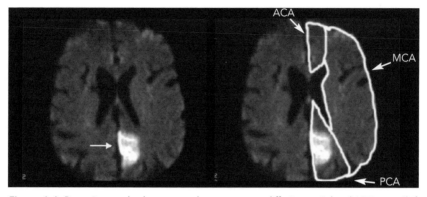

Figure 1-6 Posterior cerebral artery stroke as seen on diffusion-weighted MRI scan (*left arrow*). Vascular distributions of ACA, MCA, and PCA are outlined by arrows at right.

inferior cerebellar artery (PICA) that feeds blood to the cerebellum and the lateral part of the medulla in the brainstem. Occlusion of the vertebral artery can lead to stroke involving both the cerebellum and brainstem. Vertigo, hiccups, ipsilateral Horner's syndrome, ipsilateral facial sensory loss with contralateral body sensory loss, hemiataxia, and palatal weakness can result.

Basilar Artery

The basilar artery is one of the most important arteries in the brain and comprises most of the blood flow in the posterior circulation. It is formed by the joining of the two vertebral arteries. It divides to form multiple arteries at the level of the pons and midbrain (brainstem). It also divides to form both the anterior inferior cerebellar artery (AICA) and the superior cerebellar artery (SCA), which feed the cerebellum not supplied by the PICA. At the distal portion, the basilar artery divides again to form two PCAs. Basilar artery strokes are extremely dangerous and can be difficult to diagnose.

Because the single basilar artery divides downstream and supplies both sides of the brainstem and cerebellum, occlusion of the single basilar artery can lead to bilateral brainstem and cerebellar strokes. The PCAs arise from the basilar artery and feed the bilateral occipital lobes and thalamus. The thalamus does many things but is vital in keeping people awake. Damage to the thalamus can result in coma. Thus a basilar artery occlusion can result in bilateral large cerebellar strokes, bilateral pontine and midbrain strokes, and bilateral thalamic strokes. Clinically, this is an unresponsive, comatose person with disconjugate gaze, poor swallow, and inability to protect the airway. Patients with complete basilar artery occlusion often die from cerebellar edema and cranial nerve dysfunction. See Chapter 12 for details of vertebral and basilar artery stroke (Figure 1-7).

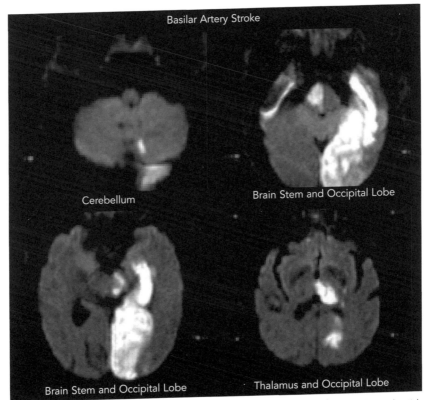

Figure 1-7 Diffusion weighted MRI of a classic basilar artery distribution stroke with midbrain, cerebellar, and occipital lobe involvement.

Clinical Anatomy of the Brain

The brain is separated into lobes of the cerebrum: frontal, temporal, parietal, and occipital. The cerebellum is in the back of the brain below the occipital lobe and behind the brainstem. The brainstem is made up of a midbrain, pons, and medulla (Figure 1-8). Different parts of the brain serve different functions. By examining a patient one can determine what areas of the brain are damaged and what cerebral artery must be involved. The larger the stroke, the more likely is a poor prognosis and the more likely a cerebral edema will occur. So localization is not just an academic exercise.

Frontal Lobe

The frontal lobe of the brain is the largest lobe in human beings. It begins in the frontal pole back to the central sulcus. The frontal lobe is where higher cortical function occurs. Frontal lobe damage can result in personality changes, aggression, irritability, or lethargy.

The damage to the far frontal poles may be almost clinically silent. The patient may have no weakness or aphasia because the damage is anterior

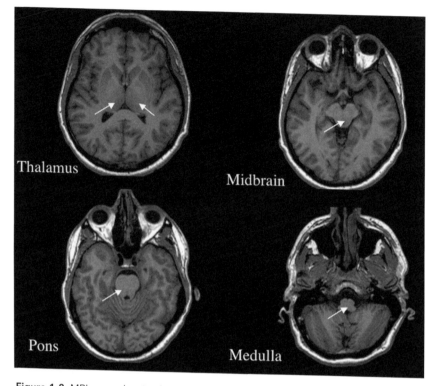

Figure 1-8 MRI scans showing basic anatomy of the brainstem.

to these "eloquent" areas. Frontal pole lesions can present with depression or abulia when damaged. Abulia is defined as a lack of spontaneity. Classically these patients are described as "like a bump on a log." Patients will often be awake but not answer questions. In fact, they can comprehend and speak but require time to answer. Sometimes as much as 30 seconds between question and answer pass, so if the examiner does not give the patient enough time, his response may be missed and the patient labeled as mute. The ACA feeds the frontal pole.

The frontal eye fields are found in the frontal lobes. Damage to the frontal eye fields leads to weakness in horizontal gaze. Therefore when a patient presents with left frontal lobe damage, there can be conjugate gaze forced deviation toward the side of the lesion. This occurs because the right eye field pulls the eyes toward the left. If the right frontal lobe is damaged, there is an inability to move eyes to the left, and the eyes drift conjugately to the right. Another way to remember this concept is that frontal lobe damage causes the eyes to look away from the hemiplegia in cortical stroke. The frontal artery branch of the MCA feeds this area.

Pre-frontal cortex damage can result in problems with praxis. *Apraxia* is defined as having normal strength and sensation but being unable to produce a motor pattern correctly. For instance, an apractic patient may have normal hand strength and sensation and can move the hand normally but be unsure how to salute, use a doorknob, or pretend to use a hammer. Apraxia can occur with damage to either frontal lobe. Oral apraxias also occur, with patients having normal motor strength in the face and mouth but inability to blow a kiss or use a straw. The MCA typically feeds the prefrontal cortex.

The posterior frontal lobe on the left is where speech is produced (Table 1-4). Broca's aphasias can occur with left frontal lobe damage. The left frontal lobe is most often the speech-dominant lobe in right-handed people. Therefore, left Broca's area strokes present with aphasia in right-handed people. This may not be the case in left-handed people. Patients with Broca's aphasia (or expressive aphasia) cannot produce language normally. Patients who communicate with sign language cannot sign. Patients with Broca's aphasia cannot write. This is an important trick in differentiating severe slurred speech from aphasia. Broca's aphasia patients do not have fluent speech. They cannot string five words together, they stutter, and they become frustrated with their inability to produce speech. They cannot name objects. They cannot repeat phrases. A typical sentence used for testing of expressive aphasias is "There are no ifs, ands, or buts." Patients with Broca's aphasia can understand normally and can read and comprehend written language.

In the most posterior aspect of the frontal lobe is the motor cortex. Damage to this area results in weakness or hemiplegia. Typically there will be weakness in the face and arm and leg with motor cortex damage. There will often be increased tone, reflexes, and an up-going toe (Babinski sign) after the acute setting has passed. The ipsilateral brain controls motor strength in the contralateral body. Left-brain controls right body. Therefore,

Table 1-4   Aphasias by Type, Location, and Presentation

Type	Area Involved	Clinical Picture
Broca's aphasia (expressive aphasia)	Frontal lobe	Non-fluent speech Cannot repeat Cannot write Can understand well
Wernicke's aphasia (receptive aphasia)	Temporal/parietal lobe	Fluent speech, nonsensical Cannot repeat Cannot write Cannot understand
Global aphasia	Frontal/temporal/parietal	Non-fluent speech Cannot repeat Cannot write Cannot understand

Adapted from Damasio AR. Aphesia. N Engl J Med. 1992; 326:531–9.

right-handed patients with a left frontal stroke will often have Broca's aphasia and a right face-arm and some leg weakness.

Temporal Lobe

The temporal lobe of the brain serves to organize hearing and memory. It has no clear sensory or motor finding, so lesions of the temporal lobe can often be missed. The temporal lobe is separated into lateral and medial areas. The medial and lateral temporal lobes have different vascular distributions and different functions.

The damage to the lateral temporal lobe results in cortical deafness, which is rare. It primarily presents with inability to hear sound simultaneously in both ears. Some forms of neglect can also occur with temporal lobe damage. Within the temporal lobes also run the optic radiations. These are the fiber tracts where the visual information passes back from the eye to the occipital lobe. Thus interruption of these fibers can result in a visual field cut. Branches of the MCA feed the lateral temporal lobes.

The medial temporal lobes primarily are the center for memory. Medial temporal lobe damage leads to the inability to lay down new memory. The medial temporal lobes have a different vascular distribution than the lateral temporal lobe. Medial temporal lobes are fed by the PCAs.

Parietal Lobe

The parietal lobe lies behind the central sulcus, in front of the occipital lobe, and above the temporal lobe. It has several complex functions. The most clinically relevant neurologic problems that present with damage to these areas are sensory loss and neglect. The sensory cortex lies within the parietal lobe. Loss of the ability to feel on one side of the body is typical of parietal lobe lesions. Neglects often occur with parietal lobe damage. This is particularly the case in the right parietal lobe but can occur on the left also. Neglects refer to the propensity for patients to ignore visual or somato-sensory input. Patients with parietal lobe lesions will ignore stimuli, visual or otherwise, when presented contralateral to the stroke. The optic radiations run through the parietal lobe also. Damage to the deep white matter in the parietal lobe can present with visual field cuts. A posterior aphasia or Wernicke's aphasia (Table 1-4) can occur with damage to the temporal/parietal area. The parietal lobe is primarily fed by the MCA.

Occipital Lobe

Occipital lobe lesions primarily present with vision loss. Occipital lobe strokes present with a homonymous hemianopia, meaning that the visual field will be lost on one side. Patients will lose vision on the right-hand side of both eyes, for instance. It does not present with monocular blindness, although patients may describe not being able to see out of one eye. Even a cursory examination of the affected eye reveals that the patient can see but has lost vision in just one field. It is common for patients with occipital strokes to have hallucinations within the affected field. A less common syndrome that is caused by occipital strokes is alexia without agraphia (patient cannot read but can write normally). The occipital lobe is primarily fed by the PCA.

Brainstem

The brainstem is divided into three major components: the midbrain, pons, and medulla. The key to brainstem lesions is that patients present with crossed findings. The findings can be sensory or motor. The classic brainstem presentation is of ipsilateral cranial nerve deficits with a contralateral motor or sensory loss. The ipsilateral deficits are due to the cranial nerve nucleus damage, and the contralateral motor or sensory findings are due to damage to descending/ascending tracts.

The midbrain is where the nucleus of the oculomotor nerve (cranial nerve III), trochlear nerve (cranial nerve IV), and the top of the reticular activating system are located. Motor, sensory, and coordination tracts also run through the midbrain. Cranial nerve III pulls the eye in toward the nose, up toward the forehead. It also constricts the pupil. A CN III palsy presents with a large, poorly reactive pupil that cannot pull in toward the nose or look up. Double vision is a typical presentation given the lack of normal yoking of the two eyes. Cranial nerve IV turns the eye in and down. Damage to CN IV presents with diplopia looking down and a head tilt. The reticular activating system mediates wakefulness, and damage to this area can result in coma. Thus, a typical midbrain lesion may present with ipsilateral CN III palsy and a contralateral hemiplegia. The midbrain is fed from small perforating arteries from the basilar artery and PCAs.

The pons is below the midbrain and is where the abducens nerve (CN VI) and the facial nerve (CN VII) reside. Cranial nerve VI pulls the eye out toward the temple. Lesions of CN VI present with diplopia and inability to look all the way out with one eye. Cranial nerve VII moves the face on the ipsilateral side. Facial nerve lesions at the pons can present with facial weakness of the upper and lower face. This is different than the typical facial weakness with cortical stroke that presents with lower facial weakness only. Again, contralateral numbness and/or weakness can also occur.

The medulla is below the pons. It is where the lower cranial nerves (VIII, IX, X, XII) are found. Vestibular cochlear nerve (CN VIII) damage presents with vertigo. The glossopharyngeal nerve (CN IX) presents with reduction in ability to lift the ipsilateral palate. Vagus nerve (CN X) damage presents with reduced gag as well as cardiac arrhythmias. Hypoglossial nerve (CN XII) damage presents with ipsilateral tongue weakness. Thus medullary strokes can present subtly with vertigo, hiccups, and inability to move the palate normally. There is often ipsilateral facial numbness, contralateral body numbness, and ataxia due to damage to cerebellar fibers. The medulla is fed by perforating small arteries from the vertebral artery.

Cerebellum

The cerebellum is above the brainstem and below the occipital lobes. The cerebellum primarily allows smooth movements. Thus ataxia is the primary problem with cerebellar strokes. Vertigo, ataxia, and falling to one side can often be the only presenting symptoms for large cerebellar strokes. Ataxia is tested through finger-to-nose and heel-to-shin testing. More sensitive is mirror testing, where a patient is asked to point her finger at the examiner's finger as if the patient is pointing into a mirror. The examiner moves his finger and the patient follows. Quick movements with quick stops will cause the patient to overshoot the target and then re-correct on one side more than the other.

It is important to recall that the fibers from the cerebellum are double-crossed. While motor and sensory fibers cross once and lead to, for instance, a left-sided stroke causing right-sided symptoms and signs, cerebellar lesions cause deficits on the same side of the stroke. Thus, left cerebellar strokes lead to left-sided ataxia. The primary concern is swelling of the cerebellum, which can lead to closing of the fourth ventricle and obstructive hydrocephalus. This is a potentially fatal complication from a stroke that may have subtle findings and symptoms. The cerebellum is fed by branches of the basilar artery, superior cerebellar artery, anterior inferior cerebellar artery, and posterior inferior cerebellar artery.

Case Study 1-1

A 72-year-old man with atrial fibrillation presents with acute onset of problems speaking. On examination he has an inability to produce language; he can understand but not repeat. He cannot write. He has weakness on the right-hand side with increased tone and reflexes. His right toe goes up in a Babinski sign.

Discussion

This is a fairly typical presentation of a stroke. The patient has a history of atrial fibrillation and presents with acute onset of neurologic deficits. Examination shows an aphasia. Because the patient cannot write, this is not a severe dysarthria or other speech issue but is typical for most aphasias. Most right-handed people have speech in the left hemisphere of the brain. The patient has trouble repeating and is not fluent, but he can understand. These findings make this a *Broca's aphasia*, also called an *expressive* or *anterior aphasia*. These aphasias usually occur from strokes in the frontal lobe. The patient has weakness on the right side with increased tone, increased reflexes, and an up-going toe. This confirms the left hemisphere involvement. There is no sensory involvement; there is no neglect or visual field cut. Therefore, we can assume that the entire MCA was not involved, just a branch supplying blood to the frontal lobe. History and physical exam are consistent with a left MCA stroke likely involving the superior division of that artery which feeds just the anterior part of the MCA distribution.

Case Study 1-2

A 67-year-old woman with hypertension and diabetes presents to your office with acute onset of unsteadiness and vertigo. She says that it occurred acutely and that at first there was severe spinning, which is less severe now. She is mildly nauseated only. Movement makes her dizzier, but there is not one direction or type of movement that makes the dizziness worse. She has direction-changing nystagmus, and her walking is very unsteady, with no ability to walk in a tandem fashion. There is ataxia on the left on finger-to-nose testing.

Discussion

Vertigo is a complex issue. It can be very hard to differentiate vertigo from central causes versus vertigo from Meniere's disease or benign positional paroxysmal vertigo. In general, vertigo from central causes is milder. There is usually less severe spinning and vomiting in the acute stages. Nystagmus is often direction changing and seen in multiple directions of gaze. The gait in both peripheral vertigo and central vertigo may be abnormal. Both causes can lead to patients listing to one side or the other. In general, patients with central vertigos list to one side much more than than expected for their mild vertigo. Lastly, ataxia is a crucial diagnostic clue. Peripheral vertigo never has ataxia as part of the exam complex. Finger-to-nose testing and heel-to-shin should be normal in peripheral vertigo. Given the isolated vertigo and ataxia without description of cranial nerve defects, this patient likely has had an isolated cerebellar stroke involving the left cerebellum. It is difficult to say which artery is involved in this particular case given the limited description; imaging will answer that question.

Case Study 1-3

A 78-year-old right-handed man with a significant history of elevated cholesterol, hypertension, and diabetes presents to an emergency room with his wife. His wife says that there has been something wrong with his left-hand side over the last 4 hours, but the patient denies this. On examination he is found to ignore visual and tactile stimuli presented on the left. He continues to deny his own deficits. He has a left facial weakness. There is reduced sensation on the left face, arm, and leg. There is, in fact, profound weakness on the left affecting the upper and lower extremity. He has increased reflexes and an up-going toe on the left. CT scan is normal. Carotid Dopplers in the ER are normal.

Discussion

This man has numerous stroke risk factors and presents with a hemiplegia and three kinds of neglect. The first is anosagnosia, which is neglect of one's own weakness or neurologic deficits. He neglects visual stimuli, which can resemble a visual field cut very closely. He also neglects somatosensory input. He is unaware of being touched. (Patients will often think they are being touched in a different area if a painful stimulus is applied.) Neglects of these kinds typically localize to frontal or parietal areas. There is a hemiplegia, weakness with increased tone, reflexes, and up-going toe. This is consistent with frontal lobe damage specifically to the motor strip in the frontal lobe. This stroke likely lies with within the frontal and parietal lobe. These areas are fed by the MCA. The CT scan is normal because the onset of the stroke occurred less than 6-24 hours before. The carotid Doppler is normal, but this could be an embolic stroke from the heart or a thrombotic stroke secondary to atherosclerotic disease and occlusion within the MCA.

Case Study 1-4

A 55-year-old woman presents to your office describing loss of vision in one eye. She states that, when walking, she noted blurred vision in the right eye and then couldn't see anything on that side. She began walking into things on the right side. She noted that she could only read one half of sentences in the newspaper. She often missed the right half of sentences on road signs. Her examination shows no significant neglect or aphasias. There is a normal strength and coordination exam. Her reflexes and tone are normal. Her cranial nerve exam shows that she cannot see a moving finger on the right field in either eye. The right eye can see but only in the left half of the visual field.

Discussion

Monocular blindness is a fairly classic presentation for ocular stroke from an embolus from the ipsilateral carotid artery. But this is not such a case. This woman does not have right eye blindness. She has lost the right half of vision in both eyes. This is a right visual field cut. Clues in the history are that she loses half of words and signs that do not occur with monocular blindness any more than you lose the ability to read sentences on this page when you close one eye. Field cuts can occur in the occipital lobe, as well as in the parietal and temporal lobes, but the latter two tend to present with quadrant defects. The most likely area to have been damaged and to present with a visual field cut without other findings is an occipital lobe lesion from a posterior cerebral artery occlusion.

Case Study 1-5

A 45-year-old man is brought to the ER comatose. He was well 4 hours before, but complained of double vision, dizziness, nausea, vomiting, and right-sided weakness. He progressed quickly to an unresponsive state. He is intubated in the ambulance due to poor ability to control secretions. On examination he is unresponsive to vocal or tactile stimuli. His cranial nerve exam shows a large unresponsive right pupil and a left facial weakness. His gaze is very dysconjugate. He moves the left side better to pain than the right side, but both are weak. His arterial blood gas, electrolytes, and liver function panel are normal. CT scan is normal.

Discussion

This man presents with vertigo, nausea, and right-sided weakness and lapses into coma. His exam shows crossed finding with left facial weakness and right-body weakness and an unreactive pupil due to midbrain damage. There is a dysconjugate gaze. This is consistent with brainstem dysfunction in the pons, midbrain, and probably medulla. There is reticular activating system damage presenting with coma from the midbrain damage or possibly from bilateral thalamic damage. There is evidence of bilateral brainstem damage at several levels. A single arterial occlusion can cause this syndrome. It would be a basilar artery occlusion causing bilateral brainstem and thalamic strokes. The strokes are too acute to see on CT, although they would be evident on MRI.

Case Study 1-6

A 79-year-old woman presents to the ER with acute onset of weakness. The deficits began 6 hours ago. She is awake but is unable to speak or understand spoken or written language. She makes only moaning sounds. She responds poorly to tactile or visual stimuli presented on the right. Her eyes are deviated to the left, and she cannot bring her eyes to or past the midline. There is a dense facial weakness on the right. Her right side is completely hemiplegic; there is no movement to painful stimuli in the right arm and only trace movement in the right leg. There are increased reflexes and an up-going toe on the right. She is unresponsive to painful stimuli applied anywhere on the right side.

Discussion

This woman presents with multiple signs, which can be confusing. She has an aphasia that is expressive (cannot speak) and is receptive (cannot comprehend). In this case it is because she has a global aphasia due to damage to both frontal temporal and parietal lobes. She has a visual and somatosensory neglect ignoring stimuli presented on the right. This is due to parietal lobe damage from stroke. She has forced gaze deviation. She cannot move her eyes to the right at all, so the eyes deviate to the left. This is due to damage to the frontal eye fields on the right in the frontal lobe. The dense hemiplegia on the right is due to damage to the motor strip in the frontal lobe. The absent tactile sensation is due to damage to the sensory cortex in the parietal lobe. Thus, we have a patient with frontal, temporal, and parietal lobe damage. This is consistent with entire-distribution MCA stroke.

REFERENCES

1. Sacco RL, Wolf PA, Gorelick PB. Risk factors and their management for stroke presentation: outlook for 1999 and beyond. Neurology. 1999;53(Supp4):S15-S24.
2. American Heart Association. 2000 Heart and Stroke Statistical Update.
3. Pulsinelli WA. Cerebrovascular diseases. In: Cecil Textbook of Medicine. New York: Elsevier; 1996.
4. Hall MJ. 1998 Summary: National Hospital Discharge Survey. Advance Data, National Center for Health Statistics; 30 June 2000; No. 316.

Chapter 2

Risk Factors and Primary and Secondary Prevention of Stroke

RAFAEL H. LLINAS, MD
CHRISTOPHER EARLEY, MD, PHD

Key Points

- Non-modifiable risk factors for stroke include age (>55 years), sex (greater incidence for men than women), race (greater incidence for African-Americans and Hispanics than whites), and family history.
- Modifiable risk factors for stroke include high blood pressure, smoking, high cholesterol, diabetes, and atrial fibrillation.
- Blood pressure should be reduced to <140/90 mm Hg and to <130/85 mm Hg in patients with heart failure, chronic renal failure, or diabetes.
- LDL cholesterol should be reduced to <100 mg/dL in patients with more than two risk factors; in patients with prior diagnosis of heart disease, LDL cholesterol should be reduced to <70 mg/dL.
- ACE inhibitors have been shown to reduce stroke rates in patients with diabetes.
- For patients older than 65 years with atrial fibrillation, warfarin with INR of 2.0 to 3.0 is usually given.
- Aspirin has not been shown to be useful in primary prevention of stroke in men.
- Asymptomatic carotid stenosis surgery is not recommended for patients older than 80 years, patients with significant operative risk, or patients with contralateral carotid artery occlusion. The surgeon should be experienced with the procedure (performing at least 12 operations per year), because low case volume has been associated with increased morbidity and mortality.

- Secondary stroke prevention depends on the etiology of the stroke.
- Prevalence of sleep apnea among those with stroke or transient ischemic attack is estimated at between 50% and 80%.

Primary Prevention of Stroke

The American Heart Association (AHA) suggests that the major risk factors for stroke are hypertension, smoking, high cholesterol, diabetes, and coronary artery disease. Control of these risk factors can reduce the incidence of stroke and reduce the rate of death and dependence. The risk factors for stroke are the same as the risk factors for cardiac disease and, as a general rule, a patient who has all the cardiac risk factors under control will have good stroke prevention also. Risk factors can be categorized as modifiable and non-modifiable.

In the case of non-modifiable risks (Table 2-1), intervention is not applicable. People with non-modifiable stroke risks are at a higher rate of stroke, so more aggressive control of modifiable risk factors might be indicated. Non-modifiable risk factors for stroke are:

- *Age over 55 years.* The risk of stroke doubles each decade after 55 years. With advancing age, the rate of co-morbidities increases, as does the rate of specific risk factors such as atrial fibrillation. Atrial fibrillation incidence increases from 2 to 3 cases per 1000 between ages 55 and 64 years to 35 cases per 1000 between ages 85 and 94 years (1,2).

- *Family history of stroke on both maternal and paternal sides.* Stroke rate increases significantly in individuals with a twin who

Table 2-1 Non-Modifiable Stroke Risk Factors

Risk Factor	Comments
Age > 55 years	Incidence doubles every 10 years after age 55
Male	Greater incidence for men than women
African American	Greater incidence than Caucasians May have greater incidence of intracranial stenosis May have greater incidence of hemorrhagic stroke
Hispanic	Greater incidence than Caucasians May have greater incidence of intracranial stenosis May have greater incidence of hemorrhagic stroke
Family history	Stroke or TIA in father increases relative risk by a factor of 2.4 Stroke or TIA in mother increases relative risk by a factor of 1.4

TIA = transient ischemic attack.
Adapted from Goldstein LB, Adams R, Becker K, et al. Primary prevention of ischemic stroke: a statement for healthcare professionals from the Stroke Council of the American Heart Association. Stroke. 2001;32:280.

has had stroke (1). Family history includes less common genetic predispositions to cerebrovascular disease such as accelerated atherosclerosis secondary to homocysteinuria, familial cavernomas, hypercoagulable states in families with autoimmune disease, CADASIL (cerebral autosomal dominant ateriopathy with subcortical infarcts and leukoencephalopathy), Fabry's disease, and mitochondrial disorders (1).

- *Sex.* Men have a higher incidence of stroke as they age, whereas women have a higher incidence of stroke in youth. This is likely secondary to oral contraceptive use, predispositions to autoimmune disease, higher incidence of migraine, and pregnancy, all of which can increase the incidence of stroke. Furthermore, women are more likely to die from strokes when they have them: women account for 60.8% of stroke fatalities (3-5).

- *Race.* African Americans, self-described Hispanics, and Asians of Chinese and Japanese descent have higher rates of both ischemic and hemorrhagic stroke (6–9). This holds true above and beyond the greater prevalence of modifiable risk factors among African Americans (10).

Evidence varies regarding the role modifiable risk factors play in the cause of stroke; it also varies regarding the benefit of controlling them. Some modifiable risk factors have strong evidence indicating their role in causing stroke, and some have evidence showing that their control can reduce incidence of stroke (Table 2-2).

Table 2-2 Modifiable Stroke Risk Factors

- Lower blood pressure
  Reduction of blood pressure below 140/90
  Below 130/90 if
  — Congestive heart failure
  — Chronic renal failure
  — Diabetes
- Smoking cessation
- Reduction of cholesterol with a statin medication
  — Reduce LDL cholesterol if total < 160 *or*
  — <100 if two stroke risk factors *or*
  — <70 if coronary heart disease is present
- Coumadin for atrial fibrillation for patients age 65 and older
- Carotid endarterectomy for patients with good operative risk with surgeon <3% morbidity/mortality

---

The study of risk factors has led to the following clinical recommendations by the AHA. Table 2-3 lists the levels of evidence and the strength of recommendation grades.

Reduction of Blood Pressure

There is level I grade A evidence that reducing blood pressure (BP) reduces the incidence of stroke (1). Hypertension is the single most important stroke risk factor. High blood pressure was previously defined as systolic >160 mm Hg and diastolic >90 mm Hg, but more recently the definition of hypertension has changed. It is now recommended that blood pressure be reduced to <140/90 mm Hg, and to <130/85 mm Hg in patients with heart failure, chronic renal failure, or diabetes (1). Control of isolated systolic blood pressure reduces risk of stroke by 42%, as demonstrated by the Syst-Eur trial (11). A meta-analysis of 18 ß-blocker trials showed the efficacy of this drug treatment in stroke reduction (12).

The PROGRESS Trial suggested that a combination of ACE inhibitors with diuretics was effective in reducing stroke rate, even though the drugs reduced blood pressure only slightly (13). In this study, 3054 subjects were randomized to a placebo study arm and 3051 to therapy with perindopril, with the addition of the diuretic indapamide if recommended by the treating physician. Similar benefits were seen in patients with and without hypertension. Over 4 years of follow-up, subjects on combination therapy experienced a drop in mean blood pressure of 12/5 mm Hg and reduced stroke risk by 43%. Single-drug therapy reduced blood pressure by 5/3 mm Hg and did not significantly reduce risk of stroke. Overall, the therapy was well tolerated, and blood pressure reduction in the active treatment group

---

Table 2-3 Lack of Evidence and Strength of Recommendation

Level of Evidence

Level I	Data from randomized trials with low false-positive and low false-negative errors
Level II	Date from randomized trials with high false-positive or high false-negative errors
Level III	Data from nonrandomized concurrent cohort studies
Level IV	Data from nonrandomized cohort studies using historical controls
Level V	Data from anecdotal case series

Strength of Recommendation

Grade A	Supported by level I evidence
Grade B	Supported by level II evidence
Grade C	Supported by level III, IV, or V evidence

Adapted from Adams HP Jr, Brott TG, Crowell RM, et al. Guidelines for the management of patients with acute ischemic stroke: a statement for healthcare professionals from a special writing group of the Stroke Council, American Heart Association. Stroke. 1994;25:1901–14.

was about 9/4 mm Hg, with a stroke risk reduction of 28% (95% CI, 17-38). Subgroups that benefited the most included those receiving dual therapy, Asians, and hypertensives. Evidence for reduction in stroke and coronary artery disease led the Joint National Committee on Prevention, Detection, Evaluation and Treatment of High Blood Pressure in their 7th report (JNC-7) to recommend strict blood pressure control parameters (14). According to its criteria, normal is considered a systolic BP of less than 130 mm Hg and a diastolic BP of less than 80 mm Hg. Pre-hypertension is defined as a systolic BP of 120-139 or a diastolic BP of 80-89.

Stage 1 hypertension is defined as systolic BP of 140-150 or diastolic BP of 90-99. Stage 2 hypertension is defined as systolic BP of greater than 160 or diastolic BP greater than 100. According to JNC-7 guidelines, patients with stage 1 hypertension may require lifestyle modification treatment only, whereas patients with pre-hypertension and diabetes or chronic kidney disease may require pharmacologic treatment as well (Figure 2-1).

JNC-7 recommends initial lifestyle changes in patients without compelling indications for medication. These changes include weight loss, dietary changes, exercise, and only moderate alcohol consumption. ACE inhibitors and diuretics in patients with stroke or stroke risk are recommended for prevention of cerebrovascular disease (14).

Smoking Cessation

There is level III grade C evidence that cessation of smoking reduces the risk of stroke (the evidence is level III grade C due to a lack of evidence from randomized controlled trials) (1). Given the considerable medical evidence on the harmful effects of smoking, a prospective, placebo-controlled trial is unlikely to be done, but the primary data regarding smoking and heart disease is probably sufficient to support the case for smoking cessation to reduce stroke risks. In addition, a meta-analysis of possible risks of stroke from cigarette smoking suggests that smokers are at double the relative risk for stroke compared with non-smokers (15). Some stroke neurologists have estimated that 18% of strokes are attributable to smoking (16). One of the most disconcerting statistics shows that there is a 1.82-fold increase in the risk of stroke among non-smokers and long-term ex-smokers exposed to environmental tobacco smoke (17). Therefore, the cessation of smoking, by the patient as well as by the patient's housemates, appears to be called for to reduce stroke risk.

Reduce LDL Cholesterol

Level I grade A evidence exists that shows that cholesterol lowering with a statin medication reduces chances of stroke and is effective in the primary and secondary prevention of stroke. It is recommended that LDL cholesterol be reduced to <100 mg/dL or to <70 mg/dL in patients with more than

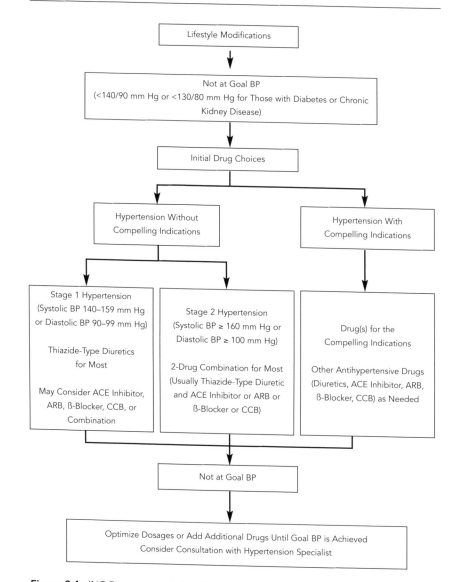

Figure 2-1 JNC-7 recommendations for blood pressure control. (From the National High Blood Pressure Education Program Coordinating Committee. The Seventh Report of the Joint National Committee on Prevention, Detection, Evaluation, and Treatment of High Blood Pressure. JAMA. 2003;289:2560–71; with permission.)

two risk factors; in patients with previous diagnosis of heart disease, LDL cholesterol should be reduced to <100 mg/dL (18). Lowering cholesterol a priori through diet or non-statin pharmacologic agents has not been shown to be effective in reducing stroke (19). It is likely that stroke reduction results primarily from effects of the statin medications. Multiple trials show an overall relative risk reduction in stroke with the use of statins of 31% (20). Stroke reduction was demonstrated with the use of pravastatin in the LIPID trial, and with simivistatin in the 4S trial, suggesting a class effect (19,20). Moreover, basic science research and cardiologic data suggest that lovastatin, fluvastatin, and atorvastatin may all have similar effects (21). The greatest benefit in stroke risk reduction was found in subjects with elevated cholesterol and coronary artery disease. Patients with previous stroke should have LDL reduced to 100 mg/dL or less.

ACE Inhibitors for Stroke Prevention in Diabetic Patients

There is level I grade A evidence that ACE inhibitors in diabetic patients reduce stroke rates (1). The HOPE trial took 3577 diabetic high-risk patients and administered ramipril. This resulted in a reduction of stroke by 33% in the treatment group. The results were unchanged when the data was controlled for small blood pressure decreases. By itself, rigid glucose control has not been shown to reduce stroke over the long term, but it has shown short-term benefit (1). Control of hyperglycemia does seem to reduce the incidence of microvascular disease. Consequently, ramipril is recommended for high-risk diabetic patients (10 mg qd) (1,22).

Atrial Fibrillation and Use of Anticoagulation

Atrial fibrillation with non-valvular atrial fibrillation is often treated with the anticoagulant warfarin. There is level I evidence from a meta-analysis that warfarin significantly reduces risk of first stroke in those with atrial fibrillation. Risk factors that tend to increase risk of stroke are age older than 65 years, transient ischemic attacks, and other cardiac/stroke risk factors (1). Other cardiac disorders often treated with anticoagulation are low left ventricular ejection fraction <25% and post-myocardial infarction with mural thrombus, although, as of yet, prospective randomized data do not exist to support this practice. In general, patients are best treated with warfarin with INR 2.0-3.0. Special consideration is often given to patients with unacceptable bleeding risks, unsteadiness, and compliance issues. In many instances, those younger than 65 years with no stroke risk factors can receive aspirin (1). Special circumstances and details of recommendations are discussed in Chapter 10.

Aspirin Not Recommended for Primary Prevention of Stroke in Men

Although low-dose aspirin has been shown to be beneficial in risk reduction of cardiac ischemia, it has not been shown to be of help in primary prevention of stroke. In fact, there is a higher rate of hemorrhagic stroke associated with low-dose aspirin. A meta-analysis of five aspirin prevention trials, with a total of 26,989 subjects treated with aspirin for primary stroke prevention and 25,262 with placebo, showed in all but one trial that patients who took aspirin had higher stroke rates than those in the placebo group (23). Although antiplatelet agents are powerful as secondary prevention, they have not been shown to be helpful in primary care of stroke in men. However, aspirin is effective in primary prevention of cardiac disease and can be used for this purpose.

Oddly enough, aspirin has been shown to be useful in primary prevention of ischemic strokes in women; however, in smaller, less well-done previous studies, it was suggested that there may be an increased risk of stroke in women. A study of 39,876 women receiving 100 mg aspirin on alternate days versus placebo was performed to look at primary prevention of heart disease and stroke in women. The aspirin group had a 24% risk reduction in ischemic stroke with no statistically significant difference between aspirin and placebo in fatal or non-fatal myocardial infarction. There were more gastrointestinal hemorrhages in the aspirin group. The sub-population who received the greatest benefit were women over 65 years of age (24).

Asymptomatic Carotid Stenosis Surgery

The issue of asymptomatic carotid stenosis is raised each time a carotid bruit is heard in patients without transient ischemic attacks or strokes. Although there have been numerous trials on asymptomatic carotid stenosis surgery, only one trial is clearly positive, the Asymptomatic Carotid Atherosclerosis Study (ACAS) (25). It showed that patients with 60% or greater carotid stenosis did better with carotid endarterectomy (CEA) plus 325 mg aspirin than they did with 325 mg aspirin alone. The results are less robust than the symptomatic carotid endarterectomy trial, showing a relative risk reduction for stroke of 55% with surgery and an absolute risk reduction with surgery of 5.9%. The results were much less impressive for women, for reasons that are unclear. The major issues with ACAS are that all patients in the trial were younger than 80 years old, none had significant contralateral carotid stenosis or occlusion, and there were exclusions for diabetes, hypertension, and cardiac disease. The overall operative risk in ACAS, including the 1.2% stroke risk for angiography, was >3.0%, representing the most experienced and skillful vascular surgeons and neurosurgeons (25).

In actuality, morbidity and mortality can vary highly depending on the surgeon. In one study, the morbidity/mortality was 3.7%, with bad outcomes for individual surgeons as high as 9.16%. The predictors of high morbidly and mortality were low volume, with the surgeon's 2-year volume below 30 cases; morbidity/mortality decreased with increasing years of surgical experience (26). Therefore, the authors recommend against surgery for patients with asymptomatic carotid disease who are over 80 years old, have significant operative risk, or contralateral stenosis; they suggest, instead, maximal medical treatment with antiplatelet agents, statins, and hypertension control. Many surgeons will only perform CEA for asymptomatic disease if there is 80% or greater stenosis. It is important that the surgeon chosen has a reputation for the procedure and a volume of at least 12 cases a year. More discussion is given in Chapter 9.

Diet and Exercise in Primary Stroke Prevention

Whether diet and exercise reduce stroke rates is difficult to determine. Obesity and inactivity do seem to be risk factors for stroke, but it is entirely possible that weight and physical inactivity as risk factors for stroke are primarily related to elevations in blood pressure. Additionally, although patients with healthier diets have lower incidents of stroke, such patients may have a healthier lifestyle overall, this being the real reason for lower stroke risk.

Dietary issues of interest were found in the Nurses Health Study, in which individuals who ate more fruits and vegetables had lower stroke risks: a higher amount of folic acid is found in healthier diets, which may decrease in homocysteine levels and reduce stroke risk (1). Intake of omega-3 fatty acids is felt to be protective against stroke because they may have mild antiplatelet effects, reduce fibrinogen, and lower blood viscosity. According to the Nurses Health Study, people who ate fish more frequently had fewer thrombotic strokes and their experience of hemorrhagic stroke did not increase (Table 2-4). In this trial, a serving of fish was 6-8 oz. Dosages of omega-3 fatty acids were calculated to be 1.51 g for dark fish meats, 0.42 g for canned tuna, and 0.48 g for other fish, with an average dose of 1.16 g. Typical omega-3 fatty acid supplements have 1-2 g (27).

Alcohol use appears to lead to a J-shaped curve with light-to-moderate alcohol consumption protective for stroke; heavy alcohol consumption leads to higher incidents of cerebrovascular disease. Depending on the study, protection appears at about two drinks per day; increased stroke

Table 2-4 Fish Consumption and Reduction in Stroke Risk in Women Not Taking Aspirin Compared with Those Who Ate Fish Less than Once a Month

Frequency of Fish Intake	Relative Risk for All Stroke (Multivariate)
1 to 3 times a month	0.93
Once a week	0.78
2–4 times a week	0.73
5 times a week	0.48
2 or more times a week	0.49

Adapted from Hiroyasu I, Rexrode K, Stampfer M, et al. Intake of fish and omega-3 fatty acids and risk of stroke in women. JAMA. 2001;285:304–12.

rates occur at five drinks or more a day. Moderate alcohol consumption of two or less drinks per day for men and one or less for women appears to mildly reduce blood pressure (lowers systolic by 2-4 mm Hg), increase HDL, and decrease the incidence of coronary artery disease that leads to cerebrovascular disease (1).

Adopting a low-fat diet such as the DASH eating plan, which incorporates increased amounts of vegetables and fruits, correlates with an approximate 8-14 mm Hg reduction in systolic blood pressure. Sodium reduction and potassium supplementation appear to be beneficial. Sodium reduction likely affects stroke rates by reducing blood pressure (28). Reduction of sodium intake to less than 2.4 g of sodium or 6 g sodium chloride correlates with a 2-8 mm Hg drop in systolic blood pressure (14). Interestingly, potassium seems deficient in the diet of many people who live in the United States. Whether this is a direct effect of potassium or potassium intake is a marker for a good diet is unclear. Increasing potassium intake through high-potassium fruits and vegetables lowers blood pressure mildly and may secondarily reduce stroke/coronary artery disease risks (29).

Exercise itself is beneficial in stroke and heart disease prevention. Regular, uninterrupted, aerobic exercise (e.g., uninterrupted brisk walking; running around at work with frequent breaks does not count!) for 30 minutes per day on most days corresponds to a 4-9 mm Hg drop in systolic blood pressure. The primary protection probably occurs when blood pressure is reduced from a combination of exercise and weight loss. According to JNC-7, systolic blood pressure is lowered by 5-20 mm Hg for every 10 lb lost (weight reduction ideally leading to healthy body mass index of 18.5-24.9) (14).

C-Reactive Protein in Primary Prevention of Stroke

C-reactive protein (CRP) is a serum marker for inflammation and an acute phase reactant. It is elevated during infection and in inflammatory conditions such as temporal arteritis. It can also be elevated in the low-grade inflammatory reactions seen in diffuse atherosclerotic disease. CRP has been shown to be an independent marker for cardiac disease and a marker for cerebrovascular disease. CRP levels are higher in smokers, people with obesity, and diffuse atherosclerosis (30).

The Framingham Study looked at risk of stroke and transient ischemic attack in men and women with multiple stroke risk factors and measured CRP levels. In this study, the CRP ranges were divided by quartiles: first quartile: 0–1.08; second quartile: 1.10–3.0; third quartile: 3.03–6.80; and fourth quartile: 6.90–48.30. This study found that after a 12–14 year follow-up, men in the highest quartile of CRP levels have twice the risk of ischemic stroke/transient ischemic attack versus those in the lowest quartile. This is also true of women, whose risk of stroke is three times when lowest and highest quartile of C-reactive protein were evaluated (30).

CRP measurements seem to correlate with stroke risk and with morbidity and mortality once stroke occurs. In cardiac disease, patients with a CRP of <1 are felt to be at low risk; those with a CRP of 2-3 are at moderate risk; and those with a CRP of >3 are at higher risk for cardiovascular events. Additionally, CRP measurement is a stronger predictor of disease than LDL measurement (31). Similar findings have been found in cerebrovascular disease. There are data to suggest that statin therapy (even with low LDL), smoking cessation, aspirin, and clopidogrel use can lower CRP levels. In general, risk factor modification reduces stroke, and aspirin/clopidogrel can reduce rates of secondary occurrence of stroke (32). CRP may be an important marker for poor risk factors and a way to objectively monitor risk factor modification (30). CRP measurement is becoming important in primary and secondary prevention of stroke, but it is unclear how much interventions will lower CRP levels. Elevated CRP levels in concerned patients can probably motivate patients to work harder at reducing their risk factors.

Secondary Prevention of Stroke

Approximately 25% of the 750,000 strokes that occur each year in the United States are recurrent strokes. The risk for subsequent stroke is highest during the first 30 days after presenting ischemic symptoms. The chances of stroke recurrence depend on the etiology of the stroke and on the treatments given to the patient at the time of the initial insult. The workup of stroke must include a heart-to-head evaluation because different stroke etiologies may require different interventions. Evaluations of intracranial and extracranial circulation, cardiac anatomic and cardiac rhythm studies, and hypercoagulable screens in the young should all be performed. Each etiology leads to a specific approach for secondary prevention (Table 2-5), which should begin in the acute hospital setting. It is safe to initiate therapy a few days after stroke in the absence of significant hemorrhage or

Table 2-5 Interventions for Reducing Risk of Recurrent Stroke

Stroke Etiology	Possible Intervention
Lacunar	Antiplatelet, statin, risk factor control
Intracranial stenosis	Antiplatelet, warfarin, statin, stenting
Carotid/vertebral stenosis	Surgery, stenting, antiplatelet
Aortic arch disease	Antiplatelet, warfarin, statin, risk factor control
Cardiac source embolus	Antiplatelet, warfarin, surgery
Hypercoagulable state	Warfarin
Hemorrhage	Stop antiplatelet or warfarin, surgery, risk factor control
Hypoperfusion	Increase blood pressure

very large ischemic strokes. Long-term antiplatelet therapy is the mainstay of secondary stroke prevention in patients without an indication for warfarin treatment and should be initiated promptly in all patients without contraindications during the first 48 hours of hospitalization. In large ischemic strokes, anticoagulation should be withheld for 48 hours. Primary prevention measures should be instituted regardless of etiology, but, in general, care should be taken before aggressively dropping blood pressure in patients with significant intracranial stenosis. Each etiology will be discussed in detail in separate chapters.

Cardiac Emboli

Approximately 20% of ischemic strokes result from cardiac source emboli. Atrial fibrillation, low left ventricular ejection fraction (<25%), and mural thrombi after myocardial infarction are the most common causes. Anticoagulation should be considered for all these stroke etiologies. Occasionally, one encounters a patient with no stroke risk factors or etiology other than a patent foramen ovale (PFO), and in this situation there is no consensus about proper treatment. Recent data suggest that in patients who have a simple PFO without atrial septal aneurysm, stroke recurrence is no greater than without PFO. The 4-year stroke recurrence rate for patients without PFO was 4.2% versus 2.3% in those with a PFO. Patients with a PFO combined with atrial septal aneurysm had a 4-year recurrence rate of 15.2% (33). Therefore, intervention with warfarin, surgery, or closure device should probably be reserved for PFO patients with atrial septal aneurysms. Further discussion is available in Chapters 10 and 13.

Aortic Arch Source

Patients with severe aortic atherosclerosis with 4 mm or greater wall thickness with mobile thrombus evident on transesophageal echocardiography have been shown to have increased rates of recurrent strokes. This increase in stroke is independent of carotid disease, atrial fibrillation, and peripheral vascular disease (34). No study has shown that warfarin is better than antiplatelet medications for severe atherosclerosis of aorta. These patients are often treated with statins in combination with either maximal antiplatelet medications or warfarin. More information is available in Chapter 14.

Carotid Stenosis

The North American Symptomatic Carotid Endarterectomy Trial (NASCET) defined treatment of symptomatic carotid disease (35). This trial compared 1300 mg aspirin plus carotid endarterectomy with 1300 mg aspirin alone, with results among some of the most robust in the stroke literature. The NASCET trial showed that with 70%-99% carotid stenosis with transient ischemic attack or minor stroke, there was an absolute risk reduction of 17% for recurrent ipsilateral stroke, 15% for recurrence of all strokes, and 16.5% for recurrence of all stroke or death in the aspirin-plus-surgery group (35). Strokes originating from ipsilateral carotid stenosis of 70%-99% require aspirin-plus-surgery therapy. See also Chapter 9.

Large Vessel and Small Vessel Disease

Stenosis of the large vessels of the circle of Willis will be missed if they are not imaged with MRA, CTA, or transcranial Doppler. Large artery stenosis can present with recurrent stereotyped transient ischemic attacks and strokes. Large artery stenosis also may present with transient neurologic deficits with trivial drops in blood pressure. Retrospective data suggest that warfarin may be superior to aspirin for intracranial stenosis (36), but this has not been confirmed by larger prospective studies. Most of the larger studies have not specifically examined intracranial stenosis.

The Warfarin versus Aspirin in Symptomatic Intracranial Disease (WASID) trial compared aspirin and warfarin in symptomatic intracranial stenosis in a prospective manner: 569 patients with symptomatic intracranial stenosis, 50%-99% by conventional angiography, were randomized either to 1300 mg aspirin or adjusted-dose warfarin. The study found no difference in recurrent ischemic stroke or central nervous system hemorrhage, but it did find that patients in the warfarin arm had significantly more non-vascular deaths. This study suggests that high-dose aspirin is probably as effective as warfarin, without negative side effects, and that aspirin should be the treatment for intracranial stenosis (37).

Many clinicians use warfarin or antiplatelet agents plus statins. Warfarin is frequently used for antiplatelet failures, and angioplasty is used for accessible lesions that fail maximal antiplatelet therapy and warfarin.

Lacunar stroke is caused by atherosclerotic disease of the very smallest penetrating arteries in the brain. These arteries are too small to be visualized by conventional arterial imaging. Presently, antiplatelets plus statins are often used for treatment. More detail is available in Chapters 11, 12, and 14.

Sleep Apnea and Stroke

Sleep apnea occurs as a consequence of alteration in muscular tone in the upper airway (obstructive) or as an alteration in brainstem respiratory drive (central) (38,39). Obstructive sleep apnea may present as a limited restriction in airway flow (hypopnea), a complete obstruction in airway flow (apnea), or a mixed hypopnea-apnea event (mixed) (38). In obstructive sleep apnea, respiratory effort persists to the point of creating large intrathoracic negative pressures, which then have an effect on the cardiovascular system. Central sleep apnea presents as a complete loss of respiratory effort and therefore loss of airway flow (38). Ondine's curse is the classic example of central sleep apnea. During sleep there is sudden abrupt cessation of respiratory effort, then oxygen saturation falls. Finally, the patient awakens and begins breathing again. This condition is extremely rare. The more common form of central sleep apnea is periodic breathing or Cheyne-Stokes respiration. This form of disordered breathing also occurs during waking periods. It is seen in patients with brain injury and in those with poor cardiac function. In this condition, breathing essentially oscillates between hyperventilation and hypoventilation. Although designated as a sleep-related problem, the disordered breathing events that are discussed below as "sleep apnea" can occur in any drowsy or altered-consciousness condition whether the altered state is sleep, drug-induced, post-seizure, brain injury, infection, or coma. "Sleep apnea" as used in the context of this section refers to obstructive hypopneic/apneic events; "central sleep apnea" refers to non-obstructed events of which Cheyne-Stokes respiration is the most common.

Studies have shown that during the period of apnea there are sharp sudden rises in intracranial pressures and that this rise correlates with abrupt changes in systemic blood pressure (40,41). Sleep apnea is associated with rapid increases and decreases in cerebral blood flow velocities and a decrease in cerebrovascular reactivity, which persists even during wakefulness. The suggested consequences of these findings are that the rapid alterations in cerebral blood flow may exceed the capacity of the cerebrovascular autoregulating mechanisms to protect the brain from damage. Sleep apnea is also associated with a decrease in peripheral endothelial-dependent vascular relaxation and circulating nitric oxide levels. The changes in peripheral endothelial factor may also be occurring in the cerebrovasculature and thus account for the effects on cerebral blood flow. Sleep apnea is associated with augmentation and fluctuation in sympathetic activity. Consequently, there are large and sudden changes in blood pressure, which often surges at the end of the apneic event and falls suddenly with normal breathing; this alternation recurs with each apneic event. These abrupt changes in blood pressure appear to be parallel to the changes in cerebral blood flow and intracranial pressures mentioned above and probably contribute significantly to these phenomena. There are increases in platelet aggregation, plasma fibrinogen, and blood viscosity in patients with sleep apnea, all of which are independent risk factors for cerebrovascular disease.

The prevalence of sleep apnea in patients who have had a stroke or transient ischemic attack has been reported to be 2-4 times higher than expected from case-control and normative data (39,40). It is unknown whether apnea is a consequence of the stroke or an antecedent factor in the stroke's cause. There are no longitudinal data on the prevalence of apnea in those who do and do not develop a stroke, but clinical indicators of apnea such as snoring and sleepiness have been studied in case-control populations. Snoring has consistently been shown to be a risk factor for stroke (41,42). Even when age, gender, and known stroke risk factors are taken into consideration, snoring remains a significant risk factor. The likely conclusion is that sleep apnea is the factor that is underlying the snoring risk. Consistent with this conclusion, it has been shown that the risk associated with snoring increased if apnea or daytime sleepiness were pre-stroke conditions co-existing with the report of snoring. If one takes apnea, daytime sleepiness, and obesity (body mass index >30) into account, then the risks for stroke are substantial (odds ratio, 8.0) (43).

The prevalence of sleep apnea (hypopneic/apneic events per hour >10) among those with stroke or transient ischemic attack is estimated at 50%-80% (44,45). The prevalence did not differ for transient ischemic attack versus stroke, stroke subtype, or the area of the brain affected. The prevalence of sleep apnea does drop from the acute stroke period (1-7 days) to the "stable" period (8-12 weeks), but the prevalence even in this "stable" period is still high at 40%-60%. There is also a drop in the severity (mean number of events per hour) of sleep apnea with time. This drop in prevalence and severity appears to be more common in those with transient ischemic attack than in those with stroke.

Whether sleep apnea is a cause or an effect of stroke, its presence in stroke patients may have an effect on rehabilitation. Sleep disruption for any reason will lead to decreased attention, memory, sense of well-being, and motivation; increased depression, anxiety and irritability; and increased fatigue and somnolence, all of which are likely to have a negative effect on recovery. Continued problems with increased nocturnal blood pressure, intracranial pressures, and cerebral blood flow may directly affect brain tissue recovery. Unfortunately, there are very few studies that have examined the long-term effects of sleep apnea on stroke outcomes. Available studies do suggest an association between sleep apnea and increased morbidity and mortality (46).

Sleep apnea should be suspected in anyone who snores and has disrupted sleep, has complaints of daytime sleepiness, is obese (body mass index >30), or has hard-to-control high blood pressure. Anyone who has had a transient ischemic stroke or stroke and also snores has an increased probability of having sleep apnea and therefore should be evaluated (47). An important caveat is that many people with sleep apnea do not report snoring. The diagnosis of sleep apnea, although considered likely or unlikely based on clinical assessment, is made by a quality nighttime polysomnogram.

Treatments for sleep apnea include weight loss, use of a continuous positive airway pressure (CPAP) device, use of dental appliances, and laser or radiofrequency uvulopalatoplasty. CPAP devices are the most studied, and in the face of difficulties losing weight, CPAP remains the treatment of choice. Intolerance to the CPAP mask is the biggest drawback: nasal congestion, claustrophobia, and general discomfort are common. Approximately 65%–70% of subjects will tolerate a CPAP mask. The changes in intracranial pressures, cerebral blood flow, blood pressure, platelet aggregation, plasma fibrinogen, and blood viscosity reported in patients with sleep apnea have all been shown to be treatable with CPAP. The only randomized trial of CPAP for the treatment of apnea in the subacute stroke patient showed significant improvements in depression ratings (47).

Conclusion

Stroke is a preventable, treatable, and survivable disease. Proper identification of patients at risk is crucial. Once patients are identified, risk factors should be addressed. Smoking cessation, blood pressure control, control of elevated cholesterol with statin medications, and diabetes management are all vital to keeping an individual's risk for stroke low. Testing a patient's CRP level may be a very powerful predictor of stroke risk and an indicator of when to aggressively control risk factors. Secondary prevention should be based on stroke etiology and may include warfarin for a cardiac source or an antiplatelet agent individually or in combination for atherosclerotic source strokes. Symptomatic carotid artery disease will require surgery if the symptomatic ipsilateral carotid stenosis is in the 70%-99% range. Sleep apnea is a disorder often neglected in stroke work-up but is treatable.

REFERENCES

1. Goldstein LB, Adams R, Becker K, et al. Primary prevention of ischemic stroke: a statement for healthcare professionals from the Stroke Council of the American Heart Association. Stroke. 2001;32:280.
2. Falk RH. Atrial fibrillation. N Engl J Med. 2001;344:1067-78.
3. Kittner SJ, Stern BJ, Feeser BR, et al. Pregnancy and the risk of stroke. N Engl J Med. 1996;335:768-74.
4. Levine SR, Brey RL, et al. Risk of recurrent thromboembolic events in patients with focal cerebral ischemia and antiphospholipid antibodies. Stroke. 1992;23(Suppl1):1-29,1-32.
5. Donaghy M, Chang CL, Poulter N, et al. Duration, frequency, recency, and type of migraine and the risk of ischaemic stroke in women of childbearing age. J Neurol Neurosurg Psychiatr. 2002;73:747-50.
6. American Heart Association. Stroke Statistics. Dallas, Tex: American Heart Association; 2000.
7. Gorelick PB. Cerebrovascular disease in African Americans. Stroke. 1998;29:2656-64.
8. Sheinart KF, Tuhrim S, Horowitz DR, et al. Stroke recurrence is more frequent in blacks and Hispanics. Neuroepidemiology. 1998;17:188-98.
9. He J, Klag MJ, Wu Z, et al. Stroke in the People's Republic of China. I: Geographic variations in incidence and risk factors. Stroke. 1995;26:2222-7.
10. Giles WH, Kittner SJ, Hebel JR, et al. Determinants of black-white differences in the risk of cerebral infarction: the National Health and Nutrition Examination Survey Epidemiologic Follow-up Study. Arch Intern Med. 1995;155:1319-24.
11. Systolic Hypertension in Europe Investigators. Randomised double-blind comparison of placebo and active treatment for older patients with isolated systolic hypertension. Lancet. 1997;350:757-64.

12. Psaty BM, Smith NL, Siscovick DS, et al. Health outcomes associated with antihypertensive therapies used as first-line agents: a systematic review and meta-analysis. JAMA. 1997;277:739-45.

13. PROGRESS Collaborative Group. Randomised trial of a perindopril-based blood-pressure-lowering regimen among 6,105 individuals with previous stroke or transient ischaemic attack. Lancet. 2001;358:1033-41.

14. Aram V, Bakris GL, Black HR, et al. The Seventh Report of the Joint National Committee on Prevention, Detection, Evaluation, and Treatment of High Blood Pressure. The JNC-7 Report. JAMA. 2003;289:2560-71.

15. Shinton R, Beevers G. Meta-analysis of relation between cigarette smoking and stroke. BMJ. 1989;298:789-94.

16. Whisnant JP. Modeling of risk factors for ischemic stroke: the Willis Lecture. Stroke. 1997;28:1840-4.

17. Bonita R, Duncan J, Truelsen T, et al. Passive smoking as well as active smoking increases the risk of acute stroke. Tobac Control. 1999;8:156-160.

18. Cholesterol, diastolic blood pressure, and stroke: 13,000 strokes in 450,000 people in 45 prospective cohorts: Prospective Studies Collaboration. Lancet. 1995;346:1647-53.

19. Long-Term Intervention with Pravastatin in Ischaemic Disease (LIPID) Study Group. Prevention of cardiovascular events and death with pravastatin in patients with coronary heart disease and a broad range of initial cholesterol levels. N Engl J Med. 1998;339:1349-57.

20. Pedersen TR, Kjekshus J, Pyorala K, et al. Effect of simvastatin on ischemic signs and symptoms in the Scandinavian simvastatin survival study (4S). Am J Cardiol. 1998;81:333-5.

21. Blauw GJ, Lagaay AM, Smelt AH, Westendorp RG. Stroke, statins, and cholesterol. A meta-analysis of randomized, placebo-controlled, double-blind trials with HMG-CoA reductase inhibitors. Stroke. 1997;28:946-50.

22. Heart Outcomes Prevention Evaluation Study Investigators. Effects of ramipril on cardiovascular and microvascular outcomes in people with diabetes mellitus: results of the HOPE study and MICRO-HOPE substudy. Lancet. 2000;355:253-9.

23. Hart RG, Halperin JL, McBride R, et al. Aspirin for the primary prevention of stroke and other major vascular events: meta-analysis and hypotheses. Arch Neurol. 2000;57:326-32.

24. Ridker PM, Cook NR, Lee I-M, et al. Randomized trial of low-dose aspirin in the primary prevention of cardiovascular disease in women. N Engl J Med. 2005;352:1293-1304.

25. Toole JF, Howard VJ, Chambless LE, for the Asymptomatic Carotid Atherosclerosis Study Group. Study design for randomized prospective trial of carotid endarterectomy for asymptomatic atherosclerosis. Stroke. 1989;20:844-9.

26. O'Neill L, Lanska DJ, Hartz A. Surgeon characteristics associated with mortality and morbidity following carotid endarterectomy Neurology. 2000;55:773-8.

27. Hiroyasu I, Rexrode K, Stampfer M, et al. Intake of fish and omega-3 fatty acids and risk of stroke in women. JAMA. 2001;285:304-12.

28. Graudal N, Gallone A, Garred P. Effects of sodium restriction on blood pressure, rennin, aldosterone, catecholamines, cholesterol, and triglycerides. JAMA. 1998;279:1383-91.

29. Whelton PK, He J, Cutler JA, et al. Effects of oral potassium on blood pressure: meta-analysis of randomized control trials. JAMA. 1997;277:1624-32.

30. Rost N, Wolf P, Kase C, et al. Plasma concentration of C-reactive protein and risk of ischemic stroke and transient ischemic attack. The Framingham Study. Stroke. 2001;32:2575-9.

31. Ridker P, Bassuk S, Toth P. C-reactive protein and risk of cardiovascular disease: evidence and clinical application. Curr Atheroscler Rep. 2003;5:341-9.

32. Cha J, Jeong M, Lee K, et al. Changes in platelet P-selectin and plasma C-reactive protein with acute atherosclerotic ischemic stroke treated with a loading dose of clopidogrel. J Thrombosis Thrombolysis. 2002;14:145-50.

33. Mas JL, Arquizan C, Lamy C, et al. Recurrent cerebrovascular events associated with patent foramen ovale, atrial septal aneurysm, or both. N Engl J Med. 2001;345:1740-6.

34. French Study of Aortic Plaques in Stroke Group. Atherosclerotic disease of the aortic arch as a risk factor for recurrent ischemic stroke. N Engl J Med. 1996;334:1216-21.

35. North American Symptomatic Carotid Endarterectomy Trial (NASCET) Collaborators. Beneficial effect of carotid endarterectomy in symptomatic patients with high-grade carotid stenosis. N Engl J Med. 1991;325:445-53.

36. Chimowitz MI, Lynn MJ, Howlett-Smith H, et al. Comparison of warfarin and aspirin for symptomatic intracranial arterial stenosis. N Engl J Med. 2005;352:1305-16.

37. Chimowitz MI, Kokkinos J, Strong J, et al. The Warfarin-Aspirin Symptomatic Intracranial Disease Study. Neurology. 1995;45:1488-93.

38. Isono S. Anatomy and physiology of upper airway obstruction. In: Kryger MH, Roth T, Dement WC, eds. Principles and Practice of Sleep Medicine, 2nd ed. Philadelphia: WB Saunders; 1994:642-56.

39. White D. Central sleep apnea. In: Kryger MH, Roth T, Dement WC, eds. Principles and Practice of Sleep Medicine, 2nd ed. Philadelphia: WB Saunders; 1994:630-41.

40. Franklin KA. Cerebral haemodynamics in obstructive sleep apnea and Cheyne-Strokes respiration. Sleep Med Rev. 2002;6:457-69.

41. Neau JP, Paquereau J, Meurice JC, et al. Stroke and sleep apnea: cause or consequence? Sleep Med Rev. 2005:6:457-69.

42. Mohsenin V. Sleep-related breathing disorders and risk of stroke. Stroke. 2001;32:1271-8.

43. Palomaki H, Partinen M, Erkinjunetti T, Kaste M. Snoring, sleep apnea syndrome, and stroke. Neurology. 1992;42:75-81; discussion 2.

44. Palomaki H. Snoring and the risk of ischemic brain infarction. Stroke. 1991;22:1021-5.

45. Spriggs DA, French JM, Murdy JM, et al. Snoring increases the risk of stroke and adversely affects prognosis. Q J Med. 1992;83:555-62.

46. Good DC, Henkle JQ, Gelber D, et al. Sleep-disordered breathing and poor functional outcome after stroke. Stroke. 1996;27:252-9.

47. Parra O. Sleep-disordered breathing and stroke: is there a rationale for treatment? Eur Respir J. 2001;18:619-22.

Chapter 3

Transient Ischemic Attack

LUCAS RESTREPO, MD

Key Points

- Transient ischemic attacks (TIAs) are rapidly reversible episodes of focal neurologic dysfunction that may herald stroke.
- Typical TIA patterns usually involve a cluster of symptoms that point to a specific brain region or vascular territory.
- The goals of the diagnostic work-up are to confirm the diagnosis of ischemia and to establish the underlying cause of the ischemia.
- The evaluation and treatment of TIA is essentially the same as for stroke and should be accomplished in an expeditious manner. In many cases, this may require an in-patient admission.
- Patients who experience a TIA associated with isolated sensory symptoms that resolve within 10 minutes are at risk for recurrent TIA but not for stroke. TIA associated with weakness and speech impairment, however, is a stronger risk factor for stroke.

Transient ischemic attack (TIA) is a rapidly reversible episode of focal neurologic dysfunction attributable to cerebrovascular disease. TIAs are not benign and are related to stroke the same way that angina is related to myocardial infarction. The analogy to angina is incomplete in that coronary artery disease is nearly always caused by coronary atherosclerosis, whereas cerebrovascular disease is a syndrome of diverse (and frequently undetermined) etiology. TIA can herald stroke in the near future and, if caused by atherosclerosis, is associated with a future risk of myocardial infarction and death. On the other hand, TIA presents physicians with a unique opportunity to avert grim outcomes through specific medical and surgical interventions.

Definition

The duration of TIA is a matter of controversy (1). The traditional definition requires a duration of less than 24 hours, despite the fact that about 75% of TIAs last less than 60 minutes (1,2). The average duration of TIA is 14 minutes when the carotid system is involved and 8 minutes when the vertebrobasilar circulation is affected (3). Furthermore, episodes of acute neurologic dysfunction lasting more than 60 minutes have only a 15% chance of spontaneous improvement over the next 23 hours (4). The 24-hour cutoff is based on the assumption that only symptoms persisting longer than 1 day portend irreversible brain injuries (1,2). However, we will later discuss that a substantial proportion of patients with symptoms lasting less than 24 hours have evidence of acute brain infarction on neuroimaging studies. Therefore, arbitrary time-defined boundaries between TIA and ischemic stroke lack an authentic pathophysiological basis.

Between 15% and 30% of patients with ischemic stroke have a preceding TIA (4a). The need for urgent evaluation of TIA is stressed by the fact that among patients with ischemic stroke and preceding TIA, the TIA predates the stroke by 1 week or less in 43% and occurs on the day of stroke in 17% (4a).

A new definition of TIA has been proposed, in which every patient with brain infarction (demonstrated on neuroimaging) is diagnosed with stroke instead of TIA, irrespective of the duration of symptoms (1). This definition implies that the difference between TIA and stroke is irreversible tissue damage in stroke.

Pathophysiology

Two main factors dictate whether brain tissue subjected to hypoperfusion becomes necrotic: the magnitude and the duration of cerebral hypoperfusion (5). The former is the most important factor, given that any decline of the cerebral blood flow (CBF) below 12 mL/100 g of tissue per minute is sufficient to cause infarction regardless of the duration of ischemia (5). (Normal CBF is 55 mL/100 g per minute.) For the most part, however, hypoperfused brain tissue does not immediately become infarcted (6). Mildly hypoperfused regions of the brain (flow >22 mL/100 g per min) are dysfunctional but may not become necrotic (6,7). Within an area subjected to ischemia, the more intensely hypoperfused region is usually centrally located, hence the term *ischemic core*, which is surrounded by regions of less severe hypoperfusion, called the *penumbra* (Figure 3-1). Tissue survival is mediated prominently by promptness of recanalization and availability of vascular collaterals. Collateral circulation becomes richer with chronic ischemia, permitting neural cells within the affected vascular

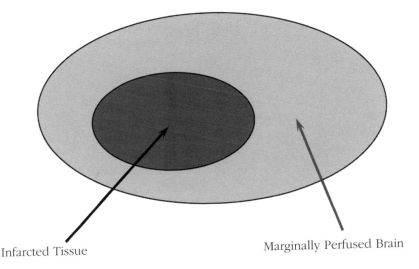

Infarcted Tissue   Marginally Perfused Brain

Figure 3-1 Diagram of the ischemic penumbra.

territory to withstand partial deteriorations of brain perfusion. Additionally, repeated ischemic insults are known to induce neuronal tolerance to ischemic injury, a phenomenon called ischemic preconditioning (8). In fact, the notion has been advanced that TIAs could be "neuroprotective," meaning that ischemic strokes preceded by TIA appear to be less severe than those not preceded by TIA (8,9).

Several lines of evidence suggest that TIA is associated with irreversible ischemic brain damage in a considerable proportion of cases (see below). A study using 1H-MR spectroscopy revealed that hemispheres affected by TIA have a decreased brain NAA/choline ratio, suggesting loss of neurons, compared with the asymptomatic hemisphere and the brains of control subjects (10).

Risk Factors

"It is much more important to know what sort of patient has a disease than what sort of disease a patient has." This ingenious adage of William Osler serves to remind us that TIAs mostly occur in the context of cardiovascular disease and its various risk factors. In fact, the absence of vascular risk factors should probably raise doubts about the validity of the diagnosis of TIA and may instead suggest a stroke "imitator." However, this paradigm may not be applicable to elderly patients with transient neurologic symptoms, which should always be taken seriously (11). Chapter 2 deals with stroke risk factors, which can be extrapolated to TIA (12).

Diagnosis

The diagnosis of TIA can be challenging because objective evidence of brain ischemia or even brain dysfunction is often lacking. Physicians usually examine patients when symptoms have resolved, and therefore may need to rely on the retrospective account of a patient who may have an acute brain injury. Whenever possible, physicians should seek the appraisal of any witnesses of the episode, particularly when the patient has a history of dementia or cognitive sequelae of prior stroke.

Symptoms

The manifestations of TIA are protean. As Toole properly points out, the symptoms of TIA are as many as there are brain functions (13). However, cerebrovascular disease is usually not manifested by isolated symptoms. Typical TIA patterns usually involve a cluster of symptoms that point to a specific brain region or a vascular territory. For example, recurrent spells of aphasia associated with right face and hand weakness and sensory loss are suggestive of left carotid artery stenosis in a right-handed individual.

Without a sophisticated knowledge of vascular anatomy, one can sort the clinical manifestations of TIA into two broad categories: anterior and posterior circulation symptoms (Table 3-1). Such classification is advantageous because it can guide management. For instance, symptoms suggestive of posterior circulation ischemia are usually the consequence of vertebrobasilar atherosclerosis. In this case, requesting a carotid ultrasound appears rather useless, whereas a computed-tomographic angiography or

---

Table 3-1 Symptoms/Signs of Transient Ischemic Attack Suggesting Specific Vascular Territory

Anterior Circulation

- Amaurosis fugax (ophthalmic artery, a branch of the internal carotid artery)
- Aphasia (language involvement—not the same as dysarthria, which is a problem with articulation)
- Unilateral cheiro-oral weakness and numbness (face and hand)

Posterior Circulation

- Dizziness (including vertigo, gait instability, drop attacks)
- Hemiparesis with contralateral facial weakness ("crossed" signs)
- Isolated hemi-anopia (occipital lobe ischemia)
- Bilateral visual field loss (top-of-the-basilar syndrome with bilateral occipital ischemia)
- Diplopia
- Bifacial, particularly perioral paresthesias

magnetic-resonance angiography are the tests of choice because they provide images of the vertebrobasilar system in addition to the carotid artery.

Another strategy of potential practical relevance is to categorize the clinical picture into "hard" and "soft" TIA. As discussed, some symptoms are strongly suggestive of TIA, whereas those listed as "soft" in Table 3-2 are less compelling. This does not mean that such transient neurologic symptoms do not need careful evaluation, particularly when they occur in the right context. For instance, transient loss of consciousness does not indicate TIA but instead points to a separate clinical entity, syncope, requiring evaluation, albeit of a different kind.

Dizziness is a common and often a perplexing symptom. The clinician first needs to determine what is the meaning of the word dizzy, which has many different connotations. Some patients mean *vertigo*, while others mean *leg weakness* or *blurred vision* or *lightheadedness*. Patients with cerebrovascular disease often assign the word *dizziness* to gait unsteadiness.

Another symptom that causes considerable uncertainty is *confusion*. Sometimes patients or observers of the TIA who report confusion are actually referring to transient aphasia. However, drowsiness, lethargy, and unusual behavior are not symptoms suggestive of TIA. Finally, cephalalgia is said to accompany about 20% of TIAs (13). Although patients with ischemic stroke frequently complain of cephalalgia, this symptom more often indicates a less grave entity such as migraine, especially in young patients. Neck pain with unilateral limb pain is not a typical symptom of TIA.

Physical Findings

It is often emphasized that the neurologic exam of patients with TIA must be normal. This appears rather deceptive if one considers that patients with TIA often have a prior history of stroke, with its wealth of confounding physical deficits. Therefore, the diagnosis of TIA should always be considered when patients report regaining baseline neurologic function. Conversely, physicians tend to disagree on the interpretation of neurologic

Table 3-2 "Hard" and "Soft" Symptoms of Transient Ischemic Attack

"Hard"	"Soft"
• Aphasia	• Hemiparesthesias
• Hemiparesis	• Vertigo
• Monocular blindness	• Lightheadedness
	• Blurred vision
	• Confusion
	• Cephalalgia
	• Cervicalgia
	• Unilateral limb pain

signs, more so if the abnormalities are subtle. An astute inquiry is to look for hemineglect or anosognosia (i.e., lack of perception of own illness). A patient with hemineglect may report being free of symptoms or deficits as a consequence of the neurologic injury, but the neurologic examination will demonstrate a deficit (e.g., focal weakness or objective sensory loss).

Evidence of cardiovascular disease can be obtained relatively quickly. The auscultation of the neck can disclose bruits. The cardiac auscultation should concentrate on the presence of S4, which may announce coronary artery disease, while S3 anticipates the presence of left ventricular dysfunction. The ophthalmologic examination does provide a unique opportunity to assess the patient's vasculature and an estimate of the bulk of systemic atherosclerosis. Furthermore, the presence of debris within the lumen of retinal arteries provides direct evidence of embolization. Occasionally, erythromelalgia (marked redness, local warmth and tenderness of the hands and feet) may precede or follow TIA in patients with myeloproliferative disorders (14).

Diagnostic Work-Up

The diagnostic work-up of TIA has two main objectives: 1) substantiate the diagnosis of brain ischemia (if possible), and 2) establish the underlying cause of brain ischemia. The point of attaining these two goals is to implement the secondary prevention of further cerebrovascular events.

General Chemistry

Metabolic abnormalities can imitate acute stroke or TIA. The most familiar stroke imitators are hypoglycemia and hyperglycemia, which can easily be ruled out using a bedside glucometer. Hyponatremia and hypernatremia can also present with focal neurologic deficits that can be confused with stroke or TIA. It is essential to keep in mind that individuals with a history of structural brain damage of any etiology can experience acute deterioration of their old focal neurologic deficits during an acute systemic illness (e.g., acute encephalopathy due to renal failure, liver dysfunction, infection, or intoxication). The clinical picture may superficially seem like an acute recurrence of a primary neurologic illness. The presence of metabolic disturbances, with the support of appropriate negative neuroimaging, may clarify the issue.

Complete Blood Cell Count

The blood cell count can provide useful clues. TIA can occasionally be associated with polycythemia, thrombocythemia, and various myeloproliferative disorders (14). Thrombocytopenia may accompany thrombotic thrombocytopenic purpura and the antiphospholipid antibody syndrome. The diagnosis of cerebrovascular disease, on the other hand, calls for an expedient correction of anemia, with a goal hematocrit of about 30%.

Neuroimaging

Every patient presenting with TIA requires prompt assessment with neuroimaging. The purpose of neuroimaging is two-fold: 1) obtain evidence of brain ischemia (acute or old), and 2) exclude structural brain lesions that may simulate stroke, including subdural hematoma, brain neoplasm (Case 3-1), arteriovenous malformation, aneurysms, and, occasionally, intracerebral hemorrhage.

Head Computed Tomography

Computed tomography (CT) is a rapid and widely available technique that can efficiently help in the assessment of TIA. CT can reliably exclude various structural brain pathologies that can produce focal neurologic deficits. It can also provide evidence of remote or even acute brain ischemia in about 20% of patients (15-17). There are no apparent differences in the clinical features and symptom duration between TIA patients who do have ischemic lesions on CT and those who do not (17). Therefore, one cannot assume that a TIA patient has a normal CT scan, and neuorimaging should still be undertaken. The addition of CT angiography can help rule out a vasculopathy as the underlying cause of TIA. Despite its various attributes, CT is not sensitive at detecting acute brain ischemia during the initial 24 hours after symptom onset and is not ideal for the assessment of the brainstem or cerebellum because of the almost universal occurrence of posterior fossa artifacts. In addition, about 50% of infarcts never become visible on CT, whereas parenchymal hemorrhages may become indistinguishable from infarcts 5-7 days after the onset of symptoms (18).

Brain Magnetic Resonance Imaging

Magnetic resonance imaging (MRI) is probably the most useful diagnostic tool available for the assessment of TIA. MRI is more sensitive than CT scan at detecting both brain ischemia and evidence of previous hemorrhage (18). The addition of magnetic resonance angiography to the conventional MRI sequences helps determine whether a vasculopathy (intra- or extra-cranial) is the cause of the TIA. However, conventional MRI may not reveal ischemic changes during the first 24 hours after the onset of symptoms. Although conventional MRI sequences may demonstrate evidence of focal, presumably ischemic, lesions in 46%-81% of patients with TIA (mostly isolated, old small infarcts) (19-21), one has to bear in mind that 28% of community-dwelling elderly subjects without known prior stroke have clinically "silent" brain infarcts on MRI scan, which are even more prevalent in individuals with cerebrovascular risk factors (22). Nevertheless, when patients are followed up with MRI 1 year after TIA, 37% develop "silent" focal lesions and more brain atrophy than controls without history of TIA (21).

Changes suggestive of acute brain infarction (e.g., evolving edema) can be demonstrated in about one third of the patients with TIA using conventional MRI sequences (20). A constraint of conventional MRI is that the differentiation between acute and chronic ischemia may be difficult, as areas of T2 hyperintensity (for instance, periventricular white matter disease) may "hide" new lesions. Such limitations can be surmounted by the addition of diffusion-weighted imaging (DWI) to the MRI protocol (see Chapter 4). DWI can detect ischemic changes earlier than conventional MRI sequences, even within 1-2 hours after the onset of symptoms. Not surprisingly, 29%-67% of patients with TIA have focal DWI abnormalities suggestive of acute brain ischemia (23-28). DWI abnormalities usually evolve into lesions appreciable on subsequent MRI, although occasionally they may regress on follow-up neuroimaging (29). Little information regarding the added value of perfusion-weighted imaging (PWI) is currently available, although some patients with TIA have presented a "mismatch" between the DWI and PWI defects (Case 3-2), whereas others present isolated regions of PWI abnormality but no acute infarction on DWI (Case 3-3) (10,30-32,32a).

Electrocardiogram

Patients with a diagnosis of reversible neurologic symptoms are at an increased risk of having cardiac events, particularly heart failure, myocardial infarction, ventricular arrhythmia, and unstable angina (33,34). The risk is greater when the electrocardiogram is abnormal. About 4% of patients presenting with TIA and electrocardiogram abnormalities may sustain a cardiac event within 90 days, whereas 0.6% of TIA cases with normal electrocardiogram have cardiac complications. Electrocardiogram evidence of left ventricular hypertrophy, atrial fibrillation, and atrioventricular conduction abnormalities appear to double the risk of cardiac events (34). The added benefits of continuous telemetry or Holter monitoring are unclear. However, both are indicated if there is suspicion of cardiac arrhythmia.

Echocardiogram

An echocardiogram should be considered for all patients with TIA because adverse cardiac outcomes are a major concern in these patients and 18%-26% of all TIAs are attributed to cardioembolism (35,36). The information provided by the echocardiogram has concrete implications for patient management. It can provide an estimate of both systolic and diastolic cardiac function and suggest the presence of coronary artery disease (e.g., show areas of ventricular hypokinesis). Diagnostic accuracy is best with transesophageal echocardiogram, which provides greater detail of valvular structures, presence of mural thrombosis, and aortic atherosclerosis. However, a transthoracic echocardiogram is almost as useful, with the advantages of being noninvasive and easier to obtain. A "bubble test" can be performed with both transthoracic and transesophageal echocardiogram, which helps rule out an intra-cardiac shunt. The treatment of up to 15% of patients with TIA is modified on the basis of the echocardiography results (37). The finding of an intracardiac thrombus or ejection fraction of less than 30% could persuade the clinician to start anticoagulation, whereas aortic atherosclerosis is a compelling reason to use statins.

Carotid Duplex and Transcranial Doppler

Ultrasound techniques are widely available and are a relatively inexpensive way to assess the craniocervical circulation. Large-artery atherosclerosis, mostly involving the extracranial portion of the internal carotid arteries, accounts for 11%-15% of all TIA cases (35,36). Duplex ultrasound is sensitive at estimating the presence and degree of stenosis compared with conventional angiography. Nevertheless, the technique may fail to detect significant abnormalities in about 20% of patients with carotid stenosis (38). Transcranial Doppler is useful for detecting intracranial vessel occlusion and stenosis (39,40). Transcranial Doppler has the added advantage that it can detect microembolic signals and suggest the presence of collateral circulation (40). The disadvantages of the technique are the occasional impossibility of finding a suitable window of insonation through the temples and its dependence on the technical skill of the operator.

Other vascular techniques such as magnetic resonance angiography, CT angiography, and conventional catheter angiography are discussed in detail in Chapter 4. All patients with TIA should have vascular evaluation of the appropriate cerebral vessels, guided by the localization of the TIA symptoms.

Differential Diagnosis

TIA is not a diagnosis of exclusion or an act of faith. The unveiling of an underlying pathology associated with brain ischemia is essential for the diagnosis to make sense. Without the pursuit of a sensible diagnostic work-up and a careful consideration of the differential diagnosis, the label "TIA" becomes *caveat emptor*. The following is a discussion of stroke and TIA imitators.

Migraine with Focal Neurologic Signs

The term *complicated migraine* refers to attacks of severe cephalalgia associated with significant focal neurologic deficits. The neurologic deficits typically precede the headache ("migraine aura"), and the most common manifestation is visual disturbance, ranging from a spot in the vision (scotoma) to frank hemianopia. Patients with hemiplegic migraine have prolonged but reversible episodes of unilateral weakness. Other manifestations include focal neurologic deficits limited to the perioral region and ipsilateral hand (i.e., cheiro-oral distribution), migratory paresthesias, and sometimes aphasia (42). Although the attacks often involve the same side, the sides may be alternately involved. Other prolonged focal neurologic deficits associated with migraine include sudden episodes of monocular visual loss or photopsias (retinal or ophthalmic migraine). The diagnosis can only be considered after a meticulous attempt to rule out a structural cerebral or ophthalmic pathology (see Case 3-3).

Migraine without Cephalalgia

Migraine auras without headaches are not uncommon and may be very difficult to differentiate from TIA. TIA has a prevalence of about 1% of the population, while almost 40% of migraineurs report auras without headache (42). In contrast to migraine with cephalalgia, acephalgic migraines usually have their onset during adulthood and become more frequent with advancing age, often referred as late-life migrainous "accompaniments." The typical story is of a patient with a history of migraine at a younger age (e.g., 20s and 30s) who has disappearance of the headaches later in life, but then who has a resurgence of migraine aura without headache in their 60s. To make matters worse, some individuals with acephalgic migraine may not have a history of headaches.

The classic paradigms of Fisher are useful in distinguishing migraine from TIA (Table 3-3) (5,42). In particular, recurrent stereotypical episodes of focal neurologic dysfunction without permanent neurologic sequelae are suggestive of migraine. Classically, a focal "spread" or "march" of symptoms has been regarded as an indication of either seizure activity or migraine. The spread of symptoms to contiguous body parts occasionally occurs at the onset of stroke or TIA, but the leisurely spread of symptoms over 20 to 30 minutes is more suggestive of migraine (43). Therefore, migraine is a diagnosis of exclusion, and the term should only be considered when cerebral ischemia and other structural brain pathologies have been duly ruled out.

Focal Seizures

Focal neurologic deficits are well-recognized consequences of seizures, although the preceding convulsive movements almost always prevent any confusion with stroke. Although ictal seizure activity is classically associated with "positive" motor phenomena such as abnormal movements and flashing lights, "negative" ictal phenomena, such as weakness or aphasia, have been described on rare occasions (44,45). Seizures should be suspected when tonic-clonic movements precede the focal neurologic deficit, when the episodes of neurologic dysfunction are stereotyped, or when alterations

---

Table 3-3 Features Suggestive of Migrainous "Accompaniments"

- Unexplained reversible neurologic episodes after thorough work-up
- Several recurrences without neurologic sequelae
- Episodes stereotypical
- Simple "positive" visual symptoms (e.g., scintillating scotoma)
- Gradual enlargement of visual symptoms over 5 to 30 minutes
- "March" of paresthesias through one side of the body over 5 to 30 minutes
- Succession of symptoms (e.g., visual aura followed by paresthesia)

of consciousness resembling a postictal period occur. At any rate, a first seizure does require thorough assessment because seizures can be the symptom of an underlying structural lesion of the brain, including stroke. The use of electroencephalography is not routine in the diagnostic work-up of TIA but should be considered in certain cases (Case 3-1).

Vertigo

Isolated vertigo is on rare occasions the presenting symptom of cerebrovascular disease (46). Nevertheless, vertigo requires a careful assessment, particularly in elderly individuals, to determine whether it corresponds to a cerebrovascular or vestibular pathology. The vertigo associated with cerebrovascular disease tends to last longer than the short bouts of symptoms associated with paroxysmal positional vertigo. In addition, evidence of cerebellar or brainstem dysfunction can often be observed in patients with cerebrovascular disease who complain of vertigo. Finally, the clinician can induce vertigo and horizontal nystagmus in patients with paroxysmal positional vertigo, whereas persons with brain ischemia have relatively persistent symptoms and nystagmus on primary gaze. Evidence of orthostatic hypotension needs to be specifically investigated. The presence of unilateral hearing loss and tinnitus should suggest inner ear pathology such as Meniere's disease. Nevertheless, the differential diagnosis of intermittent vertigo is large and one of the most challenging neurologic symptoms to evaluate.

Cataplexy-Narcolepsy Syndrome

Approximately one out of 10 patients with vertebrobasilar insufficiency may experience falls without loss of consciousness (47). Patients with TIA may report sudden weakness of the legs, which buckle at the knees as if lacking muscle tone, sometimes precipitated by extensor or rotational movements of the neck. On the other hand, patients with cataplexy usually experience falls in association with strong emotions such as laughter. In addition, they may report the other three classic components of the syndrome: short and irresistible attacks of inappropriate sleep (narcolepsy), sleep paralysis, and hallucinations at the beginning or end of sleep. The differential diagnosis of drop attacks also include cardiac syncope and "atonic" seizures (45). Patients with atonic seizures usually have a longstanding history of severe epilepsy.

Other Entities

On rare occasions, mitochondrial encephalopathies can present with brief episodes of focal neurologic dysfunction. These patients may have a history of hearing or visual impairment, diabetes, short stature, and myopathy.

Increased levels of plasma lactic acid, presence of white matter disease on MRI, and a muscle biopsy showing ragged-red fibers can be used to support the diagnosis. Specific genetic testing can also be considered. Steroid-responsive encephalopathies, such as Hashimoto's, can occasionally present with intermittent or transient neurologic signs, usually associated with drowsiness or confusion. Thyroid-stimulating hormone levels are usually high but can be normal. The presence of elevated titers of serum anti-thyroglobulin and anti-microsomal antibodies are useful to support the diagnosis. Finally, peripheral neuropathies can occasionally be confused with TIA, particularly carpal tunnel syndrome. It is always useful to remember that brain problems are almost never manifested by isolated hand paresthesia or pain.

Management

Management of TIA is probably best accomplished as an in-patient service, not only for safety but also for pragmatism (i.e., speed of work-up). Nevertheless, an outpatient work up is acceptable when symptoms are unlikely to represent brain ischemia (particularly young persons with cephalalgia, sensory symptoms, or vertigo), provided that a follow-up as an outpatient can be reliably arranged within a short period of time (e.g., 1 week). Referral to a neurologist or a neurology center is recommended for most patients with TIA, particularly if the consultant can see the patient in a timely manner and advise with the initial steps of the evaluation.

The treatment of TIA is essentially the same as for stroke. Some recommendations are nonetheless pertinent. Like in stroke, the clinician needs to observe caution at managing the blood pressure. Recurrence of TIA coinciding with the implementation of antihypertensive medication suggests there may be a hemodynamically sensitive stenosis in the cerebral arterial tree. After vascular assessment has been performed, patients with TIA caused by atherosclerotic disease benefit from risk factor control (see Chapter 2). Patients with TIA caused by high-grade carotid artery stenosis should be rapidly assessed for carotid endarterectomy because a delay of surgical treatment exposes the patient to a period of high risk of stroke and reduces the benefit of surgery (see Chapter 9).

Prognosis

Potential cardiovascular death and ischemic stroke are the paramount concerns in patients presenting with TIA. Contemporary estimates suggest that 15% of patients with TIA die within 1 year after their discharge from the hospital (48). However, some simple clinical characteristics are associated with recurrent TIA rather than subsequent stroke, which may help determine which patients need to be admitted to the hospital and receive careful follow-up (33).

One study showed that spells lasting more than 10 minutes were associated with a low risk of recurrent TIA but increased risk of stroke (49). Symptoms lasting longer than 1 hour are associated with evidence of infarction on neuroimaging (25). A history of multiple TIAs, particularly if featuring sensory symptoms, predict recurrent TIA but not subsequent stroke. For example, patients presenting with isolated sensory symptoms resolving within 10 minutes had a 90-day risk for recurrent TIA of 40%, but none had a stroke (33). On the other hand, weakness and speech impairment with the spell and history of diabetes are risk factors for stroke but not for recurrent TIA (33). Motor deficits and aphasia are also correlated with acute infarction on neuroimaging (25). When the CT shows an infarction, patients may have increased mortality, although this was not substantiated by another study (16,17). The underlying mechanism of brain ischemia also has important connotations. The most powerful predictor of early recurrent stroke (within 30 days after stroke) appears to be large-artery atherosclerosis with >50% stenosis, whereas the strongest predictor of stroke recurrence over 5 years is diabetes (50).

Conclusion

Transient ischemic attacks are rapidly reversible episodes of focal neurologic dysfunction attributable to cerebrovascular disease. TIAs are not benign and may herald menacing complications, including ischemic stroke, myocardial infarction, congestive heart failure, and death. However, physicians have the opportunity to avert these complications with the help of a detailed history taking, neurological examination, and the selection of certain tests, particularly MRI, to stratify the risk of patients and subsequently plan specific medical or surgical interventions.

Case Study 3-1

A 48-year-old right-handed woman with history of breast cancer presented with a 10-minute episode of word-finding difficulties. She had noted a recent recurrent frontal cephalalgia, which she attributed to sinusitis. The physical and neurologic examinations were completely unremarkable, as was head CT. She was admitted for work-up of possible TIA.

Another episode of speech difficulty lasting 20 minutes was witnessed by a medical student, who noted non-fluent aphasia, anomia, and intact ability to follow complex commands. No hemiparesis or facial asymmetry was reported. An electroencephalogram was normal. The patient's brain MRI is shown in Figure 3-2. A spinal tap showed 1 RBC, 1 WBC, protein of 86, and glucose of 45 mg/dL. Cerebral spinal fluid cytopathology analysis revealed adeno-carcinomatous cells.

The patient was treated with IV dexamethasone and whole-brain radiation. She had another episode of aphasia, this time lasting almost 40 minutes. She underwent 48-hour video electroencephalogram monitoring, which was normal, although no episodes of aphasia occurred during the recording. One week later, the patient had a focal motor seizure involving the right upper extremity and was treated with IV phenytoin. She died 1 month later.

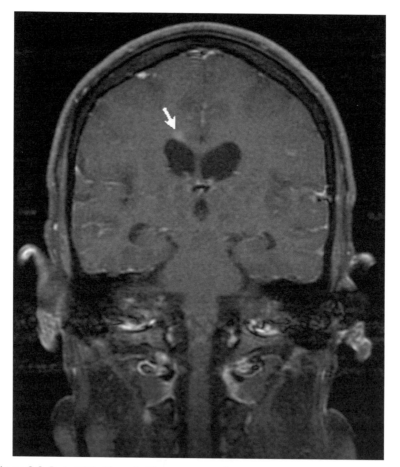

Figure 3-2 Brain MRI with and without contrast of patient in Case 3-1, showing a small, rounded enhancing lesion on the right frontal lobe vertex and multiple areas of contrast enhancement in the periventricular region and cerebellum. No acute infarction was noted. The magnetic resonance angiogram (not shown) was normal.

Discussion

This patient with carcinomatous meningitis likely had ictal aphasia despite the negative electroencephalogram studies. In this condition, a focal seizure affects only the language area of the brain, causing temporary dysfunction.

Case Study 3-2

A 64-year-old man with history of hypertension, coronary artery disease, and hyperlipidemia suddenly experienced a 10-minute episode of right-sided weakness and word-finding difficulties. He suffered a similar episode while en-route to the emergency department. Once in the hospital, a fluctuating non-fluent aphasia accompanied by severe right hemiparesis was noted by his physicians for almost 12 hours. The episodes resolved completely after therapy with intravenous fluids and heparin were initiated. Interestingly, the patient had noted a subjective bruit on the left side of the neck over the 2 preceding weeks, which suddenly disappeared before the onset of focal neurologic symptoms.

On exam, the blood pressure was 144/63 and the pulse rate was 70. The neck auscultation revealed no bruits. The neurologic examination was essentially unremarkable, except for subtle cupping of the right hand when closing the eyes while holding the arms outstretched. The carotid duplex suggested complete occlusion of the left internal carotid artery. A brain MRI obtained several days after the onset of symptoms (Figure 3-3) showed acute infarction in the deep left middle cerebral artery territory. The perfusion scan showed hypoperfusion in the left middle cerebral artery territory in a similar region as the infarction, but perhaps a more extensive lesion than the infarction. Such "mismatch" between the perfusion and diffusion-weighted images is thought to indicate the presence of a brain at risk of becoming infarcted (the area of hypoperfusion without infarction) and therefore may signal the presence of salvageable tissue.

Transthoracic echocardiography was unremarkable. A conventional angiography demonstrated critical left internal carotid artery stenosis with "trickle of flow" (99%). The patient was taken to the operating room for a carotid endarterectomy 4 days after the onset of his symptoms. He had an excellent recovery and was discharged home on aspirin and simvastatin.

Discussion

This case demonstrates that although the patient met criteria for the traditional definition of TIA (with resolution of symptoms within 24 hours), the patient actually had a significant infarction on MRI.

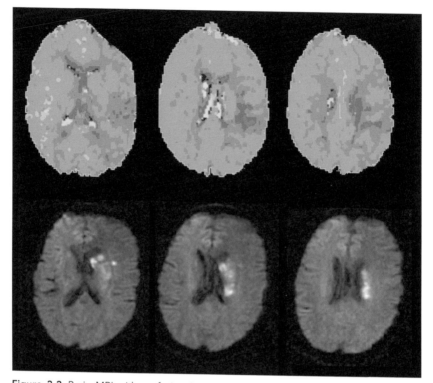

Figure 3-3 Brain MRI with perfusion (*upper sequence*) and diffusion-weighted images (*lower sequence*) of Case 3-2, demonstrating several acute subcortical infarcts, suggestive of artery-to-artery embolization. The perfusion scan shows ipsilateral regions of relative hypoperfusion (*darker grey area*), which do not match the acutely infarcted tissue (*bright signal on the diffusion scan*). The most affected region on the diffusion sequence, the caudate nucleus, appears reperfused. Such "mismatch" between the perfusion and diffusion-weighted images is thought to indicate the presence of a brain at risk of becoming infarcted and therefore may signal the presence of salvageable tissue.

Moreover, the presence of a persistent perfusion defect was found to be caused by high-grade carotid stenosis, and the patient was at risk of further infarction due to the precarious degree of perfusion in the left carotid territory. These findings led to admission of the patient and relatively quick surgical treatment of the carotid artery stenosis.

Case Study 3-3

A 42-year-old woman with a history of migraines experienced a 20-minute episode of right-sided weakness and paresthesias associated with speech difficulties during what appeared to be a typical migraine. The patient had had a similar episode, also associated with headache, 1 year before. Otherwise, the recurrent episodes of cephalalgia never

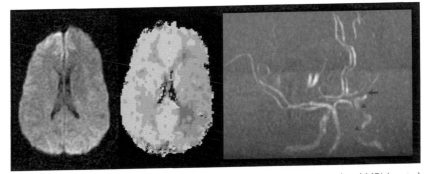

Figure 3-4 Brain MRI with diffusion-weighted MRI (*left*), perfusion-weighted MRI (*center*) and magnetic resonance angiogram (*right*) of Case 3-3, showing a large area of relative hypoperfusion affecting the left middle cerebral artery territory (*darker grey area in the middle image*). The magnetic resonance angiogram demonstrates an occlusion of the M1 segment of the left middle cerebral artery (*arrow*) and poor flow in the left internal carotid artery (*arrowheads*). The other MRI sequences, including T_1, T_2, fluid-attenuated inversion recovery (FLAIR), and diffusion-weighted imaging (DWI), were all normal.

featured focal neurologic symptoms, except for fortification spectra. The headaches began at age 38, with a frequency of 2 per week and duration of 2-24 hours, usually associated with photophobia, sonophobia, nausea, and intolerance to movements. The past medical history was also significant for hypertension, type 2 diabetes, hyperlipidemia, and hypothyroidism after radioablation for Graves' disease.

The patient reported that a new medication for blood pressure had been prescribed 1 week before the latest episode of reversible hemiparesis. She was a former smoker, with a 20-pack-year history. The physical exam was unremarkable, except for central obesity (weight was 245 lb). The blood glucose was 132 mg/dL, hemoglobin was 10 g/dL, and hematocrit was 33.1%. The thyroid-stimulating hormone level was within normal limits. Total cholesterol was 201 and LDL was 110 mg/dL. Electrocardiogram was normal.

MRI and magnetic resonance angiogram (Figure 3-4) showed no evidence of infarction but showed hypoperfusion in the left middle cerebral artery territory. Magnetic resonance angiography suggested left middle cerebral artery occlusion, which was subsequently confirmed on conventional angiography. Angiography also showed extensive small collateral vessels that helped to supply the distal left middle cerebral artery territory, which suggested that this was a slowly progressive occlusion of the vessel due to atherosclerosis.

Discussion

This patient had migraine with aura, but a change in the type of neurologic symptom prompted further evaluation, revealing intracranial atherosclerotic disease as the underlying cause. The recent addition of a new antihypertensive medication probably triggered the TIA in an already compromised hemisphere.

REFERENCES

1. Albers GW, Caplan LR, Easton JD, et al. Transient ischemic attack: proposal for a new definition. N Engl J Med. 2002;347:1713-6.
2. Marshall J. The natural history of transient ischaemic cerebro-vascular attacks. QJM. 1964;33:309-24.
3. Dyken ML, Conneally M, Haerer AF, et al. Cooperative study of hospital frequency and character of transient ischemic attacks, I: background, organization and clinical survey. JAMA. 1977;237:882-6.
4. Levy DE. How transient are transient ischemic attacks? Neurology. 1988;38:674-7.
4a. Rothwell PM, Warlow CP. Timing of TIAs preceding stroke. Neurology. 2005;64:817-20.
5. Adams R, Victor M, Ropper AH. Cerebrovascular diseases. In: Adams R, Victor M, Ropper AH. Principles of Neurology, 6th ed. New York: McGraw-Hill; 1997:781-5.
6. Heiss WD. Imaging in cerebrovascular disease. Curr Opin Neurol. 2001;14:67-75.
7. Heiss WD. Ischemic penumbra: evidence from functional imaging in man. J Cerebral Blood Flow Metab. 2000;20:1276-93.
8. Schaller B, Graf R. Cerebral ischemic preconditioning: an experimental phenomenon or a clinical important entity of stroke prevention? J Neurol. 2002;249:1503-11.
9. Moncayo J, de Freitas GR, Bogousslavsky J, et al. Do transient ischemic attacks have a neuroprotective effect? Neurology. 2000;54:2089-94.
10. Bisschops RHC, Kappelle LJ, Mali WPTM, van der Grond J. Hemodynamic and metabolic changes in transient ischemic attack patients: a magnetic resonance angiography and 1H-magnetic resonance spectroscopy study performed within 3 days of onset of a transient ischemic attack. Stroke. 2002;33:110-5.
11. Bots ML, van der Wilk EC, Koudstaal PJ, et al. Transient neurological attacks in the general population. Prevalence, risk factors, and clinical relevance. Stroke. 1997;28:768-73.
12. Whisnant JP, Brown RD, Petty GW, et al. Comparison of population-based models of risk factors for TIA and ischemic stroke. Neurology. 1999;53:532-6.
13. Toole JF. TIA: pathogenesis and clinical features. In: Toole JF, ed. Cerebrovascular Disorders, 5th ed. Philadelphia: Lippincott Williams & Wilkins;1999:60-70.
14. Michiels JJ, van Genderen PJ, Jansen PH, Koudstaal PJ. Atypical transient ischemic attacks in thrombocythemia of various myeloproliferative disorders. Leuk Lymphoma. 1996;22(Suppl 1):65-70.
15. Davalos A, Matias-Guiu J, Torrent O, et al. Computed tomography in reversible ischaemic attacks: clinical and prognostic correlations in a prospective study. J Neurol. 1988;235:155-8.
16. Evans GW, Howard G, Murros KE, et al. Cerebral infarction verified by cranial computed tomography and prognosis for survival following transient ischemic attack. Stroke. 1991;22:431-6.
17. Dennis M, Bamford J, Sandercock P, et al. Computed tomography in patients with transient ischaemic attacks: when is a transient ischaemic attack not a transient ischaemic attack but a stroke? J Neurol. 1990;237:257-61.
18. Wardlaw JM. Radiology of stroke. J Neurol Neurosurg Psychiatr. 2001;70(Suppl I):7-11.
19. Bhadelia RA, Anderson M, Polak JF, et al. Prevalence and associations of MRI: demonstrated brain infarcts in elderly subjects with a history of transient ischemic attack. The Cardiovascular Health Study. Stroke. 1999;30:383-8.
20. Fazekas F, Fazekas G, Schmidt R, et al. Magnetic resonance imaging correlates of transient cerebral ischemic attacks. Stroke. 1996;27:607-11.

21. Walters RJ, Fox NC, Schott JM, et al. Transient ischaemic attacks are associated with increased rates of global cerebral atrophy. J Neurol Neurosurg Psychiatr. 2003;74:213-6.

22. Price TR, Psaty B, O'Leary D, et al. Assessment of cerebrovascular disease in the Cardiovascular Health Study. Ann Epidemiol. 1993;3:5047.

23. Kidwell CS, Alger JR, Di Salle F, et al. Diffusion MRI in patients with transient ischemic attacks. Stroke. 1999;30:1174-80.

24. Ay H, Oliveira-Filho J, Buonanno FS, et al. 'Footprints' of transient ischemic attacks: a diffusion-weighted MRI study. Cerebrovasc Dis. 2002;14:177-86.

25. Crisostomo RA, Garcia MM, Tong DC. Detection of diffusion-weighted MRI abnormalities in patients with transient ischemic attack: correlation with clinical characteristics. Stroke. 2003;34:932-7.

26. Marx JJ, Mika-Gruettner A, Thoemke F, et al. Diffusion weighted magnetic resonance imaging in the diagnosis of reversible ischaemic deficits of the brainstem. J Neurol Neurosurg Psychiatr. 2002;72:572-5.

27. Kastrup A, Schulz JB, Mader I, et al. Diffusion-weighted MRI in patients with symptomatic internal carotid artery disease. J Neurol. 2002;249:1168-74.

28. Rovira A, Rovira-Gols A, Pedraza S, et al. Diffusion-weighted MR imaging in the acute phase of transient ischemic attacks. Am J Neurolradiol. 2002;23:77-83.

29. Lecouvet FE, Duprez TPJ, Raymackers JM, et al. Resolution of early diffusion-weighted and FLAIR MRI abnormalities in a patient with TIA. Neurology. 1999;52:1085.

30. Darby DG, Barber PA, Gerraty RP, et al. Pathophysiological topography of acute ischemia by combined diffusion-weighted and perfusion MRI. Stroke. 1999;30:2043-52.

31. El-Koussy M, Lovblad KO, Steinlin M, et al. Perfusion MRI abnormalities in the absence of diffusion changes in a case of moyamoya-like syndrome in neurofibromatosis type 1. Neuroradiology. 2002;44:938-41.

32. Neumann-Haefelin T, Wittsack HJ, Wenserski F, et al. Diffusion- and perfusion-weighted MRI in a patient with a prolonged reversible ischaemic neurological deficit. Neuroradiology. 2000;42:444-7.

32a. Restrepo L, Jacobs MA, Barker PB, Wityk RJ. Assessment of transient ischemic attack with diffusion- and perfusion-weighted imaging. Am J Neuroradiol. 2004;25:1645-52.

33. Johnston SC, Gress DR, Browner WS, Sidney S. Short-term prognosis after emergency-department diagnosis of TIA. JAMA. 2000;284:2901-6.

34. Elkins JS, Sidney S, Gress DR, et al. Electrocardiographic findings predict short-term cardiac morbidity after transient ischemic attack. Arch Neurol. 2000;59:1437-41.

35. Sempere AP, Duarte J, Cabezas C, Clavería LE. Etiopathogenesis of transient ischemic attacks and minor ischemic strokes: a community-based study in Segovia, Spain. Stroke. 1998;29:40-5.

36. Weimar C, Kraywinkel K, Rödl J, et al. Etiology, duration, and prognosis of transient ischemic attacks: an analysis from the German Stroke Data Bank. Arch Neurol. 2002;59:1584-8.

37. Strandberg M, Marttila RJ, Helenius H, Hartiala J. Transoesophageal echocardiography in selecting patients for anticoagulation after ischaemic stroke or transient ischaemic attack. J Neurol Neurosurg Psychiatry. 2002;73:29-33.

38. Johnston DC, Goldstein LB. Clinical carotid endarterectomy decision making: noninvasive vascular imaging versus angiography. Neurology. 2001;56:1009-15.

39. Alexandrov AV, Demchuck AM, Wein TH. Yield of transcranial Doppler in acute cerebral ischemia. Stroke. 1999;30:1604-9.

40. Babikian VL, Feldmann E, Weschler LR, et al. Transcranial Doppler ultrasonography: Year 2000 update. J Neuroimaging. 2000;10:101-15.

41. Johnston DC, Chapman KM, Goldstein LB. Low rate of complications of cerebral angiography in routine clinical practice. Neurology. 2001;57:2012-4.

42. Davidoff RA. Unusual forms of migraine, variants and equivalents. In: Davidoff RA, ed. Migraine: Manifestations, Pathogenesis and Management. 2nd ed. New York: Oxford University Press; 2002:68-89.

43. Cohen SN, Muthukumaran A, Gasser H, El-Saden S. Symptom spread to contiguous body parts as a presentation of cerebral ischemia. Cerebrovasc Dis. 2002;14:84-9.

44. So NK. Atonic phenomena and partial seizures: a reappraisal. In: Negative Motor Phenomena. Fahn S, Hallett H, Luders HO, Marsden CD, eds. Advances in Neurology, vol. 67. Philadelphia: Lippincott-Raven; 1995:29-39.

45. Lee MS, Marsden CD. Drop attacks. In: Negative Motor Phenomena. Fahn S, Hallett H, Luders HO, Marsden CD, eds. Advances in Neurology, vol 67. Philadelphia: Lippincott-Raven; 1995:41-52.

46. Gomez CR, Cruz-Flores S, Malkoff MD, et al. Isolated vertigo as a manifestation of vertebrobasilar ischemia. Neurology. 1996;47:94-7.

47. Brust JCM, Plank CR, Healton EB, Sanchez GF. The pathology of drop attacks: a case report. Neurology. 1979;29:786-90.

48. Bravata DM, Ho SY, Brass LM, et al. Long-term mortality in cerebrovascular disease. Stroke. 2003;34:699-704.

49. Johnston CS, Sidney S, Bernstein AL, Gress DR. A comparison of risk factors for recurrent TIA and stroke in patients diagnosed with TIA. Neurology. 2003;60:280-5.

50. Hankey GJ. Long-term outcome after ischaemic stroke/transient ischaemic attack. Cerebrovasc Dis. 2003;16(Suppl 1):14-9.

Chapter 4

Diagnostic Testing

ROBERT J. WITYK, MD

Key Points

- Imaging studies are useful not only for diagnosis but for assessing for therapeutic interventions.
- Computed tomography is the imaging study most frequently used for acute stroke evaluation.
- The resolution and sensitivity of MRI for the detection of ischemia is higher than that of CT.
- Diffusion-weighted imaging can detect an infarct within 30 minutes after onset of focal ischemia and allows acute infarcts to be distinguished from chronic ischemic changes.
- Perfusion-weighted MRI demonstrates the region of cerebral hypoperfusion. When there is a diffusion-perfusion "mismatch," the area of hypoperfusion without infarction may be salvageable with reperfusion.
- Catheter cerebral angiography is the gold standard for the evaluation of the cerebral vessels.

In most stroke patients, a careful history and neurologic examination provide enough information to localize the lesion and develop several hypotheses of etiology. In situations where the clinical presentation is non-specific or examination findings are uncertain, diagnostic testing is useful to confirm the presence of an ischemic lesion and identify a mechanism of stroke. However, diagnostic tests should be primarily used to confirm or refute hypotheses generated by the history and neurologic examination. Blind reliance on diagnostic testing without an adequate history and neurologic examination can lead to therapeutic misadventures. Unfortunately, it is not unusual to come across patients who present to the hospital with symptoms of vertebrobasilar ischemia who wind up having carotid artery endarterectomy before discharge, simply because a carotid artery lesion was found on a test. It is dangerous to miss a basilar artery stenosis because the carotid artery lesion was easier to find. Current neuro-imaging techniques are extremely sensitive in detecting abnormalities, but not always specific as to the etiology or significance. A substantial portion of the author's outpatient practice consists of evaluation of patients with "abnormalities" on magnetic resonance imaging (MRI) studies obtained to evaluate headaches or other non-specific symptoms. Ironically, the first step in determining the significance of these MRI findings is to take a careful medical history and examine the patient.

Diagnostic tests can be grouped according to the information that they provide. Brain imaging studies such as computed tomography (CT) and MRI show the cerebral anatomy and reveal structural lesions. They can confirm the diagnosis of stroke and localize the lesion and should be performed in all patients in whom stroke or transient ischemic attack (TIA) is suspected. Newer brain imaging techniques also allow assessment of cerebral perfusion, providing functional information. Vascular studies such as ultrasound (carotid duplex and transcranial Doppler [TCD]), magnetic resonance angiography (MRA), CT angiography (CTA), and catheter cerebral angiography assess the cerebrovascular tree in the neck and inside the skull. Cardiac assessment includes electrocardiogram (EKG), echocardiography, and monitoring for cardiac arrhythmias. Laboratory tests assess risk factors (as described in Chapter 2) and focus on hematologic disorders that can contribute to ischemic or hemorrhagic stroke.

In the past, imaging studies focused upon diagnosis, but with the advent of thrombolytic therapy for ischemic stroke we now appreciate that diagnostic imaging plays a critical early role in assessing the patient for therapeutic interventions. These diagnostic imperatives have led to new CT and MRI techniques at an increasing pace. A critical balance currently exists between the need for treatment as early as possible and the time delay associated with increasingly complex diagnostic tests. Although the capabilities of MRI in acute stroke are impressive, factors such as logistics, expense, and availability of testing equipment outside of major centers are recognized as important in determining the acute stroke diagnostic paradigm of the future.

Brain Imaging
Computed Tomography

Computed tomography is the modality most frequently used for acute stroke evaluation due to its availability and sensitivity for detecting intracranial hemorrhage. The initial CT scan may not show a lesion in the early

stage of ischemic stroke and may be insensitive to small infarcts (particularly in the brainstem). Large strokes will be easily visible several days after
stroke onset, but subtle signs may be present even in the first few hours
(see below). CT is extremely reliable in detecting acute intracerebral hemorrhage. CT can also detect old strokes or mass lesions that aid with the differential diagnosis. Because of this high sensitivity to acute bleeding and
ability to detect subacute stroke and other mass lesions, CT provides critical information in assessing patients for thrombolytic therapy. It is also a
rapid test that is available in most hospitals and emergency rooms in the
United States.

Acute hemorrhage is dense (white) on CT, whether in the parenchyma
or in the subarachnoid or subdural space (Figure 4-1). Bone, calcium, and
iodine contrast dye are also dense on CT. Small calcium deposits can occur
in tumors, old strokes, and arteriovenous malformations. Some tumors,
such as meningiomas, may be extensively calcified and mimic bleeds. In
general, a hemorrhage appears as a dense mass exerting pressure on the
surrounding brain and is often surrounded by an area of hypodense edema.

Until recently, the traditional teaching was that an ischemic infarct does
not show up on CT until after 1 to 2 days. Recent studies of patients in
thrombolytic trials reveal that subtle ischemic changes can be identified in
some patients as early as a few hours after stroke onset. The water content
of ischemic brain tissue changes, leading to subtle changes in intensity. These
can be detected by looking for the normal differences between gray matter
(e.g., the cortical ribbon and basal ganglia structures) and the white matter tracts. In the normal brain, gray matter appears slightly brighter (hyperdense) on CT, whereas white matter appears slightly darker (hypodense).

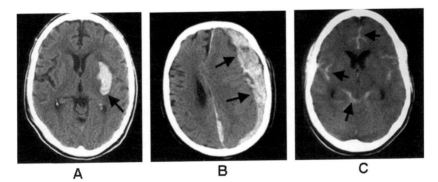

A   **B**   **C**

Figure 4-1 CT images of acute intracerebral blood. **A,** Acute left basal ganglia hemorrhage (*arrow*) limited to the region of the putamen. There is a mild degree of mass effect
with narrowing of the left anterior horn. **B,** Acute left subdural hematoma (*arrows*) throughout the left convexity with mass effect and compression of the ipsilateral brain. **C,** Acute
subarachnoid hemorrhage with blood in the cerebrospinal fluid spaces. Note blood as
bright areas in the anterior interhemispheric fissure (*top arrow*), in the right sylvian fissure
(*middle arrow*), and around the upper brainstem (*bottom arrow*). Subarachnoid blood
does not extend into the ventricles, which remain dark.

A loss of distinction between gray and white matter is a hallmark of early ischemic change. Typical early CT signs of acute cerebral infarction include 1) blurring of the internal capsule, 2) loss of the insular ribbon (a white matter band adjacent to the insular cortex) (Figure 4-2), 3) loss of differentiation between the cortical gray and subcortical white matter, 4) swelling of the cortical gyri, and 5) sulcal effacement.

Another useful sign in acute embolic stroke is the hyperdense middle cerebral artery (MCA) sign. A clot lodged in the MCA is bright and correlates with angiographically demonstrated thrombus (Figure 4-3). This common finding is associated with poor patient outcome.

Despite the important role conventional CT has and will continue to play in acute stroke, some notable deficiencies exist. Despite the examples listed above of early CT changes in ischemic stroke, detection of these changes is difficult in routine practice, and inter-observer agreement is limited even among experts.

Magnetic Resonance Imaging

Acute cerebral ischemia is characterized by changes in water and protein content of brain tissue. MRI takes advantage of the fact that water protons have different biophysical properties depending upon the local environment. The resolution and sensitivity of MRI for the detection of ischemia is higher than CT, particularly for strokes in the brainstem and cerebellum, where CT is limited due to artifact from the adjacent skull base (Figure 4-4). Lacunar infarcts and small cortical strokes are also more readily visualized with MRI. The fluid-attenuated inversion recovery (FLAIR) sequence is especially sensitive to ischemic lesions. FLAIR is essentially a T_2-weighted image in which cerebrospinal fluid signal is suppressed and rendered dark, so that even small infarcts in the cortex can be seen without interference with bright signal from cerebrospinal fluid (Figure 4-5).

A challenge for MRI is the exclusion of intracerebral bleeding in the patient with acute stroke. Spin echo techniques are sensitive for the detection of subacute and chronic blood. In the hyperacute stages of hemorrhage, however, there has been minimal conversion of oxyhemoglobin to breakdown products, and no mature clot formation. Conventional MR sequences are less sensitive under these circumstances, but when combined with hemosiderin-sensitive sequences (e.g. gradient recall echo), hyperacute hemorrhage can be identified. (Figure 4-6). If the sensitivity and specificity of this approach can be confirmed in clinical trials, MRI could be used instead of CT as the initial brain-imaging technique in acute stroke patients.

Diffusion-Weighted Imaging

Diffusion-weighted imaging (DWI) is an exciting new development that capitalizes upon diffusion of water molecules. The technique can be performed on clinical MRI scanners using appropriate software. Within ischemic tissue,

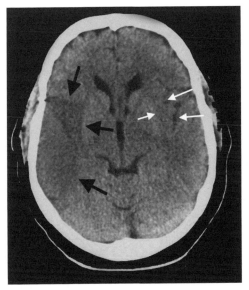

Figure 4-2 Subtle CT signs of acute ischemia. The patient has an acute infarct in the right temporal lobe seen as a region of subtle hypodensity (*black arrows*). Note loss of the insular ribbon, a region of hypodensity between the relatively brighter putamen and insular cortex (*bounded by the white arrows*).

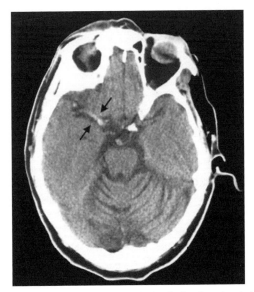

Figure 4-3 Hyperdense MCA sign. Acute embolus lodged in the right middle cerebral artery (*arrows*) appears bright on CT and can be seen immediately, before infarction develops on the remainder of the scan.

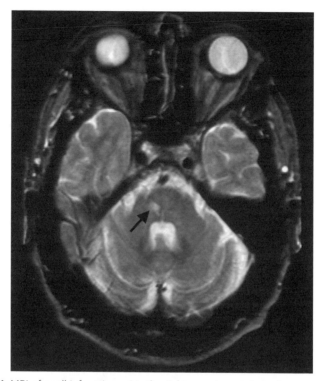

Figure 4-4 MRI of small infarct (*arrow*) in the right pons in a patient who presented with dizziness, dysarthria, and mild left-sided clumsiness. The acute lesion was not visible on the admission CT scan.

water molecule diffusion is decreased, and water molecules are trapped inside of neurons. Restricted diffusion of water molecules results in a conspicuously bright signal on a DWI image. An infarct can be recognized on DWI within 30 minutes after onset of focal ischemia when both conventional MRI and CT images are normal (Figure 4-7). In clinical studies, areas abnormal on DWI almost always progressed to infarction, and for practical purposes, the DWI lesion represents the completed infarct. (Some recent studies, however, suggest that DWI lesions may be partially reversed under circumstances of very early reperfusion.)

The bright signal on DWI of an acute ischemic stroke will fade (pseudo-normalize) over 7 to 10 days if a repeat MRI is obtained. This time-dependent phenomenon is particularly useful because it allows one to distinguish acute infarcts (those occuring within 7 to 10 days) from chronic ischemic changes. In patients with old infarcts or extensive periventricular white matter changes, one can pick out the small focus of acute ischemic damage amidst a region of chronic changes on the MRI (Figure 4-8).

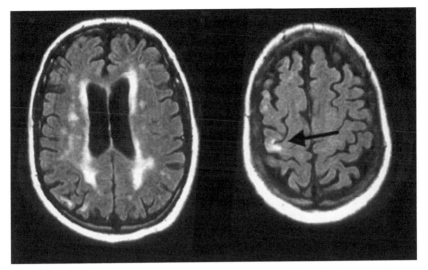

Figure 4-5 MRI FLAIR image. This sequence shows abnormal tissue as bright, with suppression of background spinal fluid bright signal as seen on T_2-weighted images. On the left, there is extensive periventricular white matter ischemic change. On the right, a small cortical infarct is seen (*arrow*), which would be difficult to detect on the standard T_2-weighted image due to adjacent bright spinal fluid signal.

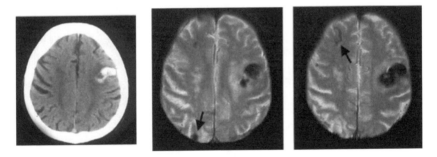

Figure 4-6 Hemosiderin-sensitive MRI sequences. The patient presented with right hand clumsiness and was found to have a small left frontal hemorrhage on CT scan (*left*). Hemosiderin-sensitive MRI (*middle and right*) revealed several other areas of previous occult bleeding in the right parietal and frontal regions (*arrows*), raising the diagnosis of amyloid angiopathy.

Magnetic Resonance Perfusion Imaging

A key component in the treatment of acute ischemic stroke is the concept of the ischemic penumbra (see Chapter 7). In brief, hypoperfusion of the brain results in deficit, but irreversible infarction does not develop immediately. This situation is analogous to "hibernating myocardium" after cardiac ischemia. Irreversible infarction tends to start in the center of a hypoperfused

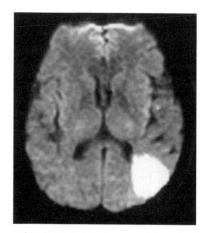

Figure 4-7 Diffusion-weighted MRI (DWI). An acute infarct in the left posterior temporal-parietal region appears as a bright wedge (indicating restricted water diffusion) on the DWI scan.

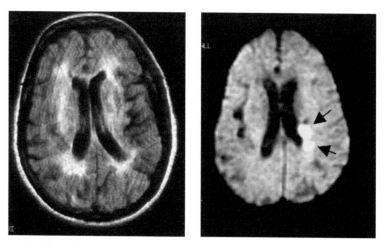

Figure 4-8 Chronic versus acute ischemia. This elderly patient presented with subtle gait deterioration over several days and minimal focal abnormality on examination. FLAIR image (*left*) shows extensive chronic white matter ischemic changes, but no clear lesion suggesting an acute infarction. The clinician was concerned about an occult infection or other metabolic disturbance as the cause of the deterioration. DWI study (*right*) shows an acute subcortical infarct in the white matter adjacent to the ventricle (*arrows*), confirming the presence of an acute infarct sometime in the past week which was hidden by the chronic ischemic changes seen on the FLAIR.

region of brain and enlarge over time. The region of brain that is hypo-perfused but not yet infarcted can potentially be salvaged by reperfusion and is operationally referred to as the "ischemic penumbra." For practical purposes, DWI serves to mark areas of infarction, and perfusion-weighted MRI (PWI) can demonstrate the region of cerebral hypoperfusion.

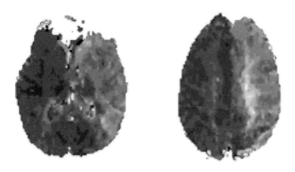

Figure 4-9 Magnetic resonance perfusion imaging (MRPI) using a "time-to-peak" analysis. MRPI in a patient with symptomatic left internal carotid artery stenosis reveals an extensive region of delay of gadolinium transit throughout the left hemisphere (*region of lighter gray and white signal*). Although this represents hypoperfusion from the carotid artery lesion, the measurements are relative to the right hemisphere and do not allow for absolute cerebral blood flow measurements.

PWI is performed using a bolus injection of contrast agent (gadolinium-diethylenetriamine pentaacetic acid) and measuring the change in MRI signal in the brain as contrast passes through. This time-dependent signal change is proportional to the amount of blood flow and can be analyzed by a number of mathematical models to produce maps of relative cerebral blood volume and cerebral blood flow. PWI maps reveal regions of hypoperfusion, particularly in the hemispheres, where blood flow in one hemisphere can be compared with the other (Figure 4-9). This technique does not reliably allow measurement of absolute cerebral blood flow at this time, although this may change with development of newer MRI techniques.

Areas of hypoperfusion correspond to dysfunctional brain and are usually due to a vascular lesion, like a thrombo-embolic occlusion. For example, focal hypoperfusion in the left temporal lobe can be seen in a patient with Wernicke's aphasia due to an embolus to a branch of the left middle cerebral embolism. If the embolus dissolves (either spontaneously or due to thrombolysis), then one often sees resolution of the perfusion defect on repeat imaging. One can imagine that a TIA represents one end of this spectrum, where a patient develops a focal perfusion defect (causing the neurologic symptoms) that resolves before an infarct has time to develop.

Many acute stroke patients have lesions on both DWI and PWI studies. If these lesions are matched in size and location, then the vessel is still occluded and the stroke has likely completed. In some patients with embolic stroke, the clot has lysed and there is a DWI lesion but no PWI lesion. Finally, some patients have a large area of hypoperfusion on PWI but a relatively small area of infarction on DWI. These patients are said to have a diffusion-perfusion "mismatch" and the area of hypoperfusion without infarction may be salvageable (Figure 4-10). Theoretically, patients with a

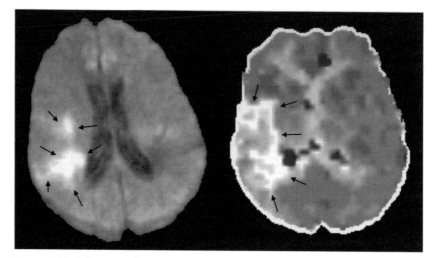

Figure 4-10 Diffusion-perfusion mismatch in acute ischemic stroke. DWI (*left*) shows an area of acute ischemia (*arrows*) in the right parietal lobe which is likely destined to infarction. PWI (*right*), however, shows a larger region of hypoperfusion (*bounded by arrows*), suggesting the brain is at risk for further infarction.

substantial diffusion-perfusion mismatch would have the most to gain from attempts at reperfusion (e.g., thrombolytic therapy), and preliminary observations in patients receiving either intravenous or intra-arterial thrombolysis suggest this may be the case.

A comprehensive evaluation of cerebral ischemia is therefore possible with advanced MRI techniques. Gradient recall echo sequences enable exclusion of intraparenchymal hemorrhage; DWI provides early delineation of the infarct; PWI demonstrates the area at risk of further infarction; and MRA (see below) can demonstrate the occluded vessel itself. These tools allow an exciting view into the cerebral physiology of patients with acute ischemic stroke and promise to improve our ability to select patients for aggressive intervention.

Vascular Assessment

Cerebral Angiography

Catheter cerebral angiography is the accepted gold standard for the evaluation of the cerebral vessels because of its superior resolution. Angiography provides the most reliable and accurate measurement of carotid artery stenosis, upon which two of the major carotid endarterectomy trials were based. Angiography also detects subtle lesions, such as minor arterial dissections, and visualizes the smaller cerebral arteries that might be affected in cerebral vasculitis (Figure 4-11). Finally, angiography remains the gold

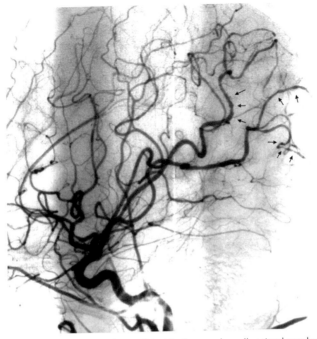

Figure 4-11 Cerebral angiogram of vasculitis. Medium and smaller sized cerebral vessels are imaged best with catheter angiography. This study shows evidence of vasculitis, with beading and irregularity of multiple distal vessels (some of which are demonstrated by *arrows*).

standard for detection of cerebral aneurysms and for the complete depiction of cerebral arteriovenous malformations.

Modern techniques of catheter angiography utilize small and highly flexible catheters which allow injection of dye selectively into the cerebral vessels, and sometimes can be navigated as far as the intracranial circulation (see Chapters 7 and 16). Use of biplane imaging with digital subtraction angiography (DSA) produces very high-resolution pictures of the cerebral vessels from a variety of angles. Rotational angiography allows for a 3-D computer reconstruction of the cerebral vessels after contrast injection. (DSA should not be confused with peripheral DSA, where digital subtraction techniques are used to visualize cerebral vessels after contrast administration through a peripheral intravenous catheter. In the author's opinion, peripheral DSA provides inadequate resolution for most diagnostic purposes in cerebrovascular disease.)

Unfortunately, invasive angiography is associated with a 1% to 2% risk of significant morbidity, which has understandably led to the development of noninvasive vascular diagnostic techniques. The risk of angiography increases with age and co-morbidities, such as hypertension and diabetes;

conversely, angiography is relatively safe in younger patients undergoing evaluation for possible aneurysms.

Duplex Ultrasound

Ultrasound studies provide a rapid and noninvasive means of assessing the cerebral arteries in the neck (carotid and vertebral artery duplex) and inside the skull (TCD). Both assessments can be performed at the bedside and are excellent screening tests, but both can suffer from operator-dependent error. Because of differences in ultrasound machines and technician skill, each laboratory should determine its own parameters for assessing degree of stenosis, and the practicing physician receiving the test reports must develop an awareness of the limitations and accuracy of the local vascular laboratory. Although the literature has suggested an accuracy of greater than 90% for carotid duplex in detecting carotid stenosis, a retrospective analysis of carotid duplex compared with angiography in centers involved in the North American Symptomatic Carotid Endarterectomy Trial found a sensitivity and specificity of only about 70% (1).

Carotid duplex scanning uses a combination of gray-scale images of the vessel with superimposed Doppler to determine flow velocities and to display waveforms. The degree of stenosis at the internal carotid artery (ICA) bifurcation can be estimated by several techniques. The most widely used approach is by analysis of Doppler velocities, particularly peak systolic velocity, end-diastolic velocity, and the ratio of ICA to common carotid artery peak systolic velocities (carotid index). It is important to realize that ultrasound velocities can be affected by systemic factors, such as cardiac output and hematocrit. Another caveat is that carotid duplex may not accurately distinguish critical ICA stenosis from ICA occlusion. When a duplex study report suggests ICA occlusion, a critical stenosis may have been missed due to very low blood flow through the stenosis. These errors are less likely with newer techniques using color imaging.

The extracranial vertebral artery can also be studied by duplex, although in a limited fashion, by insonating the vessel in the neck between vertebral bodies. Duplex can usually identify whether the artery is patent and can determine the direction of flow, such as demonstrating reversal of flow in the subclavian steal syndrome. However, given the limited window to study the artery, vertebral ultrasound is inadequate to assess the entire length of the cervical portion of the artery for disease. MRA and CTA are probably better techniques for screening this vessel.

Transcranial Doppler

Pulsed-wave TCD is a noninvasive technique designed to study the intracranial vessels. Vessels are interrogated at various depths and locations via the following "windows" into the skull: 1) through the temple (MCA, anterior cerebral artery, and distal ICA); 2) the orbit (ophthalmic artery, carotid siphon); and 3) the foramen magnum in the back of the neck (vertebral and basilar arteries). Lack of a transtemporal window due to thickness of the skull limits investigation in about 10% to 15% of patients. TCD is limited to detecting intracranial stenosis and occlusion around the circle of Willis, including the distal intracranial ICA, the proximal MCA, and the intracranial portions of the vertebral and basilar arteries (Figure 4-12). More distal branches of these vessels may not be reliably identified.

Only a few studies have compared TCD with angiography to determine the sensitivity and specificity of TCD, and further studies are needed to determine the relative accuracy of TCD compared with other non-invasive techniques. In the acute setting, however, TCD provides a unique window into the patient's vascular status and can be used to monitor vessel patency over time. For example, continuous TCD recording can be obtained in patients who receive IV thrombolytic therapy. Clinical studies show that recanalization of blocked vessels typically occur within an hour of start of therapy and are associated with better outcome than patients without recanalization.

Magnetic Resonance Angiography

MRA creates images of the cerebral vessels by capitalizing upon the differential characteristics of flowing blood. MRA studies can be ordered to assess the cervical vessels, the intracranial vessels, or both in the same setting. Several techniques are available, which continue to improve with new computing algorithms. Unfortunately, turbulent flow tends to cause dephasing and loss of signal in regions of stenosis or in tortuous segments of

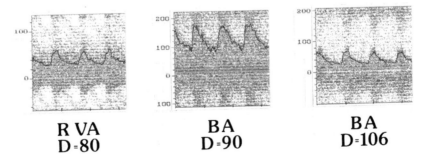

R VA
D=80   **BA**
D=90   **BA**
D=106

Figure 4-12 Transcranial Doppler (TCD) study of basilar artery stenosis. Insonation was through the foramen magnum in the back of the neck. At a depth corresponding to the right vertebral artery (*left*), the waveform and velocity are normal. As the ultrasound reading is taken deeper to the region of the proximal basilar artery (*middle*), the waveform and velocity change markedly, suggesting increased velocity due to a tight basilar artery stenosis. Further insonation at a greater depth (*right*) now shows normal or subnormal velocity in the basilar artery distal to the stenosis.

vessels. This may cause artifactual "stenosis" or overestimation of the degree of stenosis.

Compared with conventional angiography, MRA of the carotid bifurcation tends to overestimate the degree of stenosis. In general, a "flow-gap" in the internal carotid suggests a high-grade (70% or greater) stenosis. Many surgeons will consider performing carotid endarterectomy without traditional angiography if both duplex ultrasound and MRA show concordant results. The development of gadolinium-enhanced MRA reduces some of the artifact produced by turbulence (Figure 4-13). Gadolinium-MRA is increasingly used for the assessment of the carotid arteries, but only a few centers are routinely using gadolinium for intracranial MRA.

Computed Tomography Angiography

Unlike MRA, spiral CTA depicts the anatomy of the vascular lumen in a fashion similar to catheter angiography. Following acquisition of data, images are processed to generate an angiographic appearance. CTA has an accuracy of approximately 90% when correlated with conventional angiography for the detection of internal carotid artery stenosis, but heavily

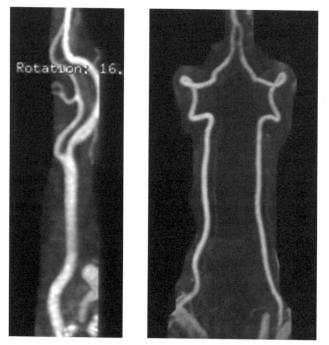

Figure 4-13 Magnetic resonance angiography (MRA) of cervical vessels. This gadolinium-enhanced MRA of the cervical vessels shows a normal right carotid artery (*left*) from its origin to the base of the skull. The right-hand image shows both vertebral arteries from the origin at the subclavian artery to the junction with the basilar artery at the top.

calcified plaque in the carotid can hinder interpretation (Figure 4-14). CTA also provides good views of the intracranial circulation, similar in accuracy to MRA. CTA is being extensively studied in the detection of intracranial aneurysms, particularly when the surgeon needs information on the relationship of the aneurysm to bony structures.

CTA can be combined with conventional CT imaging in patients with acute stroke to detect occlusion of the major cerebral vessels. A particularly attractive approach is to perform head CT along with CTA of the head and neck vessels immediately on presentation for patients with acute stroke. Thus, standard imaging for thrombolytic therapy is accomplished, but with very little added time vascular imaging from the neck to the head is available to confirm major artery occlusion.

Various techniques are being developed to assess cerebral perfusion by contrast CT, similar to PWI. An imaging paradigm of CT, CTA, and CT perfusion could provide much of the data made available by MRI techniques. The widespread availability of CT scanners as compared to MRI in most hospitals has resulted in the re-emergence of CT-based imaging protocols for acute stroke imaging.

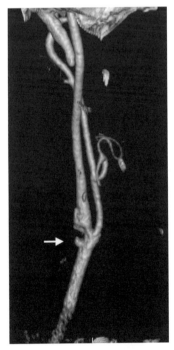

Figure 4-14 Computed tomography angiography (CTA) of carotid artery stenosis. This image shows the carotid artery from the common carotid artery through the base of the skull. There is stenosis and plaque at the internal carotid artery origin with a large ulceration (*arrow*).

Cardiac Evaluation

Cardiac embolism is the cause of approximately 15%-30% of ischemic strokes. Sources of cardiac embolism can be categorized as either "high" or "moderate" in terms of chances of recurrent stroke risk (2). For some conditions, such as atrial fibrillation, natural history studies and clinical trials provide good estimates of stroke risk, but for other conditions the data are extremely limited.

Echocardiography

Transthoracic (TTE) and transesophageal (TEE) echocardiography are the primary tools to assess for cardiac lesions that predispose to embolism. TTE is less invasive and provides excellent views of the mitral valve. TEE, on the other hand, requires conscious sedation but provides better assessment of the left atrium, intracardiac shunt (e.g., patent foramen ovale [PFO]), and aortic arch disease. Contraindications to TEE include esophageal disease (e.g., perforation, stricture, tumor), and patients with unexplained dysphagia require evaluation by a gastroenterologist because the TEE device provides no direct visualization of the esophagus during the procedure.

TEE is the only means of assessing the ascending aorta and portions of the aortic arch for atheroma or mobile adherent thrombus. Thick aortic plaque (>4 mm) and complex aortic lesions with mobile components are associated with stroke in patients without other identified causes of stroke. Advanced atherosclerotic disease of the aorta may be the source of embolism or merely an indicator of systemic atherosclerosis.

TEE also detects mitral valve strands, which are filamentous, threadlike densities arising from the mitral valve. These are generally benign, but in some studies are associated with stroke or a hypercoagulable state (3). Large, sterile vegetations arising from cardiac valves are seen in non-bacterial endocarditis associated with either malignancy or systemic lupus erythematosus (Libman-Sachs endocarditis).

An intracardiac shunt such as a PFO is optimally detected by injection of intravenous microbubbles (using agitated saline) during the TEE and observing echogenic bubbles in the left ventricle. The bubbles should appear within three cardiac cycles of injection if related to a PFO. The procedure should be done at rest (twice) and, if negative, repeated during Valsalva and cough (maneuvers which increase the pressure gradient from right to left atrium). A TEE performed without Valsalva or with an insufficient volume of agitated saline can easily miss a PFO, particularly one which only opens with increased right atrial pressures.

Occasional patients with PFO and stroke have clinical signs and positive non-invasive tests for deep venous thrombosis in the legs, strengthening the contention that the ischemic event was caused by paradoxical embolism. However, the vast majority of patients with PFO and stroke do not have clinical signs of deep venous thrombosis, and searching for venous clot by femoral vein Doppler is usually unrewarding. One report found evidence for pelvic vein thrombi by MRI and another found small calf thrombi by venography in these patients. In patients with deep venous thrombosis and pulmonary embolism, the secondary increase in pulmonary vascular resistance leads to higher pulmonary artery pressures and increased right-to-left shunting across the PFO.

TCD can also be used to detect PFO and other right-to-left shunts. Agitated saline containing microbubbles is injected intravenously as during TEE studies while one middle cerebral artery is continuously insonated by TCD. The microbubbles produce high-frequency "chirps" superimposed upon the Doppler waveform indicating passage of bubbles into the intracranial circulation. Bubbles detected within 3 cardiac cycles of injection or within 10 seconds of injection indicate an intracardiac shunt. Bubbles seen later may indicate extra-cardiac shunts, for example, as seen in patients with Osler-Weber-Rendu syndrome and pulmonary arteriovenous malformations. With careful technique, the sensitivity of bubble TCD in detecting PFO (as confirmed by TEE) approaches 90% (4).

Questions have arisen as to the yield and cost-effectiveness of TEE versus TTE in patients with stroke. Pearson and Labovitz studied 79 unselected patients admitted with stroke or TIA using both TTE and TEE (5). TEE proved superior to TTE in detecting an additional 4 patients with atrial septal aneurysm, 9 patients with PFO, 6 patients with left atrial thrombi, and 13 patients with left atrial spontaneous contrast. However, most of the patients with left atrial thrombi or spontaneous contrast had either atrial fibrillation or mitral stenosis. Two patients with apical thrombus seen on TTE were missed on TEE. In patients without clinical cardiac disease, therefore, TEE detected a further cardiac source of embolism in 20% of patients. Rauh and Fischereder reported a series of 30 patients without clear cause of stroke (e.g., atrial fibrillation or carotid stenosis) who had negative TTE studies (6). TEE revealed left atrial thrombus in 3 patients, atrial septal aneurysm in 2 patients, and PFO in 7 patients, giving an overall yield of 9/30 patients with a significant new finding. These findings led to a change in therapy (i.e., anticoagulation) in the three patients with left atrial thrombi.

McNamara and Lima used Markov decision analysis to test various strategies of TEE/TTE use in a hypothetical cohort of 65-year-old patients with new-onset stroke and in normal sinus rhythm (7). Strategies such as no cardiac imaging, TTE followed by TEE, TEE alone, or TEE restricted to patients with a cardiac history were studied. Identification of thrombus was the only finding which led to the use of anticoagulation as opposed to antiplatelet therapy. Data were used from the literature to assess stroke prevention, treatment complications, and overall costs of various approaches. Both the selected use of TEE for patients with a history of cardiac disease and the use of TEE in all stroke patients were found to be cost-effective strategies ($13,000 per quality-adjusted life-year in the "all patients" strategy), whereas the use of TTE followed by TEE was found to be substantially more expensive. At our institution, TTE with contrast is used for stroke admissions. TEE is preferred for young stroke patients and patients with suspected embolism but negative TTE.

Holter Monitor

The primary purpose of long-term electrocardiography is to detect intermittent atrial fibrillation not evident on the admission EKG. The yield of Holter monitoring is low but may result in significant change in therapy for patients who would otherwise not be put on anticoagulation. Arrhythmias are common after stroke and may be secondary to central autonomic disturbances, but they are usually benign and self-limited. Stroke causing atrial fibrillation is probably rare. Several studies have found significant arrhythmias on Holter monitoring in approximately 3% of patients with stroke or TIA (8,9). Holter monitoring should be considered in patients with suspected embolic stroke but without a defined cardiac source of embolism. Many stroke units now use cardiac telemetry for several days in stroke and TIA patients to detect intermittent arrhythmias.

Laboratory Testing
Routine Laboratory Tests

Routine laboratory tests in patients with suspected stroke should include electrolytes, chemistry profile, and a complete blood count to detect major metabolic and hematologic abnormalities that can mimic cerebrovascular disease (e.g., hypoglycemia) or be etiologic factors (e.g., polycythemia, diabetes). Other tests such as a serologic test for syphilis, antinuclear antibodies, and sedimentation rate are useful in appropriate clinical settings. Toxicological studies of blood and urine should be performed on young patients with stroke to look for drugs of abuse, particularly amphetamines and cocaine metabolites in patients with intracerebral hemorrhage. (Age may be a relative factor for drug abuse these days, as the author's recent experience with heroin- and cocaine-using grandmothers suggests.) A list of possible laboratory tests used in the evaluation of stroke patients is given in Table 4-1, with the proviso that not all tests are needed, unless there is a clinical suspicion.

The sedimentation rate is non-specific, and values must be adjusted for age. Markedly elevated sedimentation rate may be seen with endocarditis, malignancy, or vasculitis (particularly temporal arteritis or other system vasculitidies) but generally is not elevated with primary vasculitis of the central nervous system. Temporal arteritis is considered in the evaluation of

Table 4-1 Laboratory Tests in Stroke Patients

- Chemistry profile with glucose, electrolytes and creatinine
- Complete blood count, platelet count, differential
- Toxicology screen
- Sedimentation rate
- Homocysteine
- Fasting lipid profile
- ANA
- VDRL

Table 4-2 Specialized Tests for Coagulation Disorders

- Prothrombin time, partial thromboplastin time
- Platelet count
- Lupus anticoagulant screen (e.g., dilute Russell viper venom time)
- Antiphospholipid antibodies
- Protein C, protein S, free protein S
- Antithrombin III
- Activated protein C resistance
- Factor V Leiden (venous stroke)
- Prothrombin gene mutation G0210A (venous stroke)

amaurosis fugax or monocular visual loss but is a very rare cause of cerebral infarction. A low-positive titre ANA (e.g., 1:80 or 1:160) with a negative DNA titre is often a non-specific finding. Patients with cerebral ischemia, systemic signs of vasculitis, and positive serologies should have catheter cerebral angiography to look for signs of cerebral vasculitis.

Specialized Tests for Coagulation Disorders

Recent discoveries of hematologic factors associated with deep venous thrombosis and pulmonary embolism have resulted in interest in these factors as causes of stroke, particularly in young patients. Often, an extensive hypercoagulable screen is suggested for young patients without a defined cause of stroke (Table 4-2). The actual yield of this approach and cost-effectiveness is uncertain in patients with arterial ischemic stroke. In contrast, a complete hypercoagulable evaluation is necessary in patients with cerebral venous thrombosis (see Chapter 14).

There can be several pitfalls in the interpretation of the results of a hypercoagulable screen. Most of the factors assayed are involved in the fibrinolytic system, which counterbalances the activity of both the intrinsic and extrinsic clotting pathways. The thrombin-thrombomodulin complex on healthy endothelium activates circulating protein C (APC), which then binds with free protein S. This complex of APC-protein S inhibits both protein Va and VIIIa, favoring plasmin-mediated fibrinolysis. Any condition that reduces the quantity or effectiveness of protein C or S will therefore be procoagulant.

Genetic deficiencies in both protein C and S are inherited in an auto-somal dominant fashion (10). Homozygotes generally have severe disease, being lethal in childhood, but heterozygotes will generally have about 50% reduction in circulating protein C or protein S levels. Levels of protein S can also be lower by acquired factors, such as pregnancy and the use of oral contraceptives (11). In addition, about 60% of protein S in blood is bound to C4b binding protein (an inhibitor of the complement system) and only the 40% of free protein S is functionally active and able to act as a cofactor for APC. C4b is an acute phase reactant, and with inflammatory conditions and perhaps after an acute stroke, C4b will rise, causing a transient reduc-tion of free protein S. Patients with low free protein S should therefore have the test repeated in 3 to 4 months. Likewise, because pregnancy and the use of oral contraceptives often lower free protein S, tests should be repeated after these factors are no longer present. Levels of both protein C and S are reduced with warfarin, so that determinations of these factors in patients on warfarin anticoagulation are unreliable.

Activated protein C resistance has recently been found to be one of the most common causes of idiopathic deep venous thrombosis. Patients with APC resistance have reduced binding of the APC-protein S complex acti-vated factor V, and hence have lost an inhibitor of thrombosis. The most common cause for APC resistance is an inherited mutation at residue 506 of factor V, replacing an arginine with glutamine (factor V Leiden). Other less common mutations exist. Since determination of factor V Leiden can be performed on DNA extracted from peripheral blood lymphocytes, the use of anticoagulants at the time of testing is not a limiting factor. APC resistance and factor V Leiden have not been found to be convincingly associated with arterial ischemic stroke to date (12,13). In the Physician's Health Study, the prevalence of factor V Leiden was similar in patients with stroke (4.3%), myocardial infarction (6.1%), and those without clinically apparent vascular disease (6.0%) (12). The authors do not recommend routine measurement of factor V Leiden or the prothrombin gene muta-tion for patients with arterial stroke (unless paradoxical embolism via PFO is postulated).

Antiphospholipid antibodies and the lupus anticoagulant are associated with hypercoagulability in patients with systemic lupus erythematosus, but each can exist in the absence of lupus and independently of each other (13). The antiphospholipid syndrome typically includes recurrent venous thromboses, fetal wastage, high titres of IgG antiphospholipid antibodies, and livedo reticularis. A variety of neurologic syndromes are associated with antiphospholipid antibodies, including ischemic stroke (particularly in young adults), migraine, amaurosis fugax, chorea, and neuropsychiatric dis-orders (14). Antibodies against beta-2-glycoprotein, a co-factor in binding of anticardiolipin antibodies, may be more specific for thrombosis.

A large case-control study found anticardiolipin antibodies in 9.7% of pa-tients (of all ages) with first ischemic stroke compared with 4.3% of controls

(15). The presence of elevated IgG anticardiolipin antibodies (>10 GPL) was found to be associated as an independent risk factor for stroke but not necessarily an etiologic factor. IgM anticardiolipin antibodies were not reported associated with stroke and may represent an acute phase reactant. (The significance of IgA anticardiolipn antibodies in patients with stroke is unclear.) This same study followed up patients about 2 years later and found that the presence of anticardiolipin antibodies was not associated with a risk of recurrent stroke or recurrent thrombo-occlusive event (16).

Low titres of anticardiolipin antibodies (e.g., 10-20 GPL) are present in the general population and become more common in the elderly. High positive titres (e.g., >40 GPL and certainly >100 GPL) are more likely to be clinically significant, particularly in young patients with a history of thrombotic events (16,17).

Anticardiolipin antibodies are the most common antiphospholipid antibodies assayed. Patients with anticardiolipin antibodies often have false-positive serologies for syphilis (positive VDRL or RPR, but negative FTA). Antibodies directed against other phospholipid moieties may also be important in patients with negative anticardiolipin antibodies

Several screening tests are available for the lupus anticoagulant. A prolonged PTT with normal PT in the absence of heparin is suggestive. The dilute Russell venom viper time is more sensitive than the PTT and is prolonged in patients with a lupus anticoagulant. An alternative test is the hexagonal phase phospholipid neutralization test. Abnormalities on screening tests are further confirmed with mixing studies demonstrating interference with coagulation by adding the patient's serum and lack of correction with factor replacement.

While the yield of testing for coagulation abnormalities in patients with arterial ischemic stroke is low, detailed testing is essential in patients with cerebral venous thrombosis. Martinelli and colleagues studied 40 patients with cerebral venous thrombosis and found the factor V Leiden mutation in 15% (versus 3% of controls) and the G20210A prothrombin gene mutation in 20% (compared to 3% controls) (18). The combination of G20210A prothrombin gene mutation and the use of oral contraceptives led to an odds ratio of 150 for the risk of cerebral venous thrombosis. Both genes can be tested on blood DNA using commercial laboratories.

REFERENCES

1. Eliasziw M, Streifler JY, Spence JD, et al. Prognosis for patients following a transient ischemic attack with and without a cerebral infarction on brain CT. North American Symptomatic Carotid Endarterectomy Trial (NASCET) Group. Neurology. 1995;45(3 Pt 1):428-31.
2. Hart RG. Cardiogenic embolism to the brain. Lancet. 1992;339:589-94.
3. Tice FD, Slivka AP. Mitral valve strands in patients with focal cerebral ischemia. Stroke. 1996;27:1183-6.

4. Anzola G, Renaldini E. Validation of transcranial Doppler sonography in the assessment of patent foramen ovale. Cerebrovasc Dis. 1995;5:194-8.

5. Pearson AC, Labovitz AJ. Superiority of transesophageal echocardiography in detecting cardiac sources of embolism in patients with cerebral ischemia of uncertain etiology. J Am Coll Cardiol. 1991;17:66-72.

6. Rauh G, Fischereder M. Transesophageal echocardiography in patients with focal cerebral ischemia of unknown cause. Stroke. 1996;27:691-4.

7. McNamara RL, Lima JAC. Echocardiographic identification of cardiovascular sources of emboli to guide clinical management of stroke: a cost-effectiveness analysis. Ann Intern Med. 1997;127:775-87.

8. Rem JA, Hachinski VC. Value of cardiac monitoring and echocardiography in TIA and stroke patients. Stroke. 1985;16:950-6.

9. Hornig CR, Haberbosch W. Specific cardiological evaluation after focal cerebral ischemia. Acta Neurol Scand. 1996;93:297-302.

10. Engesser L, Broekmans AW. Hereditary protein S deficiencies: clinical manifestations. Ann Intern Med. 1987;106:677-82.

11. Comp PC. Laboratory evaluation of protein S status. Semin Thrombosis Hemostasis. 1987;16:177-81.

12. Ridker PM, Hennekens CH. Mutation in the gene coding for coagulation factor V and the risk of myocardial infarction, stroke, and venous thrombosis in apparently healthy men. N Engl J Med. 1995;332:912-7.

13. Love PE, Santoro SA. Antiphospholipid antibodies: anticardiolipin and the lupus anticoagulant in systemic lupus erythematosus (SLE) and in non-SLE disorders. Ann Intern Med. 1990;112:682-98.

14. Briley DP, Coull BM. Neurologic disease associated with antiphospholipid antibodies. Ann Neurol. 1989;25:221-7.

15. The Antiphospholipid Antibodies and Stroke Study (APASS) Group. Anticardiolipin antibodies are an independent risk factor for first ischemic stroke. Neurology. 1993;43:2069–73.

16. The Antiphospholipid Antibodies and Stroke Study (APASS) Group. Anticardiolipin antibodies and the risk of recurrent thrombo-occlusive events and death. Neurology. 1997;48:91-4.

17. Verro P, Levine SR. Cerebrovascular ischemic events with high positive anticardiolipin antibodies. Stroke. 1998;29:2245-53.

18. Martinelli I, Sacchi E, Landi G, et al. High risk of cerebral-vein thrombosis in carriers of a prothrombin-gene mutation and in users of oral contraceptives. N Engl J Med. 1998;338:1793-7.

Chapter 5

General Treatment Principles

JASON D. ROSENBERG, MD
REBECCA GOTTESMAN, MD
ARGYE HILLIS, MD

Key Points

- The treatment of acute stroke patients should involve integrated, multi-disciplinary inpatient care.
- Because the likelihood of worsening, recurrence, or complication of stroke is high, prompt work-up and treatment is of paramount importance.
- Patients that should be admitted to the intensive care unit include those with intracranial hemorrhage, very large strokes and cerebral edema, significant cerebellar strokes or bleeds, or cardiovascular instability, and those who have received thrombolytic therapy.
- Rehabilitation teams should be contacted soon after the patient's arrival.
- Computed tomography should be carried out in all cases of suspected stroke and transient ischemic attack. Other diagnostic testing includes cardiac monitoring, routine hematologic tests, coagulation measures, urinalysis, and toxicology screen.
- Anticoagulation generally has no benefit in the treatment of acute stroke but is reserved for patients with certain cardioembolic strokes and strokes of other uncommon causes.
- Even in hypertensive patients, lowering blood pressure during the acute stage of ischemic stroke should be avoided (with certain exceptions).
- Stroke patients need to be monitored carefully for acute neurological change.
- Complications of stroke include increased intracranial pressure, brain edema, hemorrhagic transformation, and perfusion abnormalities.

Acute stroke also carries a high risk of medical complications such as deep vein thrombosis, dysphagia, urinary tract infection, pressure ulcers, and depression.

• Most patients with moderate and severe strokes are discharged to continued inpatient rehabilitation.

A stroke, perhaps more than any other medical illness, is a life-altering event. Although the individual may feel completely well until the very moment of onset, years of silent underlying hypertension, diabetes, hypercholesterolemia, smoking, or adverse genetic background have set the stage for sudden ischemia to the brain. Whether from thrombosis of a vessel, distal embolization, or global hypotension, the outcome for the brain—and the patient—is much the same. Neuronal dysfunction is nearly immediate, and cell death follows shortly thereafter via a cascading web of failed cellular energy metabolism, excitotoxic and free radical damage, necrosis, apoptosis, and even inflammation. Strokes deprive patients of abilities that are generally taken for granted—the use of the fingers, the sense of touch, the ability to swallow. Beyond compromising sensory or motor functions, strokes may also damage any aspect of cognition, whether language, perception, memory, or executive function. In consequence, the world through which the patient formerly navigated with adaptive ease is suddenly rife with previously unimagined obstacles. No other illness is such a direct assault on the integrity of the self, both body and mind.

Strokes are usually survived (approximately 90% to 95%), and as a result they are the major source of adult disability in this country. Recovery is frequently incomplete and nearly always an uphill battle, requiring the skilled input of health care professionals from all levels. In addition to the obvious neurological manifestations, patients in the acute phase of stroke face risks of numerous potential medical complications, as well as morbidity from pre-existing ailments. Stroke is the final common pathway of a number of underlying conditions; conversely, stroke negatively affects a variety of physiologic systems, thereby exacerbating other illnesses.

In our current medical era, however, there is ample reason to hope and strive for good outcomes. While neurological symptoms are dramatic at onset, deficits typically improve over 6 months or more, provided that the patient is managed appropriately from the outset. The road to recovery begins in the hospital, from minutes to days after the onset of symptoms. During this crucial period of initial medical management the patient undergoes a rigorous diagnostic assessment. In each case, the goal is to determine why the stroke happened, how best to treat it, how to avoid complications, how best to rehabilitate, and how to prevent future events. A general approach to inpatient stroke care is the focus of this chapter (Table 5-1).

Table 5-1 General Principles for Management of Acute Stroke

- Admit all stroke or TIA patients to a hospital for assessment.
- Use an inpatient stroke unit and pathway, if possible.
- Involve a vascular neurologist, if possible.
- Assess underlying risk factors for secondary prevention (serologic, vascular, cardiac).
- Maintain normoglycemia, normothermia, and euvolemic normonatremia.
- Prophylax against aspiration, gastritis, and DVT.
- Relax blood pressure management in the acute setting.
- Use CT scan for changes in neurological exam or mental status.
- Start antiplatelet therapy in all patients without contraindications.
- Begin rehabilitation early, involving OT, PT, and speech therapy as needed.

Inpatient Stroke Management

Treatment of the hospitalized stroke patient should be a multi-disciplinary effort, aimed at preventing complications and managing specific neurological sequelae. Although there is little that can be done to salvage already infarcted brain tissue, there is much that can be done to maximize potential for recovery. While the pathology itself is limited to the central nervous system, there are multiple potential medical complications of the initial cerebrovascular injury. Aspiration pneumonia, deep vein thrombosis, pressure ulcers, and depression comprise a large portion of the initial morbidity and mortality of stroke. With due vigilance, such complications can be prevented, or at least recognized and treated early, greatly improving outcomes. Typical stroke patients should be all too recognizable to the internist: elderly, with the common co-morbidities of diabetes, hypertension, cardiac disease, and chronic obstructive pulmonary disease. Much of the subsequent secondary stroke prevention efforts should also be familiar to internists and primary care physicians, because prevention of cardiovascular and cerebrovascular disease is much the same.

One emerging consensus from the literature of the early 1990s onwards is that stroke patients are best cared for in dedicated inpatient stroke units. Due to their singular importance in improving patient outcomes, we will discuss them here in some detail. The remainder of the chapter will discuss medical management of the stroke inpatient. Topics include blood pressure management, glucose control, temperature regulation, as well as medical and neurological complications.

Stroke Units

Integrated, multi-disciplinary inpatient care has the potential to be more effective and more efficient, and this approach has been increasingly utilized in stroke management. A few stroke intensive care units (ICUs) were organized in the 1960s and 70s in Europe and the United States, and initial data collection indicated that the approach was convenient and practical if not definitively of proven outcome benefit. The implementation of stroke units has evolved over the years, with most now resembling non-critical coronary care units, utilizing an intermediate level of specialized monitoring and nursing. Organized around a designated team of physicians, nurses, and therapists familiar with acute stroke care, this approach to patient management has been shown in numerous studies to be beneficial over standard inpatient treatment models. In fact, the development of the stroke unit has improved outcomes perhaps more than any other single intervention in recent years (more than thrombolytic therapy, for example).

Stroke patients are in many ways ideally suited for "pathway" style management in dedicated inpatient units, using a template set of orders and guidelines for diagnostic work-up, medical management, and early rehabilitation. First, a limited number of common, preventable, recognizable, and treatable complications account for the majority of the morbidity of the illness. In terms of diagnostic work-up, there is a well-known, limited set of risk factors and co-morbidities, and thus a common set of laboratory and imaging tests suffices for most patients. Moreover, due to limited availability of effective interventions, there are relatively few management "branch points." Finally, specialized knowledge—of nurses as well as physicians—not only improves decision-making but also aids in the early recognition of worrisome symptoms and signs. The pathway ensures that care is streamlined and unified, with built-in assessment mechanisms to address issues specific to the stroke patient, such as new swallowing problems, communication difficulties, or immobility. Moreover, as medical knowledge advances, guidelines can be updated, ensuring system-wide uniformity of cutting-edge, evidence-based care. The Brain Attack Coalition, an umbrella association of professional, voluntary, and federal government agencies, maintains a Web site which includes a number of other current guidelines and pathways (http://www.stroke-site.org). The Coalition has also published a consensus paper on the creation of stroke units (1). The European Stroke Initiative is a similar association overseas, with online updated resources (http://www.eusi-stroke.com). The current iteration of the Johns Hopkins Hospital Stroke Pathway is summarized in the Appendix at the end of this chapter.

Proponents of this mode of care are justifiably vociferous, their advocacy backed up by studies and theoretical advantages (2). Much of the initial stroke unit data come from Scandinavia (with Norway leading the way, where nearly all major acute hospitals have stroke units), but literature review reveals that the UK, Germany, Spain, Canada, Portugal, India, Italy, and France are well on their way to making stroke units the standard of care. Numerous observational studies and several randomized controlled trials have shown that such units result in reduced hospitalization time, a larger portion of affected patients returning home, improved functional recovery, and even substantial reduction of short- and long-term mortality, without accompanying increase in long-term institutionalization (2-5). Moreover, the magnitude of the effect is not small; poor outcome—death or institutionalization—may be reduced by more than one third (6). The Stroke Unit Trialists' Collaboration and the Cochrane Reviews have periodically evaluated studies of stroke units and have concluded that the data provide overwhelming evidence that death, dependency, and need for institutional care are all reduced and that this improvement in outcome is independent of patient subgroup or specific features of the particular stroke unit (7-9).

The exact reasons for the substantial outcome benefits of stroke units are not entirely clear. Analysis of available data suggests that the mortality benefit comes largely from reduction of death associated with medical complications, particularly from those resulting from immobility (10,11). Besides early mobilization, more aggressive use of aspirin and antipyretics may also play a significant role, but there are probably many other less tangible factors, such as familiarity of the physicians and multidisciplinary staff with stroke and its effects. Early recognition and treatment of typical complications is likely facilitated by pathway management and staff experience. One of the most significant factors, however, may be the hospital presence of a cerebrovascular neurologist, as indicated in a recent multi-center retrospective study in California, which indicated that stroke mortality might be reduced by as much as half in hospitals with such a subspecialist (12). The stroke neurologists were also associated with significantly reduced lengths of stay.

Cost effectiveness data for stroke units are scarcer, but several studies have suggested potential savings, predominately arising from decreased length of stay (13). Such savings are likely to be at least partly offset by the increased numbers of diagnostic tests that tend to be performed in the more specialized setting. As it turns out, a far more important factor in the cost of stroke care than the manner in which it is delivered, however, is the size of the initial infarct, with the most severely affected patients accruing by far the longest stays and highest costs. Thus, overall savings may be relatively small, especially because stroke units tend to house sicker patients. Certainly, no studies to date have suggested that the units result in an overall increase of cost, and most authors feel that they are economically viable.

Finally, it should be noted that stroke units facilitate the design and implementation of research protocols by virtue of their carefully monitored, well-structured clinical setting. In fact, much of the recent patient recruitment into large stroke trials comes from these centers. Stroke units are ideal sites for small pilot studies, and pathways and protocols can be unified relatively easily between institutions for multi-center trials. Advances in stroke management and treatment will undoubtedly proceed more rapidly due to their inception.

Initial Assessment and Admission

The chance of early worsening, recurrence, or complication after stroke is sufficiently high that work-up and treatment should be expedited as much as possible. Once an area of the brain is infarcted, it cannot be salvaged by any means, so prevention is of utmost importance. We therefore favor admitting all acute stroke patients (and even most transient ischemic attack [TIA] patients) to a hospital, ideally to a stroke unit. In many ways, patients with the mildest symptoms at initial presentation are those with the most to lose, so even though they may look quite well overall, they should be brought in for urgent assessment, at least overnight. Outpatient management of minor strokes or TIAs is certainly feasible, but in practice scheduling difficulties may delay completion of work-up over a few weeks, which is precisely the period of highest recurrence risk. Thus, the emergency room should be utilized as a gateway to expeditious work-up and treatment of all cases, rather than a triage and diagnostic center. With a limited set of imaging, diagnostic, and laboratory studies, most of the potentially modifiable stroke risk factors (see Chapter 2) can be identified within a few days of admission, allowing early initiation of secondary preventive measures. This work-up is easily undertaken even as the acute management issues are being addressed.

After the patient is stabilized, initial imaging (see below) should be performed. With the presumptive diagnosis of stroke, the decision of whether to use thrombolytics must be made rapidly ("time is brain"), being mindful of exclusion criteria (see Chapter 7 for a complete discussion of thrombolytic therapy). The next question that must be answered is whether the patient requires critical care in a monitored setting (Table 5-2). Routine admission of stroke patients to the ICU is not warranted due to greatly increased costs without corresponding improvement in outcome, as shown in a recent trial (14). Patients appropriate for ICUs include those with intracranial hemorrhages (ICH) (which require careful blood pressure control and may worsen rapidly due to ongoing or re-bleeding in the first 6-24 hours), those with very large strokes and cerebral edema, those with significant

---

Table 5-2 Characteristics of Patients Appropriate for Initial ICU Admission

- Significantly depressed level of consciousness
- Intracranial hemorrhage (any size)
- Large or hemispheric stroke with edema
- Cerebellar strokes or hemorrhage
- Cardiovascular instability, including severe hypertension
- Post-thrombolysis
- Suspected basilar artery occlusion
- Severe dysarthria or dysphagia

cerebellar strokes or bleeds, and those with cardiovascular instability (including severe hypertension), as well as any that have received thrombolytic therapy. Posterior circulation strokes with suspected ongoing basilar artery thrombosis are best monitored in ICUs as well, because progressive and ultimately fatal brainstem involvement can occur. Any patient presenting with significantly decreased mental status (Glasgow Coma Score < 9 or so) or with severe dysarthria or dysphagia may be at risk for losing airway patency and should also be considered for a higher level of triage.

ICU treatment of stroke has become a highly specialized field in its own right, with specific strategies for management of severe edema, intracranial pressure monitoring, mechanical ventilation, and regulation of cerebral blood flow and oxygenation. This exciting and rapidly expanding area of neurology has been the subject of several recent reviews (15-17), although it is beyond the scope of this chapter. Fortunately, relatively few patients require this level of care. When judged sufficiently stable, ICU patients can be transferred to the stroke unit or regular ward for further work-up and management.

Rehabilitation teams should be contacted soon after the patient's arrival, as many of the previously discussed stroke unit trials indicate that early mobilization is likely to have a substantial role in improving outcome. All efforts should be made at the time of admission to obtain family contact information and the patient's wishes regarding resuscitation and intubation. Many patients will be unable to speak for themselves, whether from aphasia, dysarthria, or decreased level of consciousness. Between 5% and 10% of all strokes result in fatal outcome, and severe or brainstem strokes may require mechanical ventilation. Many patients with large strokes deteriorate neurologically before improving—sometimes dramatically so—due to rising intracranial pressure from worsening edema over the first few days. It is worth noting that patients with neurological disorders often require intubation, not from respiratory failure per se, but from inability to adequately protect their airways, whether due to swallowing dysfunction or decreased level of consciousness. Delay in securing and protecting the airway may lead to hypoxemia, aspiration pneumonia, and hypercapnia, resulting in poorer outcome. Should their neurological status improve, these patients are typically extubated fairly easily. Patients with devastating strokes without return to normal level of consciousness or those with ongoing severe dysphagia often require tracheostomies and gastrostomy feeding tubes.

Finally, it is worth mentioning that sudden, focal neurological deficits are not always the result of stroke. While stroke is certainly the most likely cause in those with appropriate risk factors, there remains a substantial differential diagnosis that should be considered (Table 5-3). Seizure, psychogenic deficits, migraine, toxic-metabolic derangement (e.g., hyperammonemia, intoxications, poisonings, or transient hypoglycemia), or occult infection with neurological decompensation are but a few examples.

Table 5-3 Partial List of Potential Stroke Mimics*

- Neurological: seizure or post-ictal state, complicated migraine, demyelinating disease, myasthenia gravis, Guillain-Barré, tumor or carcinomatous meningitis, hypertensive encephalopathy, subdural hematoma, other spinal cord or nerve-root process, Bell's palsy
- Toxic: medication side-effects, substance abuse
- Infectious: encephalitis, meningitis, CNS abscess, sepsis, urinary tract infection (elderly)
- Respiratory: hypoxia or hypercarbia
- Metabolic: hyperglycemia or hypoglycemia, hyperammonemia, other severe electrolyte abnormalities, intoxications, poisonings
- Psychogenic

* Many systemic conditions can cause neurological decompensation or bring out prior deficits in patients with previous strokes or dementia.

Any serious metabolic derangement or infection can lead to decompensation in a patient with pre-existing brain injury, sometimes dramatically exacerbating previous underlying deficits. It is not unusual for an elderly patient recovered from a significant hemiparesis from an old stroke to present with the same symptoms all over again in the setting of a urinary tract infection. These patients may still be best served in a stroke unit, where it is most likely that an alternative diagnosis will be made in the course of work-up and management in the hands of experienced staff.

Imaging

Diagnostic testing is discussed in more detail in Chapter 4. At minimum, an initial computed tomography (CT) (or magnetic resonance imaging [MRI] scan with gradient echo sequences to reveal blood) should be performed on all suspected stroke or TIA patients on admission. CT reveals in seconds after scan is complete whether the stroke is ischemic or hemorrhagic (Figure 5-1). CT also identifies strokes with initially significant amounts of edema or mass effect with impending herniation and can serve as a baseline should the patient subsequently decompensate. Sometimes CT scans reveal surprises as well, such as unexpected subdural hematomas, tumors with large amounts of edema, or changes suggestive of hypertensive encephalopathy. However, the size of an acute stroke may not be readily evident on initial CT scan, and in fact the CT may be normal in the early stages of a large stroke. In addition, strokes located in the brainstem or cerebellum are poorly visualized due to bony artifacts.

MRI is generally more expensive, more time consuming, and less readily available than CT. The payoff of MRI technology, however, is the generally superior image quality, the earlier detection of strokes, and ease of viewing the vascular anatomy without a dye load. MRI is also superior in detecting non-stroke lesions that might present with acute neurological

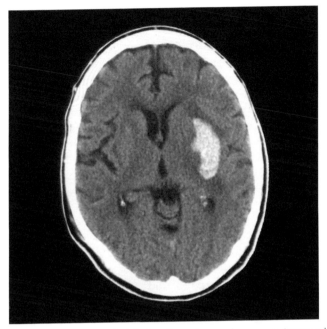

Figure 5-1 CT scan of patient with right hemiparesis reveals an acute intracerebral hemorrhage (*white area*) in the left putamen. Involvement of the left internal capsule explains the right hemiparesis.

deficit. Although some centers use MRIs as a centerpiece of their acute stroke management strategy, most institutions utilize a CT scan as the initial emergency room triage image, with an MRI being performed later, within a day or two of hospital admission. As discussed in Chapter 4, MRI and MR angiography (MRA) are sometimes quite useful, not only in determining stroke etiology but in foreseeing potential complications. Specific MRI sequences (gradient echo images) are also excellent at detecting blood, even the presence of blood products from a remote hemorrhage no longer visible on CT.

Diffusion-weighted imaging (DWI) is so sensitive for ischemia that a negative DWI scan in a patient with ongoing, new neurological deficits should cause some reconsideration for the initial diagnosis of stroke (see Table 5-3). DWI is indicated when the diagnosis of stroke is considered, but DWI negative stroke, although uncommon, can be seen. A quick DWI scan of a patient with atypical neurological findings or fluctuating exam can prevent unnecessary exposure to potentially risky thrombolytic therapy; conversely, DWI could lead to life-saving intervention when a patient has been intubated, sedated, and paralyzed in the emergency room for reduced level of consciousness before definitive diagnosis, such as in the case of a patient "found down" from acute basilar artery thrombosis.

Cardiac Monitoring

Telemetric monitoring of cardiac rhythm, blood pressure and respiration should be considered in the initial phase of hospitalization, because many patients present with significantly elevated blood pressure and accompanying cardiovascular disease. Congestive heart failure and ischemia complicate management of some cases. The rare patient with myocardial infarction or aortic dissection may present with stroke. Other patients have new-onset or intermittent atrial fibrillation as the cause of stroke, and occasional patients have neurogenic arrhythmias as a result of their infarctions. Routine diagnostic work-up should also include echocardiography because perhaps 15% to 30% of ischemic strokes are cardioembolic in origin. Chapter 4 goes into detail about echocardiography, including the question of whether to pursue a transesophageal rather than transthoracic study.

Laboratory Studies

Initial laboratory work should include routine hematological profiles, chemistries, and coagulation measures (PT and PTT) but also other tests, such as urinalysis and toxicology screen, that might point to an alternative diagnosis (see Table 5-3). Various medications and substances of abuse can cause mental status changes if taken in excess, and these may be mistaken as stroke or can worsen the appearance of neurological deficits. Heroin and cocaine are both associated with stroke, and cocaine and chronic alcohol with intracranial hemorrhage. Initial finger stick blood glucose should be measured and addressed promptly at first presentation to the emergency room (see below), and it is worth mentioning that both hyperglycemia and hypoglycemia can themselves present with stroke-like deficits. Other serologic testing identifies major treatable stroke risk factors, including hyperlipidemia, diabetes, and infectious or inflammatory disorders, within 2 or 3 days of admission, allowing prompt initiation of secondary prevention measures. Recommended routine laboratory tests are listed in Table 5-4, and are further discussed in Chapter 4.

Antiplatelet and Antithrombotic Therapy

Secondary prevention should be based on stroke etiology and may include warfarin for cardiac source or long-term antiplatelet agent individually or in combination for atherosclerotic source strokes. Studies suggest that there is a benefit to early intervention, and, for the most part, treatment should be initiated promptly in all patients without contraindications during the first 48 hours of hospitalization. The therapy does not so much treat the stroke that has already occurred but rather prevents subsequent events. When a patient who is already on antiplatelet therapy suffers a stroke, many physicians term this a "treatment failure" and switch medications or add a second

Table 5-4 Laboratory Tests in Stroke Inpatients

• Chemistry profile with glucose, electrolytes and creatinine	• Sedimentation rate
	• Homocysteine
• Complete blood count, platelet count, differential	• Fasting lipid profile
	• ANA
• Toxicology screen	• VDRL

agent. It is not clear from the data whether this practice is justified. It is important, however, to evaluate for noncompliance with prescribed therapy and for concurrent medications that could potentially interfere with the beneficial antiplatelet effects of aspirin, such as nonsteroidal anti-inflammatory drugs.

Anticoagulation is also an effective measure for secondary stroke prevention over the long term. In general, however, acute anticoagulation has no proven benefit in the treatment of acute stroke. It is generally reserved for patients with cardioembolic strokes due to atrial fibrillation, low ejection fraction, patent foramen ovale with atrial septal aneurysm, or severe wall motion abnormalities, and for certain uncommon etiologies of stroke such as sinus thrombosis and arterial dissection. There is no role for warfarin therapy in patients with noncardioembolic strokes, because antiplatelet therapy is equally effective with less potential for hemorrhagic complications. Heparin's role in most cases except venous strokes is increasingly being questioned. To minimize risk of intracranial bleeding, it is common practice to withhold initiation of anticoagulation for 48 hours or so after intracranial hemorrhage or large stroke. If necessary, it can be withheld for up to a few weeks, even in those with mechanical valves or atrial fibrillation, as the risk of cardioembolic stroke is typically measured in percentages per year, compared with a potentially much higher up-front risk of bleeding in specific cases. Further discussion of antiplatelet and antithrombotic therapy can be found in Chapter 6.

Blood Pressure Management

In normal conditions, circulation to the brain is autoregulated, such that increases in systemic blood pressure do not affect cerebral blood flow. However, in brain injuries such as acute ischemic stroke, there is a loss of this normal autoregulation, so that increases in systemic blood pressure directly cause increased cerebral blood flow. Ischemic tissue surrounding the actual infarct may depend on this additional supply for survival. The vulnerability to worsening stroke in the absence of increased blood pressure and blood flow is particularly common in patients with severe large vessel stenosis. Cerebral blood flow, often described as cerebral perfusion pressure (CPP), also varies negatively with increased intracranial pressure.

That is, CPP is equal to the mean arterial pressure minus the intracranial pressure (CPP = MAP – ICP). Any increase in intracranial pressure, such as that caused by the peaking edema 2 to 3 days after a large stroke, will reduce cerebral blood flow unless systemic blood pressure rises as well, whether as a natural response or due to therapy.

In normal, otherwise healthy adults with acute intracranial pathology, a CPP of 60-70 mm Hg is necessary to prevent worsening ischemia. However, in chronically hypertensive adults, there is a shift in the autoregulatory curve, such that higher a CPP is required to prevent ischemia. For these reasons, lowering blood pressure, at least in the first 72 hours of stroke, can increase the size of the infarct. Therefore, even in markedly hypertensive patients, lowering blood pressure in the acute phase should be avoided unless the high blood pressure is causing hypertensive encephalopathy, cardiac ischemia, congestive failure, compromise of vital organs, or if the stroke is due to aortic dissection. Typically, cerebrovascular neurologists do not routinely attempt to reduce blood pressure unless the systolic pressure exceeds some comfort threshold, typically 200-220 mm Hg or so. The patient's usual anti-hypertensive medications are generally discontinued or decreased upon admission to the hospital, although medications such as clonidine and beta-blockers generally should be tapered slowly.

There is frequently a spontaneous increase in blood pressure in the first 24 hours of a stroke, even without withdrawal of antihypertensive medications. This increase in blood pressure often gradually resolves on its own over the first week. Between baseline chronic hypertension and this acute physiologic response, it is not at all unusual to care for patients with initial systolic pressures greater than 200 mm Hg. If it is necessary to lower blood pressure in acute stroke (e.g., due to cardiac ischemia), it is preferable to use non-vasodilatory medications such as beta-blockers. Intravenous labetalol is the preferred acute medication, because the dose can be carefully titrated, avoiding a drop in blood pressure that results in worsening neurological condition. Typical doses are 10-40 mg intravenous doses repeated every 15 minutes as needed. Intravenous enalapril is another reasonable option. Sublingual nifedipine should be avoided due to the chance of precipitous drop in pressure and subsequent worsening of ischemia. If at all possible, blood pressure should be lowered gradually and cautiously.

It should be noted that blood pressure management in acute stroke is controversial, given absence of clinical trial data. Some small studies have shown that deliberately augmenting the blood pressure in the acute stroke setting (using phenylephrine or fluids, for example) can have beneficial results. There is a theoretical risk of increasing hemorrhagic transformation, edema, or hypertensive encephalopathy, but these complications have not been observed in any of the reported studies. In the International Stroke Trial, a large study of acute stroke, there was a U-shaped relationship between systolic blood pressure on admission and clinical outcome (early death, late death, or disability) (18). The best outcomes were in patients with systolic blood pressure on admission of 140-179 mm Hg. In this study, early death increased by 17.9% for every 10 mm Hg under 150 mm Hg, suggesting that patients with systolic blood pressure below 140 might benefit from blood pressure elevation. The poor outcome in patients with very high blood pressure in that study may have been a reflection of greater spontaneous increases in blood pressure in patients with large strokes (who require high blood pressure management, but nevertheless are most likely to have poor outcome). Therefore, in general, any medical treatment of high blood pressure should be withheld in the first 72 hours of ischemic stroke.

Treatment of hypertension in intracranial hemorrhage is also poorly studied, although there is more of a consensus for empiric blood pressure lowering in these patients (see Chapter 15). Due to the above reasoning about cerebral perfusion, some stroke neurologists do not treat high blood pressure even in acute hemorrhages caused by hypertension unless the systolic pressure exceeds 160-180 mm Hg or a mean arterial pressure of 110-130. However, many neurosurgeons and neuro-intensivists recommend lowering systolic blood pressure to 130-140 mm Hg in hemorrhage patients, especially for the initial 24-hour period of maximal rebleeding. In patients with subarachnoid hemorrhage, excessively high blood pressure is felt to be a risk for rupture if the aneurysm has not been clipped or temporarily secured with coils (see Chapter 17). Further studies are needed to determine the optimum blood pressure in these situations.

Finally, it should be noted that chronic hypertension is the single most important stroke risk factor. As outpatients, most stroke survivors should have their blood pressure tightly controlled in the normal range (recognizing that there is no clear cutoff for "normal," in much the same way there may be no optimal level for cholesterol). Accumulating evidence suggests that risk for adverse cardiovascular events increases across the pre-hypertensive range, well before 140/90 is reached. Thus, the only exception to strict blood pressure reduction should be in those with symptomatic orthostasis or severe large vessel stenoses with recurrence of deficits when blood pressure is lowered. Blood pressure control for secondary prevention can usually be started several weeks to months after acute stroke, but the optimal time is uncertain. The setting of acute ischemic stroke (first few days) is not the ideal time to worry about secondary prevention from hypertension, given the potential harm of rapid blood pressure reduction. In addition, there are a variety of considerations to keep in mind when choosing which anti-hypertensive medication to use, both for secondary prevention and to avoid slowing the pace of recovery. This topic is discussed in detail in Chapters 2 and 8.

Glucose Management

Diabetes is a well-known risk factor for stroke. The disease results in gradual damage to the vascular endothelium, leading to lipohyalinization of the walls of small blood vessels. These pathologic changes predispose the patient to cerebrovascular events of all types, but to lacunar infarctions in particular. While the risks of diabetes are cumulative over years, acute hyperglycemia during a stroke itself, even in a non-diabetic patient, is associated with poor outcome. The TOAST trial (Trial of ORG [a low-molecular-weight heparinoid] in Acute Stroke Treatment) found that admission hyperglycemia was associated with a poor outcome at 3 months in patients with nonlacunar strokes (19). Such hyperglycemia may be either reactive or causative; significant ischemia can result in hyperglycemia as a type of stress reaction, but the presence of hyperglycemia may also worsen ischemia or expand the ischemic penumbra. In animal models, high blood glucose has been shown to worsen lactic acidosis in the area of an infarct, which may increase free-radical formation and subsequently enlarge the area of tissue injury (20). Acute surges of hyperglycemia also likely contribute to vascular endothelial injury in the short-term.

Many studies have shown a correlation between elevated glucose and poor short- or long-term outcome after stroke, as well as increased co-morbidities. Clinical trials have not yet, however, demonstrated a causative link or shown definitive benefit of tight glycemic control in stroke. Nevertheless, there is a general consensus amongst stroke neurologists that due to the overwhelmingly probable deleterious effects of hyperglycemia and the relative ease of treatment, optimal glucose management should be exercised in the acute stroke setting, even for non-diabetics. A fairly strict regular insulin sliding scale should be initiated if there is even mild-to-moderate hyperglycemia; even serum glucose values above 120 mg/dL are considered elevated in reference to protection of brain tissue. Oral hypoglycemic medications are usually continued, although metformin may need to be withdrawn if there is an anticipated need to perform a radiologic study requiring contrast agents, due to the risk of renal compromise and subsequent lactic acidosis from reduced clearance of the drug. Precautions to avoid hypoglycemia should be taken in patients unable to eat due to neurological conditions or pending diagnostic studies.

Hyperglycemia prior to the administration of tPA is also associated with poor outcome. Several studies have also found an increased risk of hemorrhagic complications associated with either diabetes or elevated glucose at the time of thrombolytic treatment. Extreme hyperglycemia or hypoglycemia is considered a relative contraindication to giving tPA, in part due to the possibility of bleeding, but also because some of the observed neurological deficits may be related to the metabolic disturbance itself and thus reversible without thrombolysis. Although lesser degrees of hyperglycemia would not preclude thrombolytic therapy, aggressive control should still be attempted before administering the drug.

Body Temperature Management

Hyperthermia, like hyperglycemia, is associated with poor outcome after stroke. Again, the relationship may be either causative or reactive, or more likely both. Hyperthermia can lead to worsening ischemic injury and may enlarge the size of the ischemic penumbra because of increased metabolic requirements, and may ultimately worsen cerebral edema and increase intracranial pressure. Strokes, particularly large infarcts, may themselves cause some degree of hyperthermia in a reactive manner. "Central" fevers of a significant elevation are more likely to be related to hemorrhage or strokes of the brainstem or hypothalamus than to damage elsewhere, but some degree of elevation can be seen with any sizeable infarction. In one study, initially normothermic patients with the most severe strokes were the ones who tended to develop fever within the first 12 hours of onset (21). Of course, there are also a number of post-stroke complications that may lead to fever, as discussed elsewhere in this chapter, such as aspiration pneumonia, urinary tract infections, and deep vein thromboses. While it is critical to understand the cause of fever and to treat any infection or other underlying process accordingly, the pyrexia itself needs to be treated because of an association with poor outcome.

There is stronger evidence that intervention improves stroke outcome in the case of fever than in the case of hyperglycemia. Low body temperature on admission may be an independent predictor of good outcome as shown in the Copenhagen Stroke Study (22). Aggressive fever control and mild-to-moderate hypothermia have been proposed as neuroprotective measures. They have been shown to improve outcome in critically ill patients with very large strokes and in those with diffuse brain injury from cardiopulmonary arrest. The potential adverse effects from induced hypothermia include infection, coagulopathy, arrhythmias, and electrolyte disturbances, but these complications were uncommon in the numerous studies using induced hypothermia in otherwise critically ill patients.

The main clinical limitation to the use of induced hypothermia is patient comfort; any moderate decrease in body temperature causes involuntary shivering which is not tolerable for an otherwise awake patient. To suppress this reaction, anesthesia (and accompanying intubation) is often required to obtain adequate hypothermia. Evaluation of endovascular cooling is underway with promising early results, one recent trial showing that patients could tolerate the procedure with only moderate sedation. Another approach is to use the concept of "controlled low normothermia;" that is, inducing core body temperatures between 36 and 37°C. This state may be safely achievable in awake, non-ventilated patients using a combination of external cooling, vasodilators, and mild sedation, but benefit on outcome has not yet been proven. As a low-risk alternative to cooling treatments, some authors have proposed administration of prophylactic round-the-clock acetaminophen for fever prevention in all stroke patients.

In summary, while significant reductions in body temperature by induced hypothermia may not be practicable in the standard post-stroke patient, it is still critical to aggressively control any pyrexia. All patients without a contraindication should have standing orders for acetaminophen or another anti-pyretic to be given for any fever (or even, perhaps, round-the-clock); they may require cooling blankets if fever continues to be a significant problem. Although the phenomenon of central fever does exist, elevated body temperature should never be assumed to be the result of the stroke itself: an infectious or other source should be sought in all cases, at the very least with microbial cultures, urinalysis, and chest radiography.

Fluid and Electrolyte Management

There are few specific recommendations for fluid management in acute stroke. Euvolemic normonatremia should be the goal in routine cases. Outmoded ideas about utilizing dehydration to prevent swelling of the injured brain have fallen by the wayside, in part due to poor outcomes from worsening of co-morbid conditions. Hyponatremia or other hypoosmolar states can certainly lead to worsening cerebral edema by fluid shifts into the brain parenchyma, so all efforts should be made to avoid substantial reductions of serum osmolarity. For this reason, we favor using normal saline rather than a hypotonic solution as routine maintenance fluid, particularly in larger strokes, along with daily sodium monitoring. Volume trends can be assessed by periodically obtaining patient weights or by carefully monitoring fluid intake and urinary output. (Indwelling urinary catheters should be avoided as much as possible, however, to reduce agitation and chance of infection.) Care must be taken to avoid volume overload and congestive heart failure in patients with pre-existing cardiac problems or underlying oliguric renal failure. Patients able to take sufficient fluid orally to meet their requirements should be allowed to do so; provided that their homeostatic mechanisms are intact, additional fluids are not needed. Only in the instances of severe, symptomatic edema should hyperosmolar therapy with mannitol or hypertonic saline solutions be contemplated, and this level of care is typically better delivered in the ICU. Uncommonly, ICH (or, rarely, infarctions) can result in central diabetes insipidus, cerebral salt wasting, or syndrome of inappropriate antidiuretic hormone (SIADH). These conditions are all potentially fatal if left untreated and should be recognized and addressed promptly. Hypervolemic therapy for vasospasm resulting from subarachnoid hemorrhage is typically ICU-level care. In rare cases, stroke patients will develop worsening or new neurological symptoms when their blood pressure falls below a certain threshold (see below). In these instances, treatment with sodium (intravenous saline or oral salt tablets), mineralocorticoids, and the alpha-agonist midodrine may be required to improve cerebral blood flow by means of relative hypertension.

Neurological Management and Complications

The number of common reasons for neurological decompensation in acute stroke is limited (Table 5-5). Careful attention of the management team can often identify these causes before the consequences are severe. Thorough documentation of the patient's neurological deficits in the chart, at least once per nursing shift, is critical to being able to determine whether there has been an actual decline in status, given that caregivers may change frequently and that patients may be unaware of or unable to communicate their deficits. A quick chart note during the day, such as, "Patient remains somewhat sleepy but conversant, with continuing dense left hemiplegia, neglect, and right gaze preference," can save needless panic when there is question of a "new" change in the middle of the night. Routine nursing assessments should include neurological screening examinations.

The highest level of vigilance is needed during the first 3-5 days of hospitalization in cases of non-lacunar cerebellar stroke, brainstem stroke, or large hemispheric stroke. In these cases, the patient's neurological status may worsen dramatically before improving. Large strokes of the hemisphere can lead to edema with subsequently fatal transtentorial herniation or to hemorrhagic transformation with increased intracranial pressure. In strokes of the posterior circulation, progressive and fatal occlusion of the vertebrobasilar system may worsen in a stuttering fashion with progressive cranial neuropathies and obtundation; these patients should be monitored in the ICU. Even a relatively small infarct or hemorrhage of the cerebellum can cause subsequent tissue swelling and thus lead to compression of the nearby brainstem, hydrocephalus by obstruction of cerebral spinal fluid outflow, or death by herniation of the cerebellar tonsils (Figure 5-2). Importantly, there are potential interventions for each of these situations,

---

Table 5-5 Causes for Change in Neurological Exam after Stroke*

- Toxic-metabolic: medications, electrolytes
- Respiratory: hypoxia, hypercarbia
- Infections: UTI and pneumonia
- Cerebral edema (cause of high intracranial pressure or herniation)
- Hemorrhagic transformation
- Stroke recurrence or progression
- Hypoperfusion: relative lack of blood flow to at-risk brain areas
- Seizures
- Depression or delirium

---

* Any new focality or dramatic change necessitates an urgent imaging study.

but they all are critically dependent upon early recognition. In these patients, reduction of the level of consciousness may be the first sign of trouble, and rapid decompensation may follow. It is critical, therefore, that these patients be awoken periodically from sleep for routine neurological assessment.

The most common culprits of a generally decreased level of consciousness and/or worsening of baseline deficits in acute stroke are non-neurological: medication side effects and medical complications (fever, urinary tract infection, pneumonia, hyponatremia, hypoxia, hypercarbia). However, any new focality, such as weakness in a previously uninvolved limb, or a new cranial nerve deficit, or dramatic worsening of the exam with unaltered level of consciousness, is considerably more alarming and raises the possibility of edema and elevated intracranial pressure, ICH, new stroke, hypoperfusion, or seizure.

In all stroke patients with acute neurological change, the appropriate course should be 1) assessment and stabilization of airway, breathing, and circulation; 2) brief neurological exam; 3) emergency treatment of increased intracranial pressure if indicated; and 4) immediate head CT scan to assess for edema or bleeding. Neurologists often refer to this period of rapid assessment and stabilization as a "brain code" (Table 5-6). Specific neurological causes of acute decompensation are described below.

Elevated Intracranial Pressure

Signs of increased intracranial pressure (of any etiology) may include lethargy, headache, and vomiting. Increased intracranial pressure can also lead to herniation. The earliest localizing sign of temporal lobe herniation

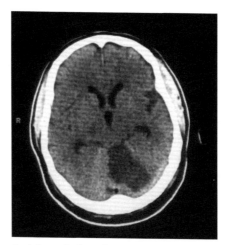

Figure 5-2 CT scan of a left cerebellar infarct with edema and mass effect. Compression of the cerebral aqueduct has led to early hydrocephalus.

Table 5-6 "Brain Code"

In the stroke patient who has become unresponsive from suspected neurological cause, especially a patient with new cranial nerve deficits:

- Intubate, hyperventilate to goal Pco_2 of approximately 30 (no less than 25)
- Mannitol 0.5-1 g/kg IV, rapidly
- CT to determine etiology after initial stabilization
- Transfer to ICU for definitive management (e.g., intraventricular catheter, craniotomy, pressor support, continued hyperosmolar therapy)

(also called "uncal herniation") is an irregular or slightly enlarged pupil, typically on the side of the herniation. A ptotic eye that is "down and out" from complete third nerve palsy is usually found only when a patient is completely obtunded and significant brainstem injury has already taken place. Similarly, papilledema of the optic disc is typically found in patients with prolonged elevation of intracranial pressure, and its absence in the acute setting does not rule out elevated intracranial pressure. Other signs of herniation include 1) a new anterior cerebral artery ischemia from subfalcine herniation that compresses the artery, causing contralateral leg weakness; and 2) new posterior cerebral artery stroke from transtentorial herniation that compresses the artery, causing contralateral visual field loss. These signs may be difficult to detect in patients with reduced consciousness.

Edema

Brain edema is a relatively common complication of non-lacunar infarcts, usually peaking at about day three after stroke onset. Avoidance of cerebral edema is difficult, because it is usually directly related to the size of the initial infarction. Appropriate fluid and electrolyte management (see above) can only do so much. Edema becomes symptomatic when the initial volume of the stroke is large or when there is little room for swelling, such as in a young person without any significant age-related atrophy. Symptomatic edema occurs in approximately 7.5% of all strokes. As long as the patient remains alert, does not develop new cranial nerve or other deficits, and can be followed clinically, expectant management is appropriate. With some large, hemispheric middle cerebral artery strokes, the edema may be rapid and relentlessly progressive, causing further brain injury. The high intracranial pressure of this so-called "malignant edema" does not respond well to even highly aggressive medical care and is most often fatal. Case series suggest that it can be treated neurosurgically with hemicraniectomy, with sometimes surprisingly good outcomes, particularly in younger patients (23-26). A bone window is temporarily removed from the skull, and the dura incised to allow the contents of the cranium to swell outwards rather than inwards toward the brainstem. Weeks later, once the edema has subsided, the bone flap can be replaced or a titanium plate put over the skull defect.

Hemorrhagic Transformation

Hemorrhagic transformation occurs in over 30% of cardioembolic stroke. Hemorrhagic transformation of an ischemic infarct is a frequently misunderstood concept. Over 80% of emboli fragment or recanalize in the first week after stroke, leading to reperfusion of the area of infarction. (Of course, because this may be taking place days later, there is no benefit to the already damaged brain.) Hemorrhagic transformation of a petechial nature (small microbleeds throughout the infracted brain tissue) is a very common autopsy finding that, depending upon the degree of hemorrhagic change, can be visualized on follow-up CT and MRI scans. This type of hemorrhagic transformation is generally benign, and patients can be continued (if deemed necessary) on anticoagulation without ill effects (27).

This transformation is in contrast to the feared complication of frank hemorrhage into an ischemic infarct, where there is a focus of bleeding causing a hematoma with mass effect and neurological deterioration. In most prospective studies, this occurs in less than 1.5% of strokes. In the NINDS trial, for example, hemorrhage rates of the control group of patients not receiving any tPA was 0.6% (28). The risk of serious bleeding is highest in larger strokes, in the presence of anticoagulation, or shortly after tPA administration (where it reaches 3% to 10% in various studies). Advanced age, hyperglycemia, and violation of NINDS inclusion criteria are associated with increased risk of hemorrhage in tPA thrombolysis patients. Specific therapies for large, symptomatic hemorrhagic infarcts are limited, but neurosurgical intervention can be lifesaving in some cases. For patients with sudden neurological deterioration while on intravenous heparin, the heparin drip should be immediately stopped and the patient sent for urgent CT scanning to look for a hemorrhage. For patients on warfarin with secondary bleeding, anticoagulation should be reversed with vitamin K and fresh frozen plasma.

Recurrence or Progression of Stroke

The risk for subsequent stroke is highest in the first days after the presenting ischemic symptoms. Second strokes in the acute setting occur in fewer than 5% of all patients. A second stroke in a completely different arterial territory is suspicious for a cardioembolic source (e.g., mural thrombus, endocarditis) or a more systemic disorder such as vasculitis. Sometimes, the territory of an initial infarct may "extend" or "progress," but there are no convincing data guiding intervention to limit these "strokes in evolution." The phenomenon is likely due to progressive medium or large vessel occlusion in many cases (which can be reflected in a large diffusion-perfusion mismatch on MRI). Anticoagulation has not been proven to prevent progressive stroke, although it is often used for this indication.

Lacunar strokes (small, end-arteriolar subcortical or brainstem strokes associated with lipohyalinosis from years of hypertension or diabetes) can also lead to fluctuation of symptoms, sometimes dramatically. Over a single day, a patient may exhibit symptoms ranging from minor motor weakness to flaccid hemiplegia. The "capsular warning syndrome" consists of staccato repetition of episodes of pure motor hemiparesis that often leads to a pure motor stroke from a lacune in the internal capsule. Once it has been established that there is no ongoing perfusion deficit, and that there is no correlation of the deficits with blood pressure, these variations can be followed with observation alone. Patients and their families should be told that the symptoms may fluctuate, but be encouraged to report any changes.

Perfusion Abnormalities

For years it has been recognized that neurological deficits in the acute stroke setting may fluctuate with variation of blood pressure. In rare, dramatic cases, patients even exhibit orthostatic positional variations (i.e., they may become entirely plegic or aphasic when sitting or standing and have few deficits when lying down). Animal studies in the 1970s demonstrated that acute stroke consists of a central core of infarcted tissue, surrounded by the "ischemic penumbra," an area of brain with a relative perfusion deficit that has not yet progressed to infarction. In other words, there is a salvageable area of brain being threatened with possible ischemic death. Sometimes, the actual area of infarction may be tiny, with the patient's more severe deficits resulting primarily from reduced blood flow. Rescue of this ischemic penumbra is the major goal of acute stroke intervention.

Patients with perfusion deficits demonstrated on MRI ("diffusion-perfusion mismatch"; see Chapter 4), by perfusion CT, or by clinical history can be considered for more aggressive treatment with hypertensive therapy utilizing hypervolemia, oral alpha-agonists, mineralocorticoids, or even intravenous pressors (phenylephrine), although this is not yet established as standard of care. The hope is that transiently supporting cerebral perfusion will allow development of collateral blood supply and thus limit tissue infarction.

Seizures

Seizures in the immediate post-stroke period are relatively uncommon, occurring in fewer than 5% of patients. The 5-year risk for single seizures may be as high as 12% (29). One large study found the risk at 34 months to be 9% for single seizures, with recurring seizures in only 2.5% (30). While the incidence is relatively low, cumulative strokes throughout the aging population are probably responsible for the majority of the late-life epilepsy.

Seizure risk is highest in patients with cortical infarctions, hemorrhages, and larger strokes, but it is not clear whether seizures in and of themselves result in higher mortality. In some cases, patients may present with status epilepticus as their initial seizure episode, requiring aggressive management.

An unexpected seizure without rapid return to baseline in the acute setting should trigger a head CT to rule out bleeding. Routine prophylaxis with antiepileptic drugs in stroke patients is not warranted due to low overall incidence and potential side effects such as sedation, but therapy should probably be initiated after even a single seizure because the post-stroke patients are at substantially higher risk for subsequent seizures than the general population. The risk of recurrence may be highest if the initial seizure occurs relatively late, a few weeks or more post-stroke (31). It is worth noting that intravenous loading of anti-epileptic medication is usually not needed for a single event; oral initiation is better tolerated. The one instance where routine prophylaxis is absolutely indicated is that of subarachnoid hemorrhage with an as-yet unsecured aneurysm, in order to avoid brief but potentially disastrous elevation of blood pressure that accompanies a seizure.

Phenytoin and valproate are easy agents to rapidly escalate to a "therapeutic" level. They can be administered orally or intravenously, although phenytoin can cause hypotension and bradycardia and may lead to severe tissue injury should an IV infiltrate. Levetiracetam, one of the newer oral antiepileptic drugs, can be initiated quickly with few drug interactions or serious side effects. Specific antiepileptic drug choice depends on the physician's familiarity with the drug, its interactions, its side-effect profile, and whether or not there is renal or liver impairment. While in the hospital, antiepileptic drug levels should be checked periodically; levels of unbound or "free" phenytoin and carbamazepine are more reliable than bound levels in patients with low albumin or renal failure. Phenytoin should not be administered within an hour of meals because the medication tends not to be well absorbed. Patients on continuous tube feeds should have the feeds held for at least an hour before phenytoin administration.

Most anticonvulsants, particularly the older agents, can cause drowsiness, ataxia, and nystagmus, especially in the period shortly after initiation, and perhaps more dramatically so in the elderly. Such side effects certainly have the potential to interfere with post-stroke rehabilitation, perhaps outweighing their potential anti-seizure benefits. Some authors have raised concerns that certain AEDs, such as phenytoin, may hinder neurological recovery through a variety of other mechanisms, but data are scarce. Patients who seem very lethargic or who are not progressing well with post-stroke rehabilitation may do better if tapered off of their antiepileptic drug or switched to a less sedating medication.

Medical Complications

Acute stroke is accompanied by a high risk of a variety of medical complications. This risk extends beyond the acute hospitalization and well into the period of rehabilitation. In a recent multi-center cohort study of nearly 4000 patients, fever (13.2%), severe hypertension (7.5%), and pneumonia (7.4%) were the most frequent significant complications of acute ischemic stroke inpatients (32). Underlying co-morbidities may also be exacerbated in the acute hospitalization: renal failure or congestive heart failure may worsen, obstructive pulmonary disease may flare, and diabetes may prove difficult to control. In general, medical complications from stroke are more common than neurological complications, and can substantially increase length of stay and worsen outcomes.

Deep Vein Thrombosis and Pulmonary Embolism

Frequently immobilized and often hospitalized for days, stroke patients are at particular risk for deep vein thrombosis (DVT) and subsequent pulmonary embolism, which may account for up to 5% or so of early deaths following stroke. In patients with ICH, the hemorrhage itself may provoke a subsequent hypercoaguable state. Although there are no definitive data showing that use of heparin affects neurological outcome in stroke patients, there are clear data demonstrating a substantial benefit in terms of DVT prevention. The benefit of low-dose heparin in DVT prevention substantially outweighs the slightly increased risk of hemorrhage, even in patients with ICH at baseline. Reductions in DVT risk are on the order of 60% or more, although too few pulmonary embolisms occurred in the stroke trials to say whether prophylaxis substantially reduces this complication.

At minimum, 5000 U of unfractionated heparin should be given subcutaneously twice daily. Low molecular weight heparins or heparanoid formulations may be of even greater benefit, but trial data lack sufficient endpoints to analyze the risk-benefit ratios and cost-effectiveness (33). Alternatively, pneumatic serial compression devices with TED stockings reduce the risk of DVT and carry few risks. It is certainly reasonable to prescribe both medical and mechanical prophylaxis, although serial compression devices can interfere with mobility and rehabilitation in ambulatory patients. Should a DVT or a pulmonary embolism occur despite prophylaxis, heparinization should be initiated cautiously, especially in patients with new or large strokes. In the first week or so post-stroke, heparin should be initiated with a maintenance dose rather than with a bolus in order to avoid "overshoot" of PTT, although all efforts should be made to reach a therapeutic level of anticoagulation within 24 hours.

Swallowing, Aspiration, and Nutrition

Due to the importance of good nutrition in recovery, and the risk of pneumonia from aspiration, all stroke patients should undergo a bedside swallow evaluation *before* the physician decides whether they should be fed. The 3-ounce Swallow Screen is a simple bedside test that involves having the patient drink a small amount of water, asking him to speak, and observing the outcome (Figure 5-3) (33a). Patients with symptoms, choking, coughing after swallowing, or a "wet" sounding voice after liquid intake should be kept NPO and undergo a formal swallowing evaluation by a speech-language pathologist, who may, in turn, recommend that videofluoroscopy be performed to determine the safety of oral alimentation and hydration. Patients with demonstrated aspiration on imaging are perhaps seven times more likely to suffer pneumonia in the acute setting than those with negative studies, and those with silent aspiration (with no cough) and a larger degree of aspiration on barium studies are at an even higher risk (34).

It is important to emphasize that aspiration pneumonia can double morbidity and mortality for stroke patients but also that it is easy to prevent with proper screening and intervention. The presence or absence of a gag reflex is not a helpful screen. However, placing all stroke patients on aspiration precautions and performing easy-to-learn bedside swallow screens are effective in minimizing this problem. After the initial evaluation for dysphagia and aspiration, there are a variety of interventions that can be recommended by the speech-language pathologist.

Adjusting the consistency of the diet can help prevent aspiration; for example, thickened liquids are often swallowed more safely than thin liquids. Upright positioning and specific swallowing techniques (e.g., tucking the chin during swallow, head turning, careful chewing, multiple successive swallows) can also reduce aspiration. One controlled trial suggested that simple patient and family teaching methods were as effective as more intensive therapy in reducing aspiration (34).

Dysphagia in stroke patients is often transient, particularly in unilateral, supratentorial stroke. In patients with severe aspiration at onset, a nasogastric tube should be placed to provide a temporary means of adequate nutrition (and oral medication administration) during the initial period. If dysphagia does not resolve or show signs of rapid improvement in the first 5 days or so, percutaneous endoscopic gastrostomy tube placement should be undertaken. This low-morbidity procedure is reversible and offers substantial benefits in terms of cosmetics, comfort, infection, reflux, and breakdown of the nasal mucosa over prolonged nasogastric tube use.

Aspiration pneumonitis, a sterile inflammatory process resulting from inhalation of caustic gastric contents, should be differentiated from aspiration pneumonia, which is an infection due to often silent inhalation of oropharyngeal flora. The former often presents acutely and dramatically,

STEP ONE

If any of the 4 following conditions are present, place a check in the box and do not continue. Do not give patient anything by mouth.

Initial Screen:
- ❑ Patient is fed enterally due to dysphagia
- ❑ Patient has a changed level of arousal/alertness
- ❑ Patient has a recent history of dysphagia with known aspiration
- ❑ Patient is unable to manage oral secretions (requiring frequent suction, drooling presistently, choking on oral secretions, or wet/gurgly vocal quality with sustained "ah")

STEP TWO

If any of the 3 boxed items below are checked, DO NOT CONTINUE. Do not give patient anything by mouth. If no items are checked, go to Step 3.

- Place patient in a chair, if possible, or sit straight up in bed
- Ensure patient's mouth is moist and clean
- Place fingers on patient's throat (specifically on the Adam's apple) to feel for laryngeal elevation
- Give 1 teaspoon of water
- Assess for:
  - ❑ No laryngeal elevation detected
  - ❑ Cough/choke response immediately after the swallow
  - ❑ Wet/gurgly vocal quality with sustained "ah" after the swallow

STEP THREE

If any of the boxed items below are checked, do not give patient anything by mouth. If no items are checked, initiate diet.
- Give patient 3 ounces (90 milliliters) of water to drink without interruption
- Assess for:
  - ❑ Cough/choke response up to a minute after the swallow
  - ❑ Wet/gurgly vocal quality with sustained "ah" after the swallow

Note: If results unclear, repeat Step 3.

Result: ❑ Pass ❑ Fail

Completed by: _____ Date _____ Time _____
    Signature/Title

Figure 5-3 Three-ounce Swallow Screen test. (Data from DePippo KL, Hotos MA, Reding MJ. Validation of the 3-oz water swallow test for aspiration following stroke. Arch Neurol. 1992;49:1259-61.)

with wheezing, coughing, and sudden hypoxia. Antibiotics may not be necessary at first, but damage to the respiratory mucosa may predispose to subsequent infection. Severe cases require intubation and have a high mortality. Silent cases may be difficult to distinguish from aspiration pneumonia and thus fever, tachypnea, reduced oxygen saturation, or chest X-ray suggestive of pneumonia in an at-risk patient should be treated with appropriate antibiotic coverage.

A recent review of aspiration pneumonia raised a number of interesting points, including the finding that hospital-acquired aspirations and community-acquired aspirations tend to have different microbial involvement, and that anaerobic coverage may not be routinely necessary (35). Its author favors the use levofloxacin for empiric coverage due to the predominance of Gram-negative organisms and suggests sampling via protected brushings or lavage to identify the involved organisms in questionable cases failing to respond. Again, the importance of fever reduction for neurological recovery should be stressed. Pneumonia itself is associated with longer hospital stays and worsened outcomes, so all efforts should be made to avoid it. It is worth noting that percutaneous endoscopic gastrostomy tubes have not been shown to reduce the incidence of aspiration pneumonia. In cases due to especially severe reflux, jejunostomy tubes may be more helpful. No feeding tube will prevent aspiration of oral secretions in the severely dysphagic patient. However, there are many advantages of percutaneous endoscopic gastrostomy tubes and jejunostomy tubes, including patient comfort and an increased ability to participate in rehabilitation. This issue is discussed in detail in Chapter 8.

Incontinence and Urinary Tract Infections

Urinary tract infections are common in hospitalized stroke patients. Due to immobility or inability to communicate, indwelling bladder catheters are often placed for convenience in patients who are not truly incontinent. These devices are clearly associated with increased risk of infection and should be avoided or removed if at all possible. Bearing in mind that soaked diapers can lead to skin rashes or breakdown, patients with impaired communication should be offered bedpans or transfer to a bedside commode every few hours while awake. As noted above, urinary tract infections in the elderly, the demented, or the stroke patient can sometimes lead to dramatic worsening of the neurological examination and should be treated aggressively with antibiotics and antipyretics if needed.

One prospective uricodynometry study of stroke patients identified three common etiologies of incontinence: the new onset of neurogenic bladder with hyperreflexia and urgency; incontinence due to poor cognition/communication ability; or overflow incontinence from underlying neuropathy (e.g., from diabetes) or medication usage (e.g., anti-cholinergics) (36). Regardless of etiology, scheduled voiding was often an effective treatment by the time of discharge from rehabilitation and generally more effective than pharmacotherapy. Further, pharmacotherapy for urinary incontinence has potential detrimental side effects such as sedation or delirium due to the anti-cholinergic mechanism of action. In our stroke unit, use of a non-invasive bladder ultrasound by nursing staff has allowed better monitoring of bladder emptying and reduced the need for urethral catheterization of patients with poor urine output.

Pressure Ulcers

Pressure ulcers (also known as bedsores or decubitus ulcers) are broken down areas of skin and tissue caused by pressure on skin and underlying tissue between bone and external surfaces such as a bed or chair. Reduced blood supply to the area of skin causes tissue necrosis, which may leave an open cavity from the body surface to the bone. The open ulcer is susceptible to secondary infection, including osteomyelitis. Pressure ulcers usually occur over bony prominences, such as the heels, sacrum, hips, or elbows, in patients who are unable to shift their own weight off of the area. It takes only 2 hours of pressure caused by immobility to cause a decubitus ulcer. Urinary incontinence, hemiplegia, reduced sensory perception, hemispatial neglect, and malnutrition are risk factors for developing bedsores.

Decubitus ulcers are notoriously difficult to treat and are therefore best prevented. Turning the immobile patient every 2 hours is essential to prevent bedsores. Identifying at-risk patients and educating them and their families is an effective preventative step as well. Sheepskin, pillows, and foam padding to relieve pressure can also be helpful. Adequate nutrition (including vitamin C and zinc), cleaning of the skin, and range-of-motion exercises for immobile patients are also important. The National Pressure Ulcer Advisory Panel (NPUAP) has developed a staging system, from stage I (a reddened, non-blanchable area) to stage IV (crater with damage to muscle or bone). Treatment is based on the stage of the ulcer. Nursing protocols for evaluating and treating pressure ulcers are critical in the care of stroke patients.

Depression

Stroke is clearly a risk factor for depression, and depression can hinder stroke recovery. One third to one half of all stroke patients show some signs of depression or other mood disorder at discharge, and similar numbers show depressive symptoms at 1 year, although the literature is somewhat difficult to interpret due to varying diagnostic criteria and methodologies (37). Depression may be both more common and more difficult to detect in the aphasic patient or the patient with limited mobility. It is likely under-recognized and under-treated. Risk is thought to be highest in patients with larger or more disabling strokes and in patients with poor social support systems. Strokes of specific cerebral locations, such as the frontal lobe, may confer higher risk. Due to the high incidence of depression, all post-stroke patients should be screened for depression before discharge, during the rehabilitation phase, and in subsequent outpatient follow-up.

Routine prophylaxis of post-stroke depression is generally not warranted, but selective serotonin reuptake inhibitors or atypical agents such as venlafaxine are recommended for symptomatic treatment, along with patient and family education and support. Older tricyclic antidepressant medications in general should be avoided due to sedation and potential adverse effect on rehabilitation. Pharmacologic therapy should be started at lower doses and advanced slowly in the elderly. Occasionally, methylphenidate may be of benefit in the abulic patient. These are patients typically with frontal lobe infarcts who may be awake but are extremely slow to respond or interact with the environment. Other patients who remain very lethargic due to large strokes may also sometimes respond to methylphenidate. Outpatient follow-up is particularly important, because depression is a chronic problem that generally does not respond to short-term therapy. Consultation with a psychiatrist is often beneficial, both for medication recommendations and long-term follow-up. This issue is further discussed in Chapter 8. Recent reviews discuss post-stroke depression in more detail (38,39).

Delirium

Characterized by a waxing and waning pattern of inattention, confusion, agitation, and even autonomic instability, delirium is common in stroke inpatients, perhaps half of whom develop the condition over the hospital stay (40). The severity of stroke symptoms (whether sensory, motor, or cognitive), old age, immobility, underlying dementia, metabolic derangement, and infectious complications are risk factors, and the results are longer hospitalizations and worsened outcomes. Although delirium may reflect the severity of the underlying brain pathology rather than be the cause of poor outcome itself, it should be treated when recognized.

Nonpharmacologic re-orienting measures are the first line of approach, and, when necessary, gentle use of low-dose neuroleptics such as risperidol, quetiapine, or olanzapine may be helpful. Attempts should be made to restore the normal sleep-wake cycle. Restraints and indwelling urinary catheters should be avoided as much as possible. Excessive sensory stimulation can exacerbate delirium (e.g., in a patient in a double room full of people talking with both TVs on). Then again, sensory deprivation can make things worse as well (e.g., for a patient alone in a room with the curtains closed and the lights off). Thus a private room, with a sitter, the TV and radio off, and the windows open and lights on can provide the right balance between the two problems and calm a delirious patient effectively without medication or restraints.

Falls

Stroke patients with decreased mental status, limb weakness, impaired balance, hemispatial neglect, and/or poor sensory feedback are all at high risk for falls. Early efforts should be made to identify and protect these patients. All patients should be assessed for their ability to ambulate and their safety awareness soon after reaching the hospital ward. Some may require a sitter to prevent climbing out of bed, even over the rails. Patients with right parietal strokes in particular often have hemispatial neglect and anosagnosia and therefore not appreciate their neurological deficits. Despite being able to talk coherently with the medical caregivers and acknowledge the need to walk only with assistance, they will then immediately try to stand up on their own the minute the physician or nurse leaves the room. Early mobilization attempts by physical therapists are crucial both in assessment and in return to a functional gait. Assistive device training can begin during the acute hospital stay.

Discharge Planning

An important part of stroke management is discharge planning. Length of hospitalization typically reflects the severity of the underlying stroke and subsequent complications, with those patients requiring mechanical ventilation, feeding tubes, and in-hospital initiation of anticoagulation obviously requiring longer courses. Determination of the most appropriate post-hospital care is generally a team effort, with input from occupational and physical therapists, speech-language pathologists, social workers, nurses, and physicians. Discharge planning also depends crucially on prognosis: whether or not the patient will likely regain use of an arm, be able to walk, be able to carry out daily activities, or require a caretaker. Although ingenious prognostic models have been developed, predicting recovery for an individual patient remains difficult. Although advanced age, medical co-morbidities, hyperglycemia, hyperthermia, and poor social support are commonly cited negative prognostic factors, it is important to note that overall patient outcome, both short- and long-term, is more dependent upon the size and severity of the initial stroke than any other factor. Optimized care can only maximize recovery, given what underlying tissue and brain function remains. Although many authors cite the first 4-6 months as the period of maximal recovery, a substantial number of patients continue to make improvements over many months or even years.

Most patients with moderate and severe strokes are discharged to continued inpatient rehabilitation or a skilled nursing facility (see Chapter 8). Rehabilitation should be begun early (second day of admission). Decisions about whether a patient might require long-term skilled nursing are often deferred until after inpatient rehabilitation. Many patients who are discharged to home benefit from home physical and occupational therapy assessments to identify alterations in the home needed to accommodate the patient's deficits. Stairs and bathrooms are typical trouble spots. The aphasic patient may require outpatient speech and language therapy for many months after returning home. Patients with significant deficits wishing to drive again should be referred to back-to-driving programs for assessment and potential rehabilitation. Some of these issues are illustrated in Case Study 5-1.

Secondary Prevention and Follow-Up

As noted above, secondary stroke prevention should begin in the acute hospital setting. Antiplatelet therapy generally begins immediately, and other modifiable risk factors are usually identified in the first few hospital days, particularly in a streamlined stroke unit. Anticoagulation will be started in specific cases. Generally, such treatment is safe to initiate a few days after stroke onset in the absence of significant hemorrhage. Carotid endarterectomy and treatment of other causes of stroke are discussed in Chapters 6, 7, and 9 through 13.

Risk factors should be addressed acutely as well. Treatment for high cholesterol and diabetes should be initiated or optimized. Lifestyle modification counseling should begin. The initial hospitalization and subsequent rehabilitation time is an excellent opportunity to attempt "cold-turkey" smoking cessation (with nicotine supplements if needed). Counseling should be offered to patients addicted to cocaine or heroin. Nutritionists may aid in helping patients plan an appropriate diet. Exercise and dietary change are the appropriate measures for those with early or mild diabetes.

Blood pressure, initially "liberalized" (allowed to go as high as the body wants), should be gradually reduced as an outpatient beginning a few weeks after stroke. Typically, optimal control is not reached until some months after discharge. At least one follow-up visit with a neurologist is highly recommended, but most secondary prevention involves modification of cardiovascular risk factors best addressed by primary care or internal medicine. Further cardiac risk stratification should be done in the outpatient setting, because coronary and cerebrovascular risk factors are similar. Because the most common cause of death after stroke is myocardial infarction, many of these patients deserve stress tests. Further discussion of stroke prevention can be found in Chapter 2 and in a recent review (41).

Case Study 5-1

A 34-year-old man who was found by his wife confused, mute, and unable to use his right side. He was diagnosed with a probable large left-hemispheric stroke, which was just becoming visible on the initial CT scan. He was admitted to the stroke unit on an ischemic stroke pathway. MRI confirmed the diagnosis of a large but patchy left middle cerebral artery territory stroke, revealed that there was no perfusion-diffusion mismatch requiring acute intervention, and hinted that the etiology was due to a left carotid dissection, which, by history, he may have suffered after a fall when waterskiing a few days before.

Based on the suspected diagnosis of dissection, he was started on a heparin drip to prevent further embolization. The PTT titrated carefully using a sliding-scale heparin dose. The dissection was verified by invasive angiography. His initially elevated blood pressure was allowed to remain high but kept below 180 with as-needed beta-blockers, a treatment verified by his nurses not to result in worsening of his deficits. Initially he was unable to swallow, requiring feeds via nasogastric tube, but re-evaluation revealed return of this function after 2 days.

When the patient's neurological examination worsened, an urgent CT scan showed expected edema of the infarcted hemisphere but no bleeding and no impending herniation. Subsequent close observation revealed intermittent complex partial seizures, and the patient was started on carbamazepine with good control.

Therapists helped maintain the range of motion of his paretic side as it slowly improved. He was turned regularly and his left side was protected, preventing bedsores and minimizing edema. The standard battery of laboratory testing revealed no other cardiovascular risk factors. Although he made some limited improvement in the hospital, his care team decided that due to the severity of his deficits, particularly poor awareness of safety and balance, he would benefit from inpatient rehabilitation. Recommendations were specifically tailored to his needs by the assessments of the inpatient occupational, physical, and speech-language therapists. He returned home within 3 weeks.

Two years later, he is still quite aphasic but can carry on simple conversations. His left arm is clumsy and his left leg drags a bit, but he jogs to work at his new job at a greenhouse. He completed a back-to-driving program and now can run errands independently. He and his wife just returned from a trip to the Grand Canyon. Vacation photos show him waving his left arm to the camera from the back of a mule.

APPENDIX

JOHNS HOPKINS STROKE UNIT CARE MAP

Physician Orders

- Initiate stroke with deficit pathway
- Diagnostic tests (check all those that apply)
    - ❑ Carotid duplex scan to r/o carotid stenosis
    - ❑ Transesophageal echocardiogram (TEE) to r/o embolic source
    - ❑ Transthoracic echocardiogram (TEE) (HCFA guideline for new-onset atrial fibrillation)
    - ❑ Magnetic resonance imaging angiography of the brain (stroke protocol)
- Transport status
    - ❑ On monitor
    - ❑ Off monitor
- Activity
    - ❑ Bed rest with HOB 30°, then dangle bid on HD#1 after orthostatic check; advance on HD#2
- Precautions
    - ❑ Fall
    - ❑ Aspiration
    - ❑ Seizure
- Tests, if not done in emergency department
    - ❑ EKG
    - ❑ CXR
    - ❑ Urinalysis
    - ❑ TSH (HCFAA guideline for new-onset atrial fibrillation)
- Admission labs, if not done in emergency department
    - ❑ Heme 8
    - ❑ Comprehensive metabolic panel
    - ❑ Toxicology screen
- Morning labs
    - ❑ Fasting lipid panel
    - ❑ Fasting homocysteine
    - ❑ ESR
    - ❑ RPR
    - ❑ Fasting glucose level
    - ❑ Hemoglobin A_{1c}
- Obtain orthostatic blood pressure on admission
- Weight within 24 hr of admission and after orthostatic check
- Vital signs q2h × 4, then q4h; on day 4, vital signs q8h
- Blood pressure goals
    - ❑ SBP _____
    - ❑ DBP _____

Continued.

- Continuous pulse oximetry, goal O_2 saturation > ___% delivered by _____
- Continuous cardiac monitoring, discontinue after 72 h if no significant rhythm abnormalities
- Neurological checks q2h × 4, then q4h; on day 4, neurological checks q8h
- Systems assessment q4h × 48h, then q8h × 48h, then q shift
- 3-oz swallowing screening upon admission (performed and documented by RN)
- If patient unable to take PO fluids, insert NG tube within 24h
- Diet
  - ❏ Strict NPO
  - ❏ NPO except medications and ice chips
  - ❏ NPO after midnight for TEE in morning
  - ❏ Advance diet on day 2 if passed Speech and Swallowing Evaluation
  - ❏ Consult GI team for placement of PEG tube if unable to swallow thickened liquids for > 5 days
- Fluid I&O q shift × 3 days
- IV fluid
  - ❏ NS @ ___ cc/hr
  - ❏ Other _____ @ ___ cc/hr
- Baseline peripheral blood glucose (PBG) upon admission unless done in emergency department; if PBG > 150 or patient known diabetic, do PBG testing q6h and follow sliding scale
- Convert to saline lock when tolerating PO intake
- Notify physician for
  - ❏ Temperature > 38.3°C
  - ❏ HR > 110 or < 50
  - ❏ SBP > 200 or < 100 mm Hg
  - ❏ DBP > 100 or < 50 mm Hg
  - ❏ Blood glucose < 50 or > 200
  - ❏ O_2 sat < 92%
  - ❏ Any decline in neurological status
- Apply TED stockings and serial compression device; discontinue when patient is ambulating > 1 hr/day
- If unable to void after 8 hr of admission, do bladder scan; if > 250 cc, straight cath; if unable to void 6–8 hr following straight cath, insert Foley catheter
- Routine medications
  - ❏ Heparin 5000 U SQ q12h (HCFA guideline)
  - ❏ ASA 325 mg PO/PGT qd
  - ❏ Docusate sodium 100 mg PO/PGT bid
  - ❏ Ranitidine 150 mg PO/PGT bid
  - ❏ Acetaminophen 650 mg PO/PGT q6h prn
  - ❏ MOM 15 cc PO/PGT qhs prn
- HCFA guideline: avoid sublingual nifedipine in patients with acute stroke
- Initiate the following if applicable
  - ❏ Physical therapy
  - ❏ Occupational therapy

Continued.

❏ Speech therapy
❏ Nutrition therapy
❏ Social work

Multi-Disciplinary/Nursing

❏ Deficit that interferes with learning (N/Y, explain)
❏ Vision problems?
❏ Hearing problems?
❏ Speech problems?
❏ Communication/cognitive deficit?
❏ Pyschomotor limitations?
❏ Language barrier?
❏ Other?

- Document assessed learning needs/plan
- Family spokesperson

Problems List

❏ Pain
❏ Altered mental status
❏ Fluid volume deficit/overload
❏ Insufficient nutritional intake
❏ Altered elimination
❏ Altered skin integrity
❏ Altered cerebral/cardiopulmonary
peripheral tissue perfusion

❏ Febrile
❏ Activity intolerance
❏ Altered mobility
❏ Knowledge deficit
❏ Self-care deficit
❏ Potential for infection/immunosuppression

Expected Outcomes

❏ Pain is absent or controlled at a pain level < _____
❏ Decision point for early discharge
    - 3-day LOS: mild hemiparesis, speech intelligible, independent swallow, eats
    - ADL, blood pressure controlled, support system in place
❏ Discharged on anti-thrombotic
❏ Alert, oriented × 3 and able to follow instruction
❏ Disorientation/anxiety absent or reduced
❏ Airway clear
❏ Breathing pattern normal/improved
❏ Hypoxemia/hypercapnia absent or reduced
❏ Cardiac output improved or at baseline
❏ Cerebral/cardiopulm/peripheral tissue perfusion adequate or improved
❏ Electrolyte balance adequate or improved
❏ Fluid volume adequate
❏ Nutritional intake meets metabolic requirements

Continued.

❑ Constipation relieved/normal bowel habits returned

❑ Urinary output adequate

❑ Skin intact or integrity improved

❑ Afebrile

❑ Able to perform ADLs without SOB or pain

❑ Able to ambulate _____ feet with _____ assist

❑ Able to verbalize understanding of discharge or self-care instructions

❑ Absence of infection

Multidisciplinary Goals

Day 1

❑ Identify location of the stroke (CT)

❑ Admission weight obtained

❑ Neurological exam at baseline or improved

❑ Blood pressure goal established

❑ Blood glucose maintained

❑ 3-oz swallowing screen (RN)

❑ Bed rest; dangle if not orthostatic

❑ Initiate appropriate protocols (fall, aspiration, DVT)

❑ Evaluate other medical problems and establish treatment plans

❑ Initiate appropriate consults

Day 2

❑ Identify location of stroke (MRI)

❑ Determine etiology of stroke and vessel blocked (MRI/A, CD, TEE, TCD, etc.)

❑ Blood pressure goal met

❑ Blood glucose maintained

❑ Advance activity

❑ No evidence of complications (aspiration pneumonia, GI bleed, DVT, PE)

❑ TSH, echocardiogram if new-onset atrial fibrillation

Day 3

❑ Neurological exam at baseline or improved (if discharged)

❑ Blood pressure goal met

❑ Blood glucose maintained

❑ PT, OT, speech evaluations completed

❑ Social work initial assessment complete

❑ Advance activity

❑ Prepare PT/family for discharge or rehab and identify needed resources

❑ Plan established for nutritional support

❑ Patient discharged?

❑ No evidence of complications (aspiration pneumonia, GI bleed, DVT, PE)

❑ Plan established for warfarin at discharge (if applicable)

Continued.

Days 4-6
- Same as Day 3

Routine Nursing Assessments

- Neurological (each shift):
  - ❑ Level of consciousness, orientation, answering questions
  - ❑ MMSE score
  - ❑ Glasgow Coma Scale (motor, verbal, eye opening, total)
  - ❑ Cranial nerves, including pupil sizes
  - ❑ Motor score (0–5) for each limb
  - ❑ Rapid alternating movements and coordination
- Pain assessment
- Respirations: pattern, cough, breath sounds
- Braden Risk Assessment score (daily) for risk of pressure ulcers
- Document the neurological deficit quantitatively daily (physician) and on each shift (nursing)
- NIH stroke scales (admission, discharge), to be performed by physician
- Modified Rankin scale (premorbid and post-stroke)

REFERENCES

1. Alberts MJ, Hademenos G, Latchaw RE, et al. Recommendations for the establishment of primary stroke centers. Brain Attack Coalition. JAMA. 2000;283:3102-9.
2. Indredavik B. Stroke units: the Norwegian experience. Cerebrovasc Dis. 2003;15(Suppl)1:19-20.
3. Jorgensen HS, Nakayama H, Raaschou HO, et al. The effect of a stroke unit: reductions in mortality, discharge rate to nursing home, length of hospital stay, and cost: a community-based study. Stroke. 1995;26:1178-82.
4. Langhorne P, Williams BO, Gilchrist W, Howie K. Do stroke units save lives? Lancet. 1993;342:395-8.
5. Ronning OM, Guldvog B. Stroke units versus general medical wards. I. Twelve- and eighteen-month survival: a randomized, controlled trial. Stroke. 1998;29:58-62.
6. Langhorne P, Williams BO, Gilchrist W, et al. A formal overview of stroke unit trials. Rev Neurol. 1995;23:394-8.
7. Organised Inpatient (Stroke Unit) Care for Stroke. Cochrane Database Syst Rev. 2002; CD000197.
8. Organised Inpatient (Stroke Unit) Care for Stroke. Stroke Unit Trialists' Collaboration. Cochrane Database Syst Rev. 2000; CD000197.
9. Collaborative Systematic Review of the Randomised Trials of Organised Inpatient (Stroke Unit) Care after Stroke. Stroke Unit Trialists' Collaboration. BMJ. 1997;314:1151-9.
10. Stroke Unit Trialists Collaboration. How do stroke units improve patient outcomes? A collaborative systematic review of the randomized trials. Stroke. 1997;28:2139-44.
11. Indredavik B, Bakke F, Slordahl SA, et al. Treatment in a combined acute and rehabilitation stroke unit: which aspects are most important? Stroke. 1999;30:917-23.
12. Gillum LA, Johnston SC. Characteristics of academic medical centers and ischemic stroke outcomes. Stroke. 2001;32:2137-42.
13. Mamoli A, Censori B, Casto L, et al. An analysis of the costs of ischemic stroke in an Italian stroke unit. Neurology. 1999;53:112-6.

14. Briggs DE, Felberg RA, Malkoff MD, et al. Should mild or moderate stroke patients be admitted to an intensive care unit? Stroke. 2001;32:871-6.

15. Ayata C, Ropper AH. Intensive care management of specific stroke treatment. Adv Neurol. 2003;92:361-77.

16. Nguyen T, Koroshetz WJ. Intensive care management of ischemic stroke. Curr Neurol Neurosci Rep. 2003;3:32-9.

17. Hanley DF. Review of critical care and emergency approaches to stroke. Stroke. 2003;34:362-4.

18. Leonardi-Bee J, Bath PMW, Philips SJ, et al. Blood pressure and clinical outcomes in the International Stroke Trial. Stroke. 2002;33:1315-20.

19. Bruno A, Biller J, Adams HP Jr., et al. Acute blood glucose level and outcome from ischemic stroke. Neurology. 1999;52:280-4.

20. Anderson RE, Tan WK, Martin HS, Meyer FB. Effects of glucose and PaO_2 modulation on cortical intracellular acidosis, NADH redox state, and infarction in the ischemic penumbra. Stroke. 1999;30:160-70.

21. Boysen G, Christensen H. Stroke severity determines body temperature in acute stroke. Stroke. 2001;32:413-7.

22. Kammersgaard LP, Jorgenson HS, Rungby JA, et al. Admission body temperature predicts long-term mortality after acute stroke. Stroke. 2002;33:1759-62.

23. Georgiadis D, Schwarz S, Aschoff A, Schwab S. Hemicraniectomy and moderate hypothermia in patients with severe ischemic stroke. Stroke. 2002;33:1584-8.

24. Wijdicks EF. Management of massive hemispheric cerebral infarct: is there a ray of hope? Mayo Clin Proc. 2000;75:945-52.

25. Schwab S, Steiner T, Aschoff A, et al. Early hemicraniectomy in patients with complete middle cerebral artery infarction. Stroke. 1998;29:1888-93.

26. Carter BS, Ogilvy CS, Candia GJ, et al. One-year outcome after decompressive surgery for massive nondominant hemispheric infarction. Neurosurgery. 1997;40:1168-75 [Discussion: 1175-6].

27. Pessin MS, Estol CJ, Lafranchise F, Caplan LR. Safety of anticoagulation after hemorrhagic infarction. Neurology. 1993;43:1298-303.

28. Tissue Plasminogen Activator for Acute Ischemic Stroke. The National Institute of Neurological Disorders and Stroke Rt-PA Stroke Study Group. N Engl J Med. 1995;333:1581-7.

29. Burn J, Dennis M, Bamford J, et al. Epileptic seizures after a first stroke. The Oxfordshire Community Stroke Project. BMJ. 1997;315:1582-7.

30. Bladin CF, Alexandrov AV, Bellavance A, et al. Seizures after stroke: a prospective multicenter study. Arch Neurol. 2000;57:1617-22.

31. Labovitz DL, Hauser WA. Preventing stroke-related seizures: when should anticonvulsant drugs be started? Neurology. 2003;60:365-6.

32. Weimar C, Roth MP, Zillessen G, et al. Complications following acute ischemic stroke. Eur Neurol. 2002;48:133-40.

33. Counsell C, Sandercock P. Low-molecular-weight heparins or heparinoids versus standard unfractionated heparin for acute ischaemic stroke. Cochrane Database Syst Rev. 2001; CD000119.

33a. Depippos, KL, Holas MA, Reding MJ. Validation of the 3-oz water swallow test for aspiration following stroke. Arch Neurol. 1992;49:1259-61.

34. Holas MA, Depippo KL, Reding MJ. Aspiration and relative risk of medical complications following stroke. Arch Neurol. 1994;51:1051-3.

35. Marik PE. Aspiration pneumonitis and aspiration pneumonia. N Engl J Med. 2001;344:665-71.

36. Gelber DA, Good DC, Laven LJ, Verhulst SJ. Causes of urinary incontinence after acute hemispheric stroke. Stroke. 1993;24:378-82.

37. **Desmond DW, Remien RH, Moroney JT, et al.** Ischemic stroke and depression. J Int Neuropsychol Soc. 2003;9:429-39.
38. **Gall A.** Post-stroke depression. Hosp Med. 2001;62:268-73.
39. **Gainotti G, Marra C.** Determinants and consequences of post-stroke depression. Curr Opin Neurol. 2002;15:85-9.
40. **Ferro JM, Caeiro L, Verdelho A.** Delirium in acute stroke. Curr Opin Neurol. 2002;15:51-5.
41. **Straus SE, Majumdar SR, McAlister FA.** New evidence for stroke prevention: scientific review. JAMA. 2002;288:1388-95.

Chapter 6

Antithrombotic Therapy

ROBERT J. WITYK, MD

Key Points

- Antiplatelet agents are effective in the secondary prevention of stroke but not in primary prevention.
- Aspirin is the most widely used antiplatelet agent for secondary prevention of stroke.
- Other antiplatelets include ticlopidine, clopidogrel, dipyrimdamole, and glycoprotein IIb/IIIa receptor antagonists.
- Considerable debate exists as to which antiplatelet strategy is best for stroke prevention; treatment should be individualized.
- The use of anticoagulation in secondary stroke prevention is limited to several specific diagnoses.
- Despite the negative results from large studies, anticoagulation with heparin or LMWH is still often used empirically.
- It is important to limit the risk of hemorrhagic complications caused by heparin.

Because most mechanisms of ischemic stroke involve thrombosis at some point, it is no surprise that antithrombotic agents play a major role in the treatment of cerebrovascular disorders. Evidenced-based medicine confirms the importance of antithrombotic therapy in the secondary prevention of stroke but maintains that its role in primary prevention is very limited. Even in secondary prevention, antiplatelet agents have the most evidence for use, with only a few specific indications for anticoagulation, such as atrial fibrillation and cardiac thombus. Finally, despite years of debate on the use of heparin in the treatment of acute ischemic stroke, there is surprisingly little evidence to support the use of anticoagulation in the acute setting.

Antiplatelet Agents

Aspirin

Antiplatelet agents are effective in the secondary prevention of stroke but not for primary prevention. Both the Physicians' Health Study in the United States (1) and a study of British physicians (2) found that regular aspirin use was associated with a small but not statistically significant increase in the rate of intracerebral hemorrhage, without a reduction in ischemic stroke risk. The Cardiovascular Health Study (3) found that low-risk women who received aspirin for primary prevention actually had a higher risk of ischemic stroke and that the overall risk of intracerebral hemorrhage in elderly subjects was increased fourfold. In contrast, the Women's Health Study reported a lower risk of stroke in women who took low-dose aspirin (100 mg every other day) compared with placebo and that this effect was particularly prominent in women over the age of 65 (3a). At this time, aspirin should not be routinely recommended for use by low-risk patients for primary prevention of stroke, but the differential effects of aspirin in men and women in terms of stroke and cardiovascular disease need further study.

Aspirin is the most widely used and studied antiplatelet agent for the secondary prevention of stroke. A meta-analysis performed by the Antiplatelet Trialists (4) found that use of aspirin reduced the risk of nonfatal stroke or myocardial infarction by 30% in patients who were at high risk for vascular disease (e.g., those with a previous history of stroke, transient ischemic attack [TIA], myocardial infarction, or unstable angina). This benefit was seen in both men and women. The appropriate dose of aspirin remains uncertain, however, and the appropriate use of newer, more expensive antiplatelet agents is a matter for debate.

The earliest antiplatelet trials studied doses of aspirin commonly used for anti-inflammatory purposes (e.g., 1300 mg/day). Later studies (e.g., the Swedish Aspirin Low-Dose Trial [5]) found that aspirin doses as low as 75 mg/day were superior to placebo in preventing vascular events. In vitro studies have shown that aspirin at a dose as low as 40 mg/day inhibits the production of thromboxane, a potent prothrombotic factor, without reducing levels of prostacyclin, an agent that promotes arteriolar dilatation and inhibits platelet aggregation. The United Kingdom Transient Ischemic Attack (TIA) aspirin trial (6) directly compared 300 mg/day and 1300 mg/day of aspirin for secondary prevention of stroke in two of the three arms of the study. No difference in efficacy was seen between these two aspirin doses; however, no statistically significant difference was found between aspirin dose and placebo, so that the study was probably underpowered to detect differences between the different aspirin doses.

On the other side of the aspirin-dose argument, however, was the observation that in vitro studies of platelet aggregation in patients taking aspirin found a significant proportion of patients on 325 mg/day of aspirin were "resistant" to the action of the drug. Even a few patients using 1300 mg/day of aspirin had no discernable in vitro antiplatelet effect (7). Recent meta-analyses of the dose of aspirin and degree of benefit have failed to find a convincing dose-response effect. At this time, aspirin doses between 81 and 325 mg/day are probably effective and equivalent, although further studies using newer platelet function assays are needed to determine whether patients who are "aspirin failures" would benefit from higher doses of aspirin.

There are two large clinical trials that show a benefit of aspirin use in the acute phase of stroke. The International Stroke Trial (8) studied the use of aspirin 300 mg/day or heparin or placebo in patients treated within 48 hours of acute ischemic stroke (see heparin section below). Aspirin use resulted in the reduction of recurrent ischemic stroke in the first 14 days by 1% without a significant increase in bleeding complications. Similarly, the Chinese Aspirin Stroke Study (CAST) (9) was another very large study which found that use of 160 mg/day of aspirin within 48 hours of acute ischemic stroke reduced death and recurrent stroke rates by 1% without significant bleeding complications. Although the effect is very modest, aspirin use should be considered as initial treatment for patients presenting to the hospital with acute ischemic stroke.

Ticlopidine

Ticlopidine is a thienopyridine drug that inhibits adenosine diphosphate activation of platelets and fibrinogen binding. Two clinical trials, one comparing ticlopidine with placebo and one with high-dose aspirin, found ticlopidine to be beneficial in the prevention of stroke in patients with prior stroke or TIA. However, ticlopidine was associated with increased side effects, including gastrointestinal upset, rash, and a 0.9% risk of severe neutropenia. In addition, a number of cases of thrombotic thrombocytopenic purpura have been reported in association with ticlopidine use, some occurring within the first 2 weeks of use. Use of ticlopidine requires close monitoring of blood counts during treatment, and because of these side effects, use of the drug in clinical practice is now limited.

Clopidogrel

Clopidogrel is a newer thienopyridine agent in the same chemical class as ticlopidine. The Clopidogrel versus Aspirin in Patients at Risk of Ischemic Events (CAPRIE) study (10) investigated the use of clopidogrel compared with 325 mg/day aspirin in a large study (19,185 subjects) of patients with either stroke, TIA, coronary artery disease, or peripheral vascular disease. Using a composite outcome event of either stroke, myocardial infarction, or vascular death, clopidogrel showed a small but statistically significant reduction of risk compared with aspirin. The relative risk reduction was 8.7% with the absolute annual risk reduction being only 0.5%. (Figure 6-1).

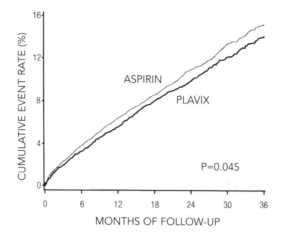

FATAL OR NON-FATAL VASCULAR EVENT

Figure 6-1 Cumulative vascular event rates in the aspirin and clopidogrel (Plavix) arms of the CAPRIE trial. (From CAPRIE Steering Committee. A randomized, blinded trial of clopidogrel versus aspirin in patients at risk of ischemic events (CAPRIE). Lancet. 1996;348: 1329-39; with permission.)

When the subgroup of patients with stroke were analyzed, no significant difference between clopidogrel and aspirin was noted, although this subgroup did not have as much power to detect a difference as in the main study. Clopidogrel was well tolerated without significant adverse events, and neutropenia was rare (0.04%).

A recent study in patients with coronary ischemia (the CURE study) suggested that the combination of aspirin and clopidogrel was superior to aspirin alone in preventing subsequent thrombotic events (11). The MATCH study was designed to test this combination in patients with TIA or ischemic stroke (12). Clopidogrel 75 mg/day was compared with clopidogrel + aspirin 75 mg/day. Unlike the CURE study, the MATCH trial found no benefit of combination therapy in preventing subsequent stroke or thrombotic events but that it was associated with an increased risk of bleeding complications. At this time, there is no routine indication for combination clopidogrel and aspirin use in secondary prevention of stroke. We do not know if the combination therapy could be useful in patients with recurrent ischemia despite adequate antiplatelet therapy or in a particular subgroup of patients (e.g., patients with high-grade atherosclerotic stenosis).

Dipyridamole

Dipyridamole had been studied in combination with moderate-dose (325 mg) or high-dose aspirin in the past, without a convincing beneficial additive effect. The most recent study, the European Stroke Prevention Study (13), compared four arms of treatment for patients with minor stroke or TIA: placebo, 50 mg aspirin, 400 mg slow-release dipyridamole, and a combination of 50 mg aspirin plus 400 mg slow-release dipyridamole. Outcome analysis included stroke, death, and combined stroke and death. Both aspirin and dipyridamole alone were more effective than placebo, but the combination was the best of all regimens. This study is different than many of the previous studies of dipyridamole in that a larger number of patients were studied (6602), the dose of aspirin was relatively low (50 mg/day), and the dose of dipyridamole was relatively high (400 mg/day).

A controlled-release formulation (Aggrenox) of 50 mg aspirin plus 200 mg of dipyridamole is now available for use, being dosed twice a day. Side effects include headache and gastrointestinal upset, so the dose is typically started at once a day for a week until the patient adjusts to the medication. Patients with a history of migraines seem to be particularly prone to developing headache problems with this medication.

Glycoprotein IIB/IIIA Receptor Antagonists

Blockage of the glycoprotein (GP) IIb/IIIa receptor on the platelet prevents crosslinking of platelets by fibrinogen, and receptor antagonists are powerful antiplatelet agents. Their use has been popularized by cardiologists as an adjunct to antithrombotic therapy for acute myocardial infarction and particularly after placement of coronary artery stents. Several trials of oral GP IIb/IIIa inhibitors have not shown superiority over aspirin and paradoxically may show harm with the risk of thrombocytopenia. Several intravenous forms of GP IIb/IIIa inhibitors are being studied currently for stroke patients, either for acute ischemic stroke treatment or for use in cerebral artery stenting.

Contraindications

There are a few contraindications for use of antiplatelet therapy in secondary prevention of stroke, including active internal bleeding and thrombocytopenia. Antiplatelet agents should be avoided in patients with a history of intracerebral hemorrhage, amyloid angiopathy, vascular malformations, poorly controlled hypertension, or a bleeding diathesis. However, some patients with a history of intracerebral hemorrhage who have well-controlled blood pressure may be treated with antiplatelet agents if the benefit in reducing stroke or myocardial infarction is felt to outweigh the risk of recurrent bleeding. Consultation with a neurologist in this setting may be helpful.

Likewise, patients with stable, unruptured cerebral aneurysms may be treated with antiplatelet agents, if the cardiovascular protective benefit is significant. Antithrombotic therapy is not felt to increase the risk of bleeding, but it may worsen the extent of bleeding if it occurs.

Other relative contraindications for specific agents include avoidance of aspirin in patients who are aspirin allergic or who have peptic ulcer disease. Use of clopidogrel is usually acceptable in these patients. (Clopidogrel does not have the ulcerogenic properties of aspirin but should be avoided in patients with active gastrointestinal bleeding.) Ticlopidine should be avoided in patients with thrombocytopenia or a history of thrombotic thrombocytopenic purpura.

Anticoagulation Agents

Anticoagulation can be thought of as preventing "red clots" as opposed to preventing "white clots" with antiplatelet therapy. Anticoagulation is an effective measure for secondary stroke prevention over the long term for the specific indications, such as atrial fibrillation and cardiac disorders, that predispose to cardiac thrombus. Current anticoagulants used in stroke include warfarin, unfractionated heparin, and low-molecular-weight heparin (LMWH) or heparinoids.

Warfarin

Warfarin antagonizes vitamin K–dependent coagulation factors, and the current accepted standard for measurement of the anticoagulant effect is the INR. The best evidence for use of warfarin comes from studies of the primary and secondary prevention of stroke in patients with atrial fibrillation. The optimal INR range is 2.0 to 3.0, with increasing incidence of embolic events when the INR dips below 1.7. In one trial, use of a target INR range of 3.0 to 4.5 led to an unacceptably high incidence of major bleeding complications. Long-term anticoagulation is generally accepted for other cardiac conditions where the risk of embolism is high, such as prosthetic heart valves and known cardiac thrombus (see Chapter 10). Ongoing studies are examining patients with low cardiac ejection fraction but without embolic complications.

Neurologists have often used warfarin empirically for patients with atherothrombotic or embolic-appearing stroke in the absence of a high-risk cardiac source of embolism. This approach has been called into question by the recent WARSS report (14). More than 2000 patients with ischemic stroke or TIA were randomized to warfarin (INR target 1.4 to 2.8) versus aspirin 325 mg/day and followed for 2 years. Patients with high-grade carotid stenosis or with high-risk cardiac sources of embolism were excluded because defined therapies exist for those conditions. In the end, there was no proven benefit of warfarin over aspirin in terms of any endpoint or for any subgroup of patients (Table 6-1). A limitation of the study is that the INR range used was low compared with current recommendations for patients with atrial fibrillation. In addition, the number of

Table 6-1 WARSS Study Results

Outcomes*	Warfarin	Aspirin
Major bleeding	2.2/100 patient years	1.5/100 patient years
Stroke or death	17.8%	16.0%
Vascular endpoint + major bleed	20.0%	17.8%

*Outcomes at two years.
Republished with permission from Mohr JP, Thompson JL, Lazar RM, et al. A comparison of warfarin and aspirin for the prevention of recurrent ischemic stroke. N Engl J Med. 2001;345:1444-51.

patients in subgroups (e.g., with intracranial atherosclerosis or with a patent foramen ovale) was small for analysis, such that a treatment effect could have been missed.

The WASID trial set out to compare high-dose aspirin with warfarin (INR target 2.0 to 3.0) in patients with high-grade intracranial atherosclerosis documented by cerebral angiography. Traditionally, this type of lesion was felt to mandate life-long anticoagulation. There was no benefit of warfarin over high-dose aspirin. Unfortunately, the recurrent stroke rate was rather high in both treatment arms.

Heparin and Heparinoids

Heparin is a glycosaminoglycan that binds and activates antithrombin III, which in turn inhibits factors II and X. Commercially available heparin consists of heterogeneous molecules with a molecular weight ranging from 5000 to 30,000 daltons, but LMWH is fractionated to use the population of smaller molecules. LMWH has a lesser antagonistic effect on thrombin but retains its ability to inhibit factor Xa. Because LMWH does not bind significantly to plasma and tissue proteins, its pharmacokinetics are more predictable and it does not require monitoring when given as a weight-adjusted subcutaneous dose, typically once or twice a day. Heparinoids are semisynthetic compounds that function similarly to LMWH.

Heparin and LMWH have a limited role in stroke prevention because of the need for intravenous or subcutaneous injections. They can be used in patients who would normally be treated with warfarin but need the oral medication stopped for a period of time (e.g., as in a patient about to undergo an invasive procedure) or in certain periods of pregnancy where warfarin is contraindicated.

The role of anticoagulation in acute ischemic stroke treatment has a long history of anecdotal use but is becoming less common given the results of recent clinical trials. Several early studies using intravenous unfractionated heparin showed no benefit of acute anticoagulation in patients with ischemic stroke, including apparent stroke-in-progression.

These studies were quite small by current standards and may have lacked the power to demonstrate an effect.

In the International Stroke Trial (8), patients were randomized to 12,500 U of subcutaneous unfractionated heparin twice daily versus placebo within 48 hours on stroke onset. The rate of recurrent ischemic stroke was about 1% higher in the placebo group, but the rate of intracerebral bleeding was also about 1% higher in the heparin group (Figure 6-2). As a result, there was no overall benefit with the use of heparin. This was a very large study (over 19,000 subjects) that included a substantial proportion of patients with atrial fibrillation as the cause of the stroke. Even in the group of patients with atrial fibrillation, the benefit of heparin for reducing recurrent stroke was balanced by an equal increase in intracerebral bleeding.

LMWH were felt to be safer in terms of bleeding complications than unfractionated heparin, and a large North American trial was conducted using the heparinoid danaparoid, with the hope of benefit without the increased intracerebral bleed risk (15). Like the IST report, patients with heparinoids did not have any significant benefit in terms of functional outcome at 3 months, and the trial was considered a negative study (Figure 6-3). Subgroup analysis, however, suggested that patients with large vessel atherosclerosis (particularly carotid artery stenosis) seemed to do better with heparinoids compared with placebo. Reports of subsequent studies using other LMWH products have likewise been unsuccessful.

Despite the negative results from large studies, anticoagulation with heparin or LMWH is still used by many neurologists in the United States on an empirical basis. Anticoagulation is often used for patients with large vessel atherosclerosis, such as critical carotid artery stenosis or basilar artery thrombosis, particularly if there is the sense of progressive deficit (suggesting

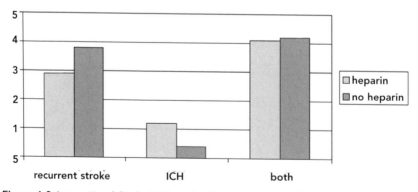

Figure 6-2 International Stroke Trial results. Rates in percent of recurrent stroke, intracerebral hemorrhage (ICH), or both events in patients who were treated with or without heparin. (Data from International Stroke Trial Collaborative Group. The International Stroke Trial (IST): a randomized trial of aspirin, subcutaneous heparin, both, or neither among 9435 patients with acute ischemic stroke. Lancet. 1997;349:1569-81.)

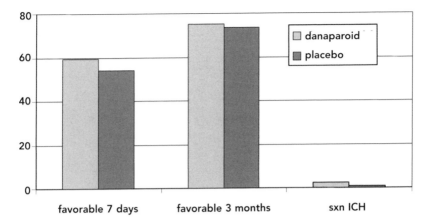

Figure 6-3 TOAST Trial Results. Percent of patients with favorable outcome at 7 days and 3 months treated with danaparoid versus placebo. Rates of symptomatic intracerebral hemorrhage (sxn ICH) were very low in both groups. (Data from the Publications Committee for the Trial of ORG 10172 in Acute Stroke Treatment (TOAST) investigators. Low molecular weight heparinoid, ORG 10172 (danaparoid), and outcome after acute ischemic stroke: a randomized controlled trial. JAMA. 1998;279:1265-72.)

propagation of thrombus) or crescendo TIAs (suggesting impending carotid artery occlusion). The benefit of anticoagulation has not been proven in these situations.

When using heparin, it is important to limit the risk of hemorrhagic complications. Our practice has been to avoid using as large a loading dose of heparin as might be used in a patient with acute pulmonary embolism and to adopt a less intense anticoagulation regime. In addition, the target PTT ratio is kept modest (1.5 to 2 times control) and adjustments to the heparin rate for IV use are small, with mandatory repeat PTT determinations at 6 hours after starting the heparin drip or after a change in dose.

LMWH theoretically may be associated with a lower rate of hemorrhagic complications, but there has been no direct trial of IV heparin versus LMWH in stroke patients. The available data suggest a similar rate of intracerebral hemorrhage in the TOAST and IST trials. LMWH has been studied in clinical practice for stroke patients being transitioned from heparin to warfarin with acceptable safety results.

Contraindications

Contraindications to anticoagulation include those discussed in relation to antiplatelet agents. However, given the higher risk of bleeding with anticoagulants, several additional factors should be considered. Patients with acute ischemic strokes are prone to hemorrhagic transformation of the infarct, and some of these patients will experience frank parenchymal hematoma formation with mass effect and neurological deterioration. Clinical observation suggests that patients with large infarcts (e.g., large and deep areas of hypodensity on CT scan) are more prone to bleeding complications.

Other relative contraindications to anticoagulant use include combination with intravenous thrombolytic therapy, intracranial dissection, and stroke due to endocarditis. Heparin may produce heparin-induced-thrombocytopenia. Long-term anticoagulation of elderly patients for secondary prevention may be risky, particularly in frail patients who are at risk of falling. In rare patients with protein S or protein C deficiency, use of warfarin loading without concomitant intravenous heparin can lead to a transient hypercoagulable state and the syndrome of warfarin skin necrosis (see Chapter 10).

Conclusion

There is still considerable debate as to which antiplatelet strategy is best for stroke prevention. For example, although the aspirin-dipyridamole combination appeared better than aspirin in the European Stroke Prevention Study, some critics believe that the dose of aspirin used was inadequate. All agents are effective in the secondary prevention of stroke, and treatment should be individualized to the patient in terms of side-effect profile and compliance (particularly in patients for whom cost of medications is a significant issue). When faced with a patient who has a further ischemic event while on aspirin (a stroke or TIA), many clinicians either switch to another antiplatelet agent or consider combination therapy. However, recurrent stroke or TIA may represent progressive vascular disease and may not be due to antithrombotic failure. No medication can completely counteract the effects of decades of atherosclerotic buildup on cerebral vessels.

The use of anticoagulation in secondary stroke prevention is limited to several diagnoses, including atrial fibrillation (other than "benign" or "lone" atrial fibrillation), cardiac thrombus, prosthetic heart valves, and certain pro-thrombotic states. In terms of acute stroke treatment, routine anticoagulation with heparin has not been shown to be beneficial in clinical trials and should be discouraged. However, there may be certain circumstances (e.g. perhaps large vessel atherostenosis or cerebral artery dissection) where empiric use of heparin may be reasonable.

REFERENCES

1. **Steering Committee of the Physicians' Health Study Research Group**. Final report on the aspirin component of the ongoing Physicians' Health Study. N Engl J Med. 1989; 321:129-35.

2. **Peto R, Gray R, Collins R, et al**. Randomized trial of prophylactic daily aspirin in British male doctors. Br Med J. 1988;296:313-6.

3. **Kronmal R, Hart R, Manolio T, et al**. Aspirin use and incident stroke in the Cardiovascular Health Study. Stroke. 1998;29:887-94.

3a. **Ridker PM, Cook NR, Lee IM, et al**. A randomized trial of low-dose aspirin in the primary prevention of cardiovascular disease in women. N Engl J Med 2005;352:1293-304.

4. **Antiplatelet Trialists' Collaboration**. Secondary prevention of vascular disease by prolonged antiplatelet treatment. Br Med J. 1988;296:320-31.

5. **SALT Collaborative Group**. Swedish aspirin low-dose trial (SALT) of 75 mg aspirin as secondary prophylaxis after cerebrovascular ischaemic events. Lancet. 1991;338:1345-9.

6. **UK TIA Study Group**. The United Kingdom transient ischaemic attack (UK-TIA) aspirin trial: final results. J Neurol Neurosurg Psychiatr. 1991;54:1044-54.

7. **Helgason CM, Bolin KM, Hoff JA, et al**. Development of aspirin resistance in persons with previous ischemic stroke. Stroke. 1994;25:2331-6.

8. **International Stroke Trial Collaborative Group**. The International Stroke Trial (IST): a randomized trial of aspirin, subcutaneous heparin, both, or neither among 19,435 patients with acute ischemic stroke. Lancet. 1997;349:1569-81.

9. **Chinese Acute Stroke Trial Collaborative Group**. CAST: randomized placebo-controlled trial of early aspirin use in 20000 patients with acute ischemic stroke. Lancet. 1997; 349:1641-9.

10. **CAPRIE Steering Committee**. A randomized, blinded trial of clopidogrel versus aspirin in patients at risk of ischemic events (CAPRIE). Lancet. 1996;348:1329-39.

11. **Albers GW, Amarenco P**. Combination therapy with clopidogrel and aspirin: can the CURE results be extrapolated to cerebrovascular patients? Stroke. 2001;32:2948-9.

12. **Diener HC, Bogousslavsky J, Brass LM, et al**. Aspirin and clopidogrel compared with clopidogrel alone after recent ischaemic stroke or transient ischaemic attack in high-risk patients (MATCH): randomised, double-blind, placebo-controlled trial. Lancet. 2004; 364:331-7.

13. **Diener HC, Cunha L, Forbes C, et al**. European Stroke Prevention Study. 2. Dipyridamole and acetylsalicylic acid in the secondary prevention of stroke. J Neurol Science. 1996;143:1-13.

14. **Mohr JP, Thompson JL, Lazar RM, et al**. A comparison of warfarin and aspirin for the prevention of recurrent ischemic stroke. N Engl J Med. 2001;345:1444-51.

15. **Publications Committee for the Trial of ORG 10172 in Acute Stroke Treatment (TOAST) Investigators**. Low molecular weight heparinoid, ORG 10172 (danaparoid), and outcome after acute ischemic stroke: a randomized controlled trial. JAMA. 1998;279:1265-72.

Chapter 7

Thrombolytic Therapy for Acute Ischemic Stroke

JAISHRI O. BLAKELEY, MD
RAFAEL H. LLINAS, MD
LOUISE D. McCULLOUGH, MD, PhD

Key Points

- Intraveneous thrombolysis has become an important part of ischemic stroke management since publication of the 1995 NINDS study.
- There are several means of reducing the risk of hemorrhage after IV thrombolysis, including strict control of blood pressure, exclusion of patients with coagulopathy, and limiting treatment to patients within 3 hours of onset of symptoms.
- For patients who meet criteria for IV thrombolysis, clinical trial evidence shows benefit of this treatment in all subtypes of ischemic stroke.
- Several newer thrombolytic agents and other reperfusion techniques are being studied.

Most strokes (approximately 80%) are ischemic and involve occlusion of blood vessels delivering essential nutrients and oxygen to the brain. As recently as less than 10 years ago, management of acute ischemic stroke consisted of diagnosis, medical support, and rehabilitation after the acute event. There are now interventions for acute revascularization, either pharmacological or mechanical, that allow blood flow to be restored promptly to the ischemic brain tissue. New strategies are also being employed based on developing pathophysiological models of stroke that emphasize the importance of factors such as glycemic control, blood viscosity, temperature, and blood pressure modulation (1-4). These developments have led to the formation of acute stroke teams and specialized intensive care settings that rapidly address the many factors that may affect stroke outcome.

Mechanism of Action of Thrombolytic Agents

Conversion of plasminogen to plasmin leads to fibrinolysis and destruction of clot. This theoretically results in revascularization of a previously occluded blood vessel and reversal of brain ischemia.

Recommendations for Clinical Practice

Thrombolytic medications in acute stroke became a significant part of stroke treatment after the publication of the National Institute of Neurological Disorders and Stroke t-PA Stroke Study Group trial (NINDS) in 1995. The use of thrombolytics like rt-PA can significantly affect the neurological status of patients, usually for the better but occasionally for the worst. Like all interventions there are risks to thrombolytic interventions in stroke. The risks are higher when used in stroke than with thrombolysis of myocardial infarcts. The most significant benefits are seen in the NINDS study, where patients were found to be 30% more likely to have little or no deficits at 3 months. There was little statistically significant benefit seen in the first 24 hours. We do know that hemorrhagic complications with rt-PA use in acute stroke occurred in 6% of patients and that of those many had worse outcomes, including death. Because of these results, care should be taken in administration of these medications. Close attention should be paid to the exclusion criteria (Table 7-1) and to the severity of the stroke best quickly evaluated through the NIH stroke scale (Table 7-2).

When a patient is evaluated for any of the thrombolytic therapies, it is vital to evaluate the patient as soon as practicable. The "Time is Brain" adage is a common expression in vascular neurology. In the acute setting, the patient should receive as quickly as possible:

1. Triage to major room
2. Airway, breathing, circulation, and fingerstick (hypoglycemia can imitate any neurological lesion)
3. Head CT scan to rule out hemorrhage and to look for early signs of infarct
4. Blood test: complete blood count, complete metabolic panel, and coagulation profile to rule out thrombocytopenia, liver failure, and recent use of anticoagulants
5. EKG
6. Evaluation of blood pressure with control using labetalol or nicardipine if systolic blood pressure is 185 or greater
7. Neurological evaluation that includes:

Table 7-1   Indications and Contraindications for Thrombolytic Management in
            Acute Stroke

Indications

1. Patient is aged 18 years or older

2. Clinical diagnosis of ischemic stroke causing a measurable neurological deficit

3. Onset of stroke symptoms well established to be less than 180 minutes (3 hours)
   before treatment would begin

Contraindications

1. Minor or rapidly resolving stroke symptoms

2. Other stroke or serious head trauma within past 3 months

3. Major surgery within 14 days

4. Known history of intracranial hemorrhage

5. Sustained systolic blood pressure >185 mm Hg or diastolic blood pressure >110 mm
   Hg at the time treatment is to begin, or patient requires aggressive blood pressure
   treatment

6. Symptoms suggestive of subarachnoid hemorrhage

7. Gastrointestinal or urinary tract hemorrhage within past 21 days

8. Arterial puncture at a noncompressible site within past 7 days

9. Patient received heparin within the last 48 hours and has an elevated PTT

10. Platelet count is <100,000 µL

Relative Contraindications

1. Seizure at the onset of stroke

2. Serum glucose <50 mg/dL or >400 mg/dL

3. Hemorrhagic eye disorder

4. Myocardial infarction in the past 6 weeks

5. Suspected septic embolism

6. Infective endocarditis

7. International Normalized Ratio (INR) > 1.7

- Time of onset (time the patient was last seen as normal, not
  the time family thinks stroke occurred)
- NIH stroke scale
- Past medical history including warfarin or heparin use and
  assessment for history of complicated migraines or seizures at
  onset

The most important exclusion criterion is not cited anywhere but is
vital: "if the history or etiology is unclear." Strokes are usually clear in onset,
presentation, and examination. It is better to withhold rt-PA in cases where
the history or time of onset is unclear than to risk poor outcome from hemorrhagic complications. Also, rt-PA requires cooperation from multiple
fields of medicine, nursing, emergency department, and radiology. If the

Table 7-2 Summary of the National Institutes of Health Stroke Score (NIHSS)*

1. Level of Consciousness
    - Alertness (0-3)
    - Orientation (0-2)
    - Ability to follow commands (0-2)

2. Gaze
    - Normal eye movements (0), gaze palsy (1), or forced eye deviation (2)

3. Vision
    - Normal vision (0), partial hemianopsia (1), complete hemianopsia (2), or blindness (3)

4. Facial Palsy
    - Symmetric face (0), mild paralysis (1), partial paralysis (2), or complete paralysis (3)

5. Motor Strength (Arms and Legs)
    - *Separate score for each limb:* No drift (can hold limb up for 10 seconds) (0), drift present (1), some effort against gravity (2), no effort against gravity (3), or no detectable movement (4)

6. Limb Ataxia
    - Only scored if out of proportion to weakness: Absent (0), present in one limb (1), or present in two limbs (2)

7. Sensory Loss
    - Measured to pin-prick/noxious stimuli: present (0), mild-to-moderate loss (1), or severe-to-total loss (2)

8. Best Language
    - The patient is shown a picture and asked to describe the events, shown objects to name, and asked to read sentences; this procedure tests for both expressive and receptive aphasia and also allows testing for dysarthria (discussed below): No aphasia (0), mild-to-moderate aphasia (1), severe aphasia (2), or global aphasia/mute (3)

9. Dysarthria
    - Normal speech (0), mild-to-moderate slurred speech (1), severe, unintelligible slurred speech (2)

10. Extinction and Inattention
    - No neglect (0), neglects visual, tactile, auditory, spatial stimuli, or self (1), has profound hemi-inattention/does not recognize own body part (2)

---

* Scores for each measure are ranked from normal (no deficits) (0) to maximal dysfunction (2, 3, or 4). Minimum score = 0; maximum score (maximal disability, i.e., coma) = 42. In general, minimal disability is reflected by a NIHSS of < 4, and severe disability is reflected by a NIHSS of > 20. (Adapted from Brott T, Adams HP, Linger CP, et al. Measurements of acute cerebral infarction: a clinical examination scale. Stroke. 1989;20:864-70.)

protocols and parameters are not in place to properly administer the medication, it can be more risky than not giving the medication at all.

Rt-PA is administered at 0.9 mg/kg dose with a maximum dose of 90 mg intravenously. Ten percent is given over 1 minute and the rest of the weight-based dose is given over 60 minutes. After rt-PA is administered, the blood pressure must be kept within the above parameters and the patient should be admitted to an intensive care unit for 24 hours at least. Arterial sticks, NG tubes, Foley catheter, and central lines should be avoided for 24 hours after thrombolytics are given.

The neurological examination should be monitored every hour. Worsening of NIH scale of 2 points or greater, decrease in consciousness, or worsening of strength or language should trigger a head CT scan quickly to rule out intracerebral hemorrhage. Hemorrhages can be seen extra-cerebrally also with bleeding into the retroperitoneal area, from the gums, into the pericardium, and brisk GI/GU bleeding. More disheartening is the patient who improves quickly, then worsens without intracerebral hemorrhage on CT scan. This usually suggests reocclusion of a recannulated artery, although hypotension, hypoglycemia, or acute anemia secondary to extracerebral hemorrhages can also be the cause. Many of the other thrombolytic medications have similar protocols.

It is important to remember that the reason the NINDS trial for the use of rt-PA was a positive trial when all others had shown no benefit before is because of its strict exclusion criteria and the rapid evaluation and administration of the drug. Protocol violations and slow time to medication delivery are important causes of poor outcomes.

Trials Evaluating Use of Thrombolytic Agents

Currently IV tissue plasminogen activator (t-PA) is the only treatment available for use in acute stroke. The seven major trials evaluating the use of thrombolytic agents in the treatment of acute ischemic stroke (Table 7-3) are discussed in this section (5-11).

Intravenous Streptokinase Trials

Intravenous (IV) thrombolytic trials have primarily used tissue plasminogen activator (t-PA). However, several of the early trials investigated the use of streptokinase. The major trials investigating streptokinase include the Multicenter Acute Stroke Trials–Italy Group (MAST-I) (5) and Europe Study Group (MAST-E) (6) and the Australian Streptokinase Trial Study Group (7). These trials used 1.5 μU of streptokinase up to 6 hours after onset of symptoms. In all three trials, there was a significant increase in the rate of symptomatic intracranial hemorrhage (ICH) and no improvement in functional outcome. In fact, all three studies were terminated early due to increased

Table 7-3 Summary of IV Thrombolytic Trials

Trial	Drug	Dose	Interval (hours)	Symptomatic ICH		Primary Outcome
				Treated	*Control*	
MAST-I, 1995 (5)	Streptokinase	1.5 µU	0-6	16%	2.6%	No difference between groups
MAST-E, 1996 (6)	Streptokinase	1.5 µU	0-6	21.2%	4.6%	No difference between groups
ASK, 1996 (7)	Streptokinase	1.5 µU	0-4	12.6%	2.4%	No difference between groups
ECASS, 1995 (8)	t-PA	1.1 mg/kg	0-6	19.8%	6.5%	No difference between groups in BI and mRS scores at 90 days
NINDS, 1995 (9)	t-PA	0.9 mg/kg	0-3	6.4%	0.6%	No difference between groups at 24 hours; significant improvement in functional status at 90 days in treated group (global odds ratio for favorable outcome, 1.7 [95% CI, 1.2-2.6])
ECASS II, 1998 (10)	t-PA	0.9 mg/kg	0-6	8.8%	3.4%	No difference between groups
ATLANTIS, 1999 (11)	t-PA	0.9 mg/kg	3-5	7.0%	1.1%	No difference between groups

mortality. It is not clear if the morbidity and mortality observed with streptokinase in these trials was due to the time interval to treatment (up to 6 hours after symptom onset), the dose of drug, or the agent itself. Nonetheless, based on these studies, streptokinase is not used clinically to treat acute ischemic stroke.

Intravenous Tissue Plasminogen Activator Trials

The Food and Drug Administration (FDA) approval of t-PA in 1996 for thrombolytic therapy for acute stroke in the United States is based on the NINDS trials (9). These trials were done in two parts and utilized t-PA at 0.9 mg/kg given within 3 hours of symptom onset. Exclusion criteria included recent surgery, history of intracerebral hemorrhage, blood pressure greater than 185/110, and glucose less than 50 mg/dL. There were no exclusions for age or ischemic changes on CT.

The first part of the trial evaluated clinical response to t-PA at 24 hours after onset of stroke. The primary outcome measure was complete resolution of symptoms or a four-point improvement on the National Institute of Health Stroke Scale (NIHSS) score. No statistically significant difference between the treatment and control groups was seen in part one, although there was a trend in favor of t-PA. Part two of the trial evaluated for continued benefit of t-PA at 90 days follow-up. A combined score on four outcome measures determined benefit: the Barthel index (BI), modified Rankin scale (mRS), NIHSS score, and Glasgow outcome scale. This is where the major benefit of t-PA was seen, as up to 53% of t-PA patients had minimal or no disability at 3 months compared with 38% of controls. The rate of symptomatic ICH was lower than what had been reported in previous trials, at 6.4% in the t-PA treated group and 0.6% in controls. There was no difference in mortality between the t-PA and control groups at 90 days (17% t-PA group, 21% placebo group).

Subsequent analysis of the NINDS trial data has shown that the benefit of t-PA was independent of severity of initial neurological deficit, age, gender, or the presumed stroke subtype. Patients with high NIHSS scores, advanced age, thrombus on early CT imaging, diabetes, and elevated admission blood pressure did less well than patients without these factors in both the control and the t-PA–treated groups (12). However, patients with these unfavorable characteristics still had benefit from t-PA; hence these factors should not be used to exclude patients from consideration of IV t-PA (13).

The NINDS trial was the first and only major trial to demonstrate clear benefit of t-PA in acute ischemic stroke. However, several other trials investigated t-PA in stroke, including two double-blind randomized trials, the European Cooperative Acute Stroke Studies (ECASS I and II) (8,10). Patients received 1.1 mg/kg (ECASS-I) or 0.9 mg/kg (ECASS-II) t-PA within 6 hours of symptom onset. While not a contraindication in the NINDS trial, exclusion criteria included infarcts involving >33% of the middle cerebral artery (MCA) territory on CT imaging because these have been associated with an increased risk of hemorrhage when t-PA is given. There was a significant increase in symptomatic ICH in the t-PA–treated group (19.8%) versus controls (6.5%) and a related increase in 30-day mortality in the t-PA–treated group in ECASS-I. However, a high percentage of protocol violations (17%) makes the results difficult to interpret. Utilizing a lower dose of t-PA (0.9 mg/kg), as well as more stringent adherence to protocol and rigid blood pressure control, the rate of symptomatic ICH in ECASS-II was reduced from that in ECASS I (8.8% t-PA–treated group versus 3.4% control group). Neither of the European studies demonstrated differences in functional outcome.

Based on the positive results of the NINDS trial, investigators have attempted to increase the time window in which patients can be treated.

Less than 5% of patients who currently have acute strokes are eligible for t-PA, and the majority are excluded for being outside the 180-minute time window. The Alteplase Thrombolysis for Acute Noninterventional Therapy in Ischemic Stroke trial (ATLANTIS) investigated extending the treatment interval for t-Pa by giving 0.9 mg/kg t-Pa within 3-5 hours of symptom onset (11). Despite rigid exclusion criteria, the mortality was increased in the t-Pa group (11% versus 6.9% in controls). The rate of symptomatic ICH was similarly higher in the t-Pa group than for controls (7% versus 1.1%). Finally, there was no difference between groups in any of the functional outcome measures. The cumulative data from this trial and from the ECASS trials suggest that the use of t-PA beyond 3 hours of symptom onset increases the risk of morbidity and mortality without increased likelihood of improved functional outcome.

Phase IV Trials of Intravenous Tissue Plasminogen Activator in Acute Stroke

Evaluation of the clinical use of t-PA for acute ischemic stroke since its FDA approval in 1996 has shown that symptomatic ICH is overall approximately 6% but can be as high as 38% when NINDS guidelines are violated (14-17). It remains unclear if this increased rate of ICH is related to violation of the time restriction or to other common infringements such as the use of warfarin or antiplatelet agents and violation of blood pressure restrictions in the peri-thrombolysis period. Several phase IV trials have demonstrated outcomes in both the rate of ICH and functional measures in patients treated with t-PA in clinical settings that are similar to those seen in the NINDS trial when guidelines are followed. For example, using data collected from a university hospital and two community hospitals in the year after the aforementioned FDA approval, Chiu et al found a rate of symptomatic ICH of 7% and a 90-day mortality rate of 20% in t-PA–treated patients. Moreover, they found that 37% of patients recovered to fully independent function (BI 100) and 30% had no disability (mRS = 0 to 1) (18). These results are remarkably similar to the results of the NINDS trial.

The Standard Treatment with Alteplase to Reverse Stroke (STARS) study is the largest prospective, multicenter, open-label study of t-PA in acute ischemic stroke patients (19). This was conducted across 57 medical centers (both academic and community-based). The rate of symptomatic ICH was 3.3% and the 30-day mortality rate was 13%. Thirty-five percent of patients had excellent outcomes (mRS = 0 to 1), and 43% were functionally independent (mRS = 0-2). These positive results were achieved despite protocol violations in 32.6% of patients. This finding emphasizes that it is unlikely all forms of protocol violation result in similar morbidity and mortality; however, it remains unclear which violations are most likely to result in poor outcome.

What is clear is that when the NINDS protocol is violated, the rates of symptomatic ICH rise considerably (15,16,20). Tanne et al reported a 6% rate of ICH overall, with rates of 11% in the patients who had violations of the NINDS trial guidelines and 4% in patients in whom protocol was observed (20). Katzan et al evaluated the use of t-PA across 29 hospitals in the Cleveland area and found a protocol violation rate of 50%. This was associated with a rate of 15.7% symptomatic ICH (15). After institution of a stroke quality-improvement program, there was a decrease in protocol violations to 19.1%. This was associated with a related drop in symptomatic ICH to 6.4% (16). More recently, Lopez-Yunez et al reviewed medical records of patients treated with t-PA in ten acute care hospitals in Indianapolis from July 1996 to February 1998 (17). Unlike the previous phase IV trials, t-PA was predominantly administered by non-stroke specialists in community hospitals. They found a rate of symptomatic ICH of 38% in patients who had protocol violations and of 5% in whom the NINDS protocol was followed.

These studies confirm that it is safe and feasible to administer t-PA in a variety of clinical settings as long as the NINDS guidelines are strictly followed (see Table 7-1). As physicians become more comfortable with the administration of lytics, protocol violations and complication rates will continue to decline. Web-based training and tutorial programs are available for physicians who may be the first to see stroke patients if no neurologist is available. The Brain Attack Coalition (www.stroke-site.org), the American Heart Association (strokeassociation.org), and the National Stroke Administration (www.stroke.org) are valuable resources for physicians, all offering copies of exclusions, dosing, and stroke scale scores. The National Institute of Neurological Disorders and Stroke (NINDS; www.NINDS.nih.gov) provides information about NIH-sponsored trials and access to stroke scales.

Desmoteplase Thrombolytic Trial

Desmoteplase is a highly fibrin-specific compound found in vampire bat saliva. The bat uses this and other substances to reduce clotting during feeding. Because of the high degree of fibrin-specific compound, it was felt to be more specific for acute thrombus and safer in acute stroke past the 3-hour window. The Desmoteplase in Acute Ischemic Stroke trial (DIAS) study was a dose-finding randomized trial designed to evaluate the safety and efficacy of intravenous desmoteplase administered within 3-9 hours of ischemic stroke. Patients were screened using MRI diffusion and perfusion imaging to determine whether there was viable tissue to salvage and to assess arterial occlusion, stenosis, and reocclusion rates.

The DIAS study had two parts. Part I assigned the first 47 patients to desmoteplase (25, 37.5, or 50 mg) or placebo. This arm of the trial showed significantly higher symptomatic hemorrhage rate, with 7 deaths, all occurring in the treatment group. Part II was conducted when it became clear that the hemorrhage rate with higher-dose medication in the treatment arm was leading to a worse outcome. A lower-dose, weight-based algorithm was used whereby patients were given 62.5, 90, or 125 µg/kg versus placebo; 57 patients were enrolled. There was only one symptomatic hemorrhage in the treatment arm after dose adjustment. The study defined a favorable outcome defined as low NIH, Rankin, and Barthel scores at 90 days much like the NINDS trial. The lower-dose trial had much better results. Favorable outcomes were seen in 22% of placebo patients at 90 days versus 13%-60% of desmoteplase-treated patients. Greater benefits were seen at the higher doses, with 125 µg/kg dose having 60% ($P = 0.0090$) favorable outcomes. The DIAS study also showed that patients who had early reperfusion of occluded or stenotic arteries were more likely to have good outcomes (52%) than those who did not (27%) ($P = 0.0028$). Additionally, patients receiving placebo were less likely to have early reperfusion. There was 71% versus 19% ($P = 0.0012$) reperfusion in the desmoteplase-treated group versus placebo (21).

A phase III trial using the lower-dose medication is presently recruiting. Expanding the thrombolysis window using highly fibrin-specific thrombolytic medications such as desmoteplase or tenecteplase, which should have lower hemorrhage rates and improved outcomes from acute stroke patients, is exciting and could potentially affect stroke treatment more than t-Pa.

Intra-Arterial Thrombolysis

The use of intra-arterial (IA) thrombolysis has become increasingly common, especially in large hospitals with the capacity to perform emergent angiogiography. This is largely due to the observation that large clots in major intracranial vessels such as the MCA, internal carotid artery (ICA), or basilar artery are less likely to have a therapeutic response to IV thrombolysis. Theoretically, administering thrombolytic agents directly to the area of clot may increase efficacy and reduce the risk of bleeding.

There have been few prospective, randomized, placebo-controlled trials of IA thrombolysis for acute stroke. Hence, there are no guidelines for the use of IA thrombolytics and there is no FDA-approved IA drug. Currently, IA thrombolysis is administered in situations deemed appropriate by experienced stroke specialists and interventional neuroradiologists. Although widely variable, indication for use includes proven large vessel occlusion in a patient that does not meet criteria for, or has failed IV thrombolysis.

The Prolyse in Acute Cerebral Thromboembolism trials (PROACT I and II) were the first large trials to investigate the efficacy and safety of IA thrombolysis with prourokinase (pro-UK) (22,23). In PROACT I, 26 patients with angiographically proven MCA occlusion received 6 mg/kg of IA pro-UK at the site of occlusion. All patients (control and pro-UK groups) also received either high (100 U/kg bolus followed by 1000 U/hr continuous infusion) or low (2000 U bolus followed by 500 U/hr continuous infusion) dose IV heparin. Recanalization occurred in 58% of the pro-UK patients and 0% of control patients. Symptomatic ICH occurred in 15% of IA patients and 7% of controls. There was no difference between groups in 90-day mortality. Although there was no significant difference between groups in functional outcome, there was a trend toward improved outcome at 90 days in the IA group.

In PROACT II, the investigators evaluated 9 mg of IA pro-UK plus low-dose heparin or low-dose heparin only in 180 patients with angiographically proven MCA occlusion. Again, there was no difference between groups in mortality, but there was an increased rate of symptomatic ICH in the heparin/pro-UK group (10%) versus heparin alone (2%). Recanalization occurred in 66% of pro-UK patients and 18% of controls. Importantly, outcome measures showed 40% of pro-UK patients had mild or no disability at 90 days (mRS < 2) compared with 25% of controls.

Subsequent studies using IA urokinase have found similar rates of symptomatic ICH (5%-17%), mortality (23%-38%), and improved functional outcome at 90 days (48%-60%) (24-26). As might be expected, the rate of recanalization is correlated with improved functional outcome in most IA thrombolysis series. However, it is important to note that angiography was not routinely performed either before or after therapy in the IV thrombolysis trials. Hence, the efficacy of IA and IV thrombolysis for recanalization cannot be compared. Cumulatively, studies suggest IA thrombolysis is an effective and relatively safe therapy, especially in patients with large vessel occlusions who are otherwise expected to have poor recanalization with IV thrombolysis. However, the majority of IA studies are small, retrospective reviews, which cannot be accurately compared with the phase II IV t-PA trials.

At this time, IA thrombolysis is limited to stroke centers with acute neurological and vascular interventional capabilities. If the decision is made to proceed with IA thrombolysis, the risks and benefits of the procedure, including the increased risk of ICH and worsening of outcome, must be frankly discussed with family members. Certainly, large hemispheric strokes with high stroke scales (NIHSS >16) should be evaluated for IA thrombolysis because the outcome is poor with no intervention. In general, CT scan is used to eliminate the possibility of hemorrhage. Patients with early ischemic changes are believed to be at higher risk for ICH with IA thrombolytic therapy. Although CT scan may not show ischemic strokes for 6-24 hours, there are some early CT findings that may be helpful (discussed later in this chapter). Patients with early ischemic changes are believed to be at higher risk of ICH with IA thrombolytic therapy. MRI is often useful in distinguishing patients who may benefit from acute treatment. If the patient has a high NIHSS (a clinically large stroke), a small diffusion lesion (implying a small area of irreversibly infarcted brain), and a large area of brain that is underperfused on perfusion imaging (tissue at risk or ischemic "penumbra"), restoration of blood flow may salvage underperfused tissue (Figure 7-1).

Combined Intra-Arterial and Intravenous Thrombolysis

One major limitation of IA therapy is the delay to treatment. Significant logistical arrangements must be made in order to initiate angiography and administer IA thrombolytics. There is additional delay from the initiation of angiography to the time of thrombolysis due to technical constraints such as tortuous and anomalous arterial anatomy. Hence, there have been several recent trials evaluating the use of IV followed by IA thrombolysis. Theoretically, this minimizes the time to treatment (with IV therapy) and maximizes the specificity of therapy and likelihood of recanalization (with IA therapy).

The Emergency Management of Stroke (EMS) bridging trial was a double-blind, prospective, randomized trial investigating IV t-PA plus IA t-PA versus placebo plus IA t-PA in acute stroke (27). Therapy with IV t-PA or placebo was given within 3 hours of symptom onset. Patients were then taken to angiography and given IA t-PA if a clot was identified. Full recanalization

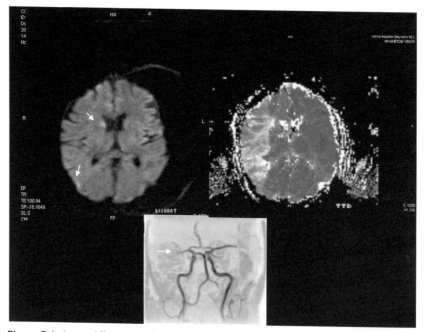

Figure 7-1 Acute diffusion, perfusion and MRA in patient with the clinical presentation of a large right MCA stroke. Diffusion imaging at 3 hours after symptom onset demonstrates two small diffusion bright lesions (*arrows*) in the right MCA distribution. Perfusion imaging demonstrates a large area of under perfusion in the entire right MCA territory. MRA demonstrates a loss of signal in the MCA (*arrow*).

was more likely in the IV/IA group (54%) than in the placebo/IA group (10%); however, this did not result in a difference in functional outcomes between the groups. There was no significant difference in the rate of symptomatic ICH (11.8% IV/IA and 5.5% placebo/IA patients). Mortality was significantly greater in IV/IA patients (45%) than in placebo/IA patients (10%), but the EMS authors felt that the increased mortality in the IV/IA group was related to adverse events not related to the study therapy.

Subsequent IV/IA trials have had variable results largely due to significant differences in study design. Ernst et al found low rates of symptomatic ICH (6.3%) and mortality (12.5%) in patients treated with IV t-PA within 3 hours of symptom onset followed by IA t-PA (28). Functional outcome was excellent in 44% of patients and good in 19% of patients. Of note, this was a retrospective, non-blinded review and patients routinely underwent clot disruption with the microcatheter in addition to local administration of IA t-PA.

Overall, use of IA thrombolysis remains rare due to several limitations. As discussed above, the most significant of these is the delay between symptom onset and initiation of treatment, and the subsequent delay between initiation of treatment and recanalization. The faster reperfusion is achieved, the better the clinical result; significant delays caused by technical difficulties and logistics hamper outcome. Conversely, because IA thrombolytic trials have shown benefit up to 6 hours after symptom onset, it may be that IA thrombolysis will be proved a safe alternative in select patients that present outside the 3-hour limit for IV t-PA. Moreover, IA thrombolysis may be the optimal therapy for patients with proven vessel occlusion who fail to respond to IV t-PA (29).

Mechanical Clot Disruption (Angioplasty)

Like IA thrombolysis, mechanical clot disruption (angioplasty) is based on the idea that large clots in the major intracranial vessels may not respond to standard doses of thrombolytic agents or may be composed of materials (e.g., cholesterol) that are resistant to pharmacologic thrombolysis. In addition, many large lesions are prone to re-occlusion after canalization.

Recent studies have investigated the safety and efficacy of mechanical disruption either alone or in conjunction with pharmacologic thrombolysis. These studies suggest that in cases involving large emboli or high-grade stenosis it may be preferable to initiate treatment with angioplasty rather than expose patients to high doses of thrombolytics that are given over several hours in order to achieve recanalization (30,31).

Nakaono et al initially demonstrated successful recanalization with percutaneous angioplasty (PTA) in 8/10 patients with MCA occlusion (30). The investigators then compared PTA with IA thrombolysis alone in patients with acute MCA trunk occlusion. Thirty-six patients were treated with IA thrombolytic therapy alone (control group) and 34 patients underwent PTA (subsequent thrombolytic therapy was given in 21 cases for distal embolism or remaining thrombus). Patients were selected for PTA based on the presence of early ischemic changes on CT or involvement of the lenticulostriate arteries because these patients were thought to have a higher risk of ICH with IA thrombolytic therapy. The rate of recanalization was significantly higher in the PTA group, 91.2% versus 63.9% in controls, and the incidence of symptomatic intracranial hemorrhage was reduced in the PTA group (2.9% versus 19.4% controls). Despite these positive results, there was no significant difference between groups in favorable outcome (mRS = 0-1); however, the 73.5% of PTA patients scored in the independent range (mRS < 2) versus 50% of the control group (31). Recent studies have supported these findings, with low rates of ICH or systemic bleeding, high rates of recanalization, and significant improvement in neurological function with combined angioplasty and thrombolysis (32,33).

Guided clot removal devices such as the MERCI (Mechanical Embolus Removal in Cerebral Ischemia) device are also under active study. A phase I study of the MERCI device showed that a clot retrieval device alone can remove clot in 43% of studied patients without additional thombolytic drugs. The recanalization rate appears higher than with thrombolysis alone, and the rate of symptomatic intracranial hemorrhage was low, occurring in none of the 30 patients studied even when combined with thrombolytic medications up to 8 hours after onset of stroke (34). However, this approach remains limited to specialized tertiary care centers and can be associated with complications such as distal emboli, residual vessel stenosis, vessel reocclusion, and traumatic injury to delicate intracranial vessels.

Basilar Artery Occlusion

One particularly troubling cause of acute stroke is vertebrobasilar artery occlusion. Interruption of the basilar artery results in brainstem ischemia and infarction that can be rapidly deadly or severely disabling (Figure 7-2). There is often a delay in diagnosis because patients present with loss of consciousness and other non-specific signs that do not immediately indicate acute stroke. Also, lesions of this vessel tend to be resistant to IV thrombolysis. Hence, IA thrombolysis has been increasingly common in acute basilar artery occlusion. In addition, because the natural history of basilar artery ischemic strokes is uniformly poor and onset of symptoms is often protracted, the treatment window for administration of IA thrombolytics may be extended to 24-72 hours after symptom onset or longer in select palliative cases.

There are no randomized, controlled trials investigating treatment options for acute basilar artery occlusion, but there have been several small series and case reports regarding the use of IA thrombolysis and angioplasty (35-37). In one of the earliest and largest series, Hacke et al evaluated 65 patients with brainstem ischemia treated with either IA thrombolysis

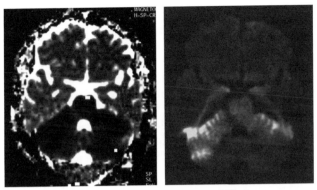

ADC   Diffusion

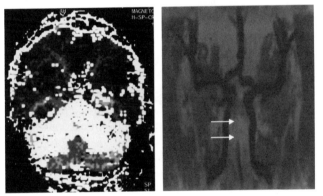

Perfusion   MRA with occluded basilar

Figure 7-2 Basilar infarction. ADC mapping and diffusion imaging show severe damage in the cerebellar hemispheres bilaterally consistent with acute basilar artery infarction. Perfusion mapping shows that the entire cerebellar hemisphere and brainstem have significantly reduced perfusion, and MRA shows loss of signal in the basilar artery (*arrows*).

or conventional antiplatelet/anticoagulation therapy. Mortality in the conventional treatment group was 86% compared with 67% in the IA thrombolysis group. Survival was correlated with the ability to recanulate the occluded vessel such that 74% of the patients in whom recanalization was achieved survived and 53% had a good clinical outcome (35).

Several studies have shown that failure to recanulate an occluded basilar artery is associated with 92%-100% mortality (38,39). Rates of recanalization with IA thrombolysis alone range between 51% and 78% (26,38,39). Because recanalization is a requirement for survival and the rates of recanalization with thrombolysis alone have been disappointing, there has been increasing interest in angioplasty or stenting of the vertrobasilar arteries. Although promising, there are significant complications from intracranial angioplasty or stenting, including arterial dissection, distal embolization, cerebral hyperperfusion leading to intracranial hemorrhage, ipsilateral hemispheric edema, and neurological deficits. Data on the safety and efficacy of basilar artery angioplasty/stenting currently remain limited to case reports.

Case Studies 7-1 (left MCA stroke, t-PA contraindicated) and 7-2 (right MCA stroke, t-PA indicated) highlight some of the major issues in thrombolytic therapy as it is currently utilized in the majority of centers (IV administration of t-PA within 3 hours of symptom onset). IA therapy as well as clot retrieval and angioplasty are still of limited use in acute stroke outside of academic stroke centers, and none are currently FDA approved. At this time, data on the possible benefit of these more aggressive therapies are limited, although interventional removal of clot has theoretical appeal. In certain situations, such as complete basilar occlusion or large hemispheric strokes with minimal damage seen on diffusion-weighted MRI, aggressive treatment is warranted if available.

Conclusion

Acute ischemic stroke is one of the leading causes of morbidity and mortality in the United States. However, newer therapies, from the established (IV thrombolysis) to the still-developing (IA thrombolysis, angioplasty, intra-arterial stenting), are promising when used in appropriate situations. All these interventions are designed to restore blood flow to ischemic brain tissue as quickly as possible. As imaging techniques become more sophisticated and more widely available and as data regarding IV t-PA, IA t-PA and mechanical clot disruption accumulate, it will become increasingly possible to identify the specific subgroups of patients who are most likely to benefit from each of these therapies with the least risk for untoward events.

Regardless of the treatment modality selected, the most important steps in the management of acute ischemic stroke remain: 1) patient education for recognition of symptoms, 2) rapid referral to an acute care center at the time of symptom onset, and 3) rapid diagnosis and evaluation by a physician experienced in acute stroke management. The importance of the rapid evaluation and treatment of acute stroke cannot be overemphasized. Once these steps are taken, options for acute intervention can be initiated and, potentially, the cascade of devastating events related to brain ischemia can be interrupted.

Case Study 7-1

Mr P is a 68-year-old white man with a history of hypertension, adult-onset diabetes mellitus, congestive heart failure, and atrial fibrillation for which he is treated with warfarin. He had been in his normal state of heath until the morning of presentation. The patient's wife reports that she woke up early and began working in the kitchen. She thought she heard Mr P get out of bed at about 8 A.M., but she wasn't certain. She returned to the bedroom at 9:30 A.M. and found her husband sitting on the side of the bed unable to speak or move his right arm. With her son's help, she was able to get Mr P out of bed to a chair. She called his primary care doctor, left a message with the emergency service, and attempted to give Mr P his morning blood pressure pills. When the physician called back, he told the wife and son to take Mr P to the emergency room immediately. After a struggle, they were able to get him into the car and to the hospital. The patient was triaged and evaluated by the emergency room staff; the neurologist on call was paged 15 minutes after his arrival. The neurologist ordered the labs and tests she wanted over the telephone and made her way to the emergency room. She examined the patient approximately 30 minutes after his arrival to the emergency department (labs and the head CT were not yet available).

The patient was taken for emergency head CT approximately 45 minutes after arrival. It showed loss of gray-white differentiation in the entire left MCA territory, with mild mass effect on the lateral ventricles (Figure 7-3). The patient continued to have deficits primarily manifest by sleepiness, right facial droop, right arm more than right leg weakness, sensory loss, severe expressive aphasia, difficulty following one-step commands, and left gaze preference. NIH stroke scale score was 18. Laboratory values showed a normal glucose, electrolyte panel, and complete blood count, but an elevated INR at 1.8.

The neurologist confirmed that the last time anyone *saw* the patient at his baseline state was the night before presentation. Additional history was taken; his wife reported that Mr P had had a lumbar laminectomy 2 weeks ago for chronic back pain but no other

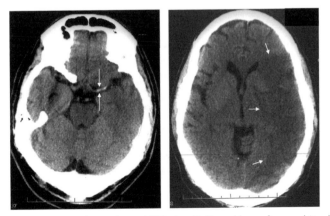

Figure 7-3 CT showing a hyperdense MCA sign (*left*), and loss of gray-white differentiation in the entire left MCA territory with mild mass effect on the lateral ventricles (*right*).

recent surgeries or procedures. He had no history of seizures, intracranial hemorrhage, or previous strokes, although the wife did recall an episode one week ago when the patient had transient difficulty speaking. No intervention was sought at that time. She also reported that he had been having difficulty controlling his blood pressure and, indeed, his blood pressure was 194/100 at the time of the neurologist's evaluation despite two doses of IV labetalol. His general exam was notable only for obesity, an irregular heartbeat, and evidence of chronic vascular changes.

The patient's family had been advised about the possible role of a "clot-buster" to "reverse the symptoms" of his stroke when they arrived at the emergency room. Now they ask you if the patient should receive this therapy.

Discussion

1. *Establishing a diagnosis.* This patient has clear risk factors for stroke, including poorly controlled hypertension, diabetes, and atrial fibrillation with a sub-therapeutic INR. In addition, his signs/symptoms are appropriate for a single vascular territory (left middle cerebral artery), and the onset/time course is consistent with a vascular event. The patient had what was likely a transient ischemic attack a week before this presentation. Hence, stroke is the most likely etiology.

2. *Time of onset.* There is no clear time of onset. The patient was last seen at his baseline the night before presentation. That Mrs P thought she *may* have heard Mr P get out of bed at 8 A.M. cannot be used to establish time of onset. There is no way to know when the event occurred between when the patient went to bed and when he was found with deficits at 9:30 A.M. The time of onset for consideration of giving t-PA must be the definitive time the patient was last seen at baseline.

3. *Emergency intervention.* The patient and his wife failed to recognize signs of a TIA the week before presentation and thus called their primary doctor as their initial intervention during the current acute episode. Patients should be counseled to immediately call 911 when they develop any acute, focal weakness, sensory changes, and difficulty with walking or speech problems. They should not drive themselves or be driven by family to the hospital because, in addition to this being unsafe, it prolongs the triage process once they arrive in the emergency department.

4. *Emergency evaluation.* Ideally the emergency room personnel will be alerted of a possible stroke patient by emergency medical services and subsequently notify the stroke team. The time from arrival to head CT should be approximately 30 minutes. Basic labs such

as a complete blood count, coagulation studies, and an electrolyte panel should be drawn immediately on arrival and sent "Stat." Initial history, including time of onset and any contraindications, should be obtained urgently.

5. *Definite contraindications.* Mr P has several contraindications to IV t-PA (see Table 7-1). He has difficult-to-control blood pressure that has not yet been brought to below the required systolic pressure of 185 mm Hg despite IV medication. In addition, he had had a lumbar laminectomy 2 weeks before presentation. Major surgery within the past 14 days is a contraindication to IV thrombolysis.

6. *Relative contraindications.* In this case, the patient has an INR that is higher than approved for t-PA (yet not high enough to be therapeutic for atrial fibrillation). An INR > 1.7 is a relative contraindication.

7. *Changes on head CT.* The patient's symptoms and the changes on head CT suggest a large territory stroke. Although involvement of greater than one third of the MCA territory was not exclusion criteria in the NINDS trials, it has been shown to be associated with an increased risk of hemorrhage when t-PA is given. In addition, the changes on CT suggest that this process is greater than 3 hours old and likely occurred at least 12 hours before evaluation. A subsequent diffusion-weighted MRI scan showed abnormality in most of the "at-risk" hemisphere, suggesting a completed infarct (Figure 7-4).

8. *Educating the family.* Although IV t-PA is the only therapy currently available for the treatment of acute stroke, its efficacy and safety are achieved only when strict inclusion and exclusion criteria are applied. Even when these criteria are used, risk remains for either

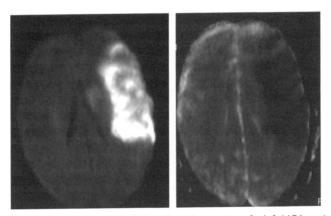

Figure 7-4 Diffusion-weighted MRI (*left*) and ADC mapping of a left MCA territory stroke (*right*).

intracranial or systemic hemorrhage, and there is no way to predict the degree of neurological improvement a patient will have with IV t-PA. Patients and families must be given realistic expectations about the treatment and be made aware of the possible complications. For all these reasons, Mr P is not a candidate for t-PA, and this should be explained to the family. However, it is appropriate for the patient to be treated at a stroke specialty center, where maximal supportive care can be offered.

Case Study 7-2

Mrs T is a 74-year-old African American woman with a history of diabetes and hypertension who was in her usual state of health until the morning of presentation. She lives with her granddaughter, who reports that the patient awoke at approximately 7 A.M. and came to the kitchen. She made her granddaughter breakfast, then sat and ate. They had a normal conversation, and the granddaughter did not note any abnormalities in Mrs T's behavior. At 7:45 by the kitchen clock, the granddaughter got ready to leave for work. Mrs T started to walk to the sink but fell to the floor. The granddaughter tried to pick her up, but Mrs T could not move her left side and was "dead weight." Mrs T was slurring her words but making sense. Her granddaughter called 911, and emergency medical services (EMS) arrived 10 minutes later. EMS notified the local stroke center of a possible acute stroke victim. Upon arrival at the emergency center, the granddaughter registered the patient while the latter was taken immediately to an acute care room. Vital signs were taken, labs were drawn, and she was taken to the CT scanner approximately 10 minutes after arrival.

The stroke pager was activated at the time of the patient's arrival to the emergency department. The neurologist on call arrived in the emergency center within 20 minutes of the patient's arrival. The granddaughter was interviewed while the patient was in the CT scanner, and acute onset of symptoms was confirmed to be between 7:45 and 7:50 A.M. She reported that Mrs T had no history of seizures, head trauma, previous strokes or transient ischemic attacks, or recent surgeries or procedures, or any known gastrointestinal or urinary tract hemorrhages. The head CT was reviewed by the neuroradiologist on call and the stroke team neurologist; it showed no acute changes.

On physical examination, the neurologist found elevated blood pressure of 170/78, pulse of 78, and pulse oximetry of 98% on room air. The patient's weight was 126 lb (57 kg). The patient was drowsy but communicative and could recall the events of the morning and confirm the time of onset of symptoms. Her NIH stroke score was 12.

Although she required verbal or gentle tactile stimulation, she was arousable and able to follow simple commands. She had moderate dysarthria and extinction to double simultaneous stimulation on the left with neglect as well as a mild right gaze preference. She also had a left facial droop and left hemiparesis. Her general exam was unremarkable. Laboratory values showed a normal glucose, normal electrolytes, normal platelets, and normal coagulation factors. At approximately 1 hour after symptom onset, the initial evaluation had been completed. The patient had stable deficits that were not improving, a normal head CT, no strong or relative contraindications to IV t-PA, and a clinical presentation consistent with stroke (acute onset of symptoms referable to the right MCA territory).

The granddaughter was confirmed as the patient's next-of-kin, and a discussion about IV t-PA was initiated with the patient and her. The purpose of IV t-PA therapy was explained. They were told that treatment with the drug increased the chance of minimal or no disability 3 months after stroke in about 10%-15% of patients and that, in some cases, patients saw immediate improvement in their symptoms. The deficits Mrs T would be expected to have from her stroke were explained, and alternative therapies such as hypertensive therapy and maximal supportive care were discussed. The patient and granddaughter were quoted a 6% risk for intracranial hemorrhage, with a 50% mortality rate for patients who develop hemorrhage. They were informed that Mrs T would require an ICU admission if given the drug.

The patient decided to undergo IV t-PA therapy. Informed consent was documented by the neurologist. At approximately 75 minutes after symptom onset, 5.3 mg of IV t-PA (10% of the total dose) was given as a bolus and 46 mg was given IV over 1 hour (for a total dose of 0.9 mg/kg or 51.3 mg). The patient's vital signs were monitored every 15 minutes, and she was transferred to the neurological critical care unit for further observation and management. Subsequent MRI scans (obtained approximately 10 hours after presentation) showed a small diffusion bright lesion in the right MCA distribution, indicating a small acute infarct (Figure 7-5).

Discussion

1. *Establishing a diagnosis.* Mrs T has risk factors for stroke, and her signs/symptoms are appropriate for a single vascular territory (right MCA). The clinical course is consistent with a vascular event, and there is no history of seizures or other paroxysmal events that may mimic stroke.

2. *Time of onset.* The patient had a witnessed change in her neurological status that was noted at a specific time. A witness corroborated the time of onset. The patient was within the 3-hour time constraint for IV t-PA.

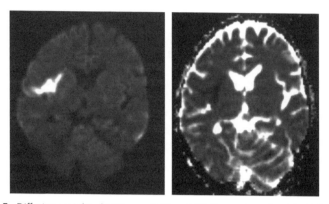

Figure 7-5 Diffusion-weighted MRI scan (*left*) and ADC mapping of a right MCA territory stroke (*right*).

3. *Emergency intervention.* The granddaughter immediately called 911, and Mrs T was taken urgently to a stroke center. In addition, there was communication between the EMS team and the emergency center staff about the arrival of a possible acute stroke victim, allowing an emergency stroke protocol to be activated.

4. *Emergency evaluation.* Due to early notification, the emergency room could clear the CT scanner and activate the stroke team in a timely fashion, ensuring that CT scan, laboratory testing, and neurological evaluation were initiated within 20-30 minutes of arrival to the emergency center.

5. *Contraindications.* The patient and her granddaughter were interviewed, and it was confirmed that the former had no definite or relative contraindications to IV t-PA.

6. *Changes on head CT.* As with most acute strokes, there were no clear changes on CT to suggest an ischemic lesion. However, an MRI obtained approximately 10 hours after presentation confirmed an acute MCA territory stroke.

7. *Educating the family.* Mrs T meets all the criteria for IV t-PA therapy and has no contraindications. Nonetheless, t-PA has known risks for intracranial and systemic bleeding, and these must be discussed with patients and their families. In addition, realistic expectations for what the likely outcome will be both with and without t-PA therapy should be discussed.

REFERENCES

1. Bruno A, Levine SR, Frankel MR, et al., for the NINDS rt-PA Stroke Study Group. Admission glucose level and clinical outcomes in the NINDS rt-PA Stroke Trial. Neurology. 2002;10;59:669-74.
2. International Society of Hypertension (ISH). Statement on the management of blood pressure in acute stroke. J Hypertens. 2003;21:665-72.

3. Schwarz S, Georgiadis D, Aschoff A, Schwab S. Effects of induced hypertension on intracranial pressure and flow velocities of the middle cerebral arteries in patients with large hemispheric stroke. Stroke. 2002;33:998-1004.

4. Kasner SE, Wein TH, Villar-Cordova CE, et al. Acetaminophen for altering body temperature in acute stroke. Stroke. 2002;33:130-4.

5. Multicentre Acute Stroke Trial-Italy Group. Randomised controlled trial of streptokinase, aspirin, and combination of both in treatment of acute ischemic stroke. Lancet. 1995;346:1509-14.

6. Multicenter Acute Stroke Trial-Europe Study Group. Thrombolytic therapy with streptokinase in acute ischemic stroke. N Engl J Med. 1996;335:145-50.

7. Donnan GA, Davis SM, Chambers BR, et al. Streptokinase for acute ischemic stroke with relationship to time of administration. Australian Streptokinase Trial Study Group. JAMA. 1996;276:961-6.

8. Hacke W, Kaste M, Fieschi C, et al. Intravenous thrombolysis with recombinant tissue plasminogen activator for acute hemispheric stroke. The European Cooperative Acute Stroke Study (ECASS). JAMA. 1995;274:1017-25.

9. National Institute of Neurological Disorders and Stroke t-PA Stroke Study Group. Tissue plasminogen activator for acute ischemic stroke. N Eng J Med. 1995;333:1581-7.

10. Hacke W, Kaste M, Fieschi C, et al. Randomised double-blind placebo-controlled trial of thrombolytic therapy with intravenous alteplase in acute ischemic stroke (ECASS II). Second European-Australian Acute Stroke Study Investigators. Lancet. 1998;352;1245-51.

11. Clark WM, Wissman S, Albert GW, et al. Recombinant tissue-type plasminogen activator (Ateplase) for ischemic stroke 3 to 5 hours after symptom onset. The ATLANTIS Study: a randomized controlled trial. JAMA. 1999;282;2019-26.

12. NINDS t-PA Stroke Study Group. Generalized efficacy of t-PA for acute ischemic stroke. Subgroup analysis of the NINDS t-PA Stroke Trial. Stroke. 1997;28:2119-25.

13. Kwiatkowski TG, Libman RB, Frankel M, et al. Effects of tissue-plasminogen activator for acute ischemic stroke at one year. National Institute of Neurological Disorders and Stroke Recombinant Tissue Plasminogen Activator Stroke Study Group. N Engl J Med. 1999;340:1781-7.

14. Grotta JC, Burgin WS, El-Mitwalli A, et al. Intravenous tissue-type plasminogen activator therapy for ischemic stroke: Houston experience 1996 to 2000. Arch Neurol. 2001; 58:2009-13.

15. Katzan IL, Furlan AJ, Lloyd LE, et al. Use of tissue-type plasminogen activator for acute ischemic stroke: the Cleveland area experience. JAMA. 2000;283:1151-8.

16. Katzan IL, Hammer MD, Furlan AJ, et al. Quality improvement and tissue-type plasminogen activator for acute ischemic stroke: a Cleveland update. Stroke. 2003;34:799-800.

17. Lopez-Yunez AM, Bruno A, Williams LS, et al. Protocol violations in community-based rTPA stroke treatment are associated with symptomatic intracerebral hemorrhage. Stroke. 2001;32:12-6.

18. Chiu D, Krieger D, Villar-Cordova C, et al. Intravenous tissue plasminogen activator for acute ischemic stroke: feasibility, safety, and efficacy in the first year of clinical practice. Stroke. 1998;29:18-22.

19. Albers GW, Bates VE, Clark WM, et al. Intravenous tissue-type plasmiogen activator for treatment of acute stroke: the Standard Treatment with Alteplase to reverse Stroke (STARS) study. JAMA. 2000;283:1145-50.

20. Tanne D, Bates VE, Verro P, et al. Initial clinical experience with IV tissue plasmiogen activator for acute ischemic stroke: a multicenter survey. The t-PA Stroke Survey Group. Neurology. 1999;53:424-7.

21. Hacke W, Albers G, Al-Rawi Y, et al. The desmoteplase in acute ischemic stroke trial (DIAS). A phase II MRI-based 9-hour window acute stroke thrombolysis trial with intravenous Desmoteplase. Stroke. 2005;36:66-73.

22. Del Zoppo GJ, Higashida RT, Furlan AJ, et al. PROACT: a phase II randomized trial of recombinant pro-urokinaseby direct arterial delivery in acute middle cerebral artery stroke. PROACT Investigators. Prolyse in acute cerebral thromboembolism. Stroke. 1998;29:4-11.

23. Furlan A, Higashida R, Wechsler L, et al. Intra-arterial prourokinase for acute ischemic stroke. The PROACT II study: a randomized controlled trial. Prolyse in Acute Cerebral Thromboembolism. JAMA. 1999;282:2003-11.

24. Jahan R, Duckwiler GR, Kidwell CS, et al. Intra-arterial thrombolysis for treatment of acute stroke: experience of 26 patients with long-term follow-up. Am J Neuroradiol. 1999;20:1291-9.

25. Gonner F, Remonda L, Mattle H, et al. Local intra-arterial thrombolysis in acute ischemic stroke. Stroke. 1998;29:1894-1900.

26. Suarez JI, Sunshine JL, Tarr R, et al. Predictors of clinical improvement, angiographic recanalization, and intracranial hemorrhage after intra-arterial thrombolysis for acute ischemic stroke. Stroke. 1999;30:2094-2100.

27. Lewandowski CA, Frankel M, Tomsick TA, et al. Combined intravenous and intra-arterial r-TPA versus intra-arterial therapy of acute ischemic stroke. Emergency Management of Stroke (EMS) Bridging Trial. Stroke. 1999;30:2598-2605.

28. Ernst R, Pancioli A, Tomsick T, et al. Combined intravenous and intra-arterial recombinant tissue plasminogen activator in acute ischemic stroke. Stroke. 2000;31:2552-7.

29. Suarez JI, Zaidat OO, Sunshine JL, et al. Endovascular administration after intravenous infusion of thrombolytic agents for the treatment of patients with acute ischemic strokes. Neurosurgery. 2002;50:251-9.

30. Nakano S, Yokogami K, Ohta H, et al. Direct percutaneous transluminal angioplasty for acute middle cerebral arerty acclusion. Am J Neuroradiol. 1998;19:767-72.

31. Nakano S, Iseda T, Yoneyama T, et al. Direct percutaneous transluminal angioplasty for acute middle cerebral artery trunk occlusion: an alternative option to intra-arterial thrombolysis. Stroke. 2002;33:2872-6.

32. Yoneyama T, Nakano S, Kawano H, et al. Combined direct percutaneous transluminal angioplasty with low-dose native tissue plasminogen activator therapy for acute embolic middle cerebral artery trunk occlusion. Am J Neuroradiol. 2002;23:277-81.

33. Qureshi AI, Siddiqui AM, Suri MF, et al. Aggressive mechanical clot disruption and low-dose intra-arterial third-generation thrombolytic agent for ischemic stroke: a prospective study. Neurosurgery. 2002;51:1319-27.

34. Gobin YP, Starkman S, Duckwiler GR, et al. MERCI 1: A phase 1 study of mechanical embolus removal in cerebral ischemia. Stroke. 2004;35:2848-54.

35. Hacke W, Zeumer H, Ferbert A, et al. Intra-areterial thrombolytic therapy improves outcome in patients with acute vertebrobasilar occlusive disease. Stroke. 1988;19:1216-22.

36. Becker KJ, Monsein LH, Ulatowski J, et al. Intraarterial thrombolysis in vertebrobasilar occlusion. Am J Neuroradiol. 1996;17:255-62.

37. Wijdicks EF, Nichols DA, Thielen KR, et al. Intra-arterial thrombolysis in acute basilar artery thromboembolism: the initial Mayo Clinic experience. Mayo Clin Proc. 1997;72:1005-13.

38. Grond M, Rudolf J, Schmulling S, et al. Early intravenous thrombolysis with recombinant tissue-type plasminogen activator in vertebrbasilar ischemic stroke. Arch Neurol. 1998;55:466-9.

39. Cross DT, Derdeyn CP, Moran CJ. Bleeding complications after basilar atery fibrinolysis with tissue plasminogen activator. Am J Neuroradiol 2001;22:521-51.

Chapter 8

Stroke Rehabilitation

ALAN LEVITT, MD
ERIC M. ALDRICH, MD, PhD

Key Points

- A rehabilitation plan is usually formulated while the stroke patient is still in the hospital.
- Rehabilitation environments may include acute rehabilitation, subacute inpatient rehabilitation, and outpatient rehabilitation.
- Functional activities initially addressed in rehabilitation include the basic activities of daily living: feeding, grooming, bathing, dressing, transfers, mobility, toileting, and continence.
- Medical management includes treating common complications and optimizing secondary prevention of stroke. Musculoskeletal pain, aphasia and communication, dysphagia, diplopia, bowel and bladder problems, spasticity, seizures, fatigue and sleep disorders, and depression and mood disorders may be addressed during rehabilitation.

Despite advances in primary and secondary prevention of stroke, as well as in emergency treatment of acute stroke, the incidence and the costs of stroke to society remain high. Furthermore, it is likely that the incidence and costs associated with stroke will continue to rise as our population ages. The sobering reality is not only that stroke is the third most common cause of death in the United States but that it is also a leading cause of disability. Some data suggest that stroke is the primary cause of disability in adults.

However, there are numerous misconceptions about life after stroke and stroke rehabilitation, both in the general population and among health

155

care providers. In some respects it depends on personal perspective in terms of interpreting the data. For example, consider the well-known saying that an optimist views a 12-ounce glass containing 6 ounces of water as "half full," whereas a pessimist views it as "half empty." Given the influence of perspective, what does the stroke recovery data show? In general, of those patients who survive their stroke, 10%-15% will recover almost completely, 25%-30% will recover with only minor impairment, 35%-40% will experience moderate-to-severe impairment, and 10%-15% will require long-term nursing home care. From a "glass is half empty" perspective, one could conclude that stroke is the leading cause of disability and that more than half of stroke survivors will end up severely impaired. Alternatively, one can also interpret these data as stating that nearly half of stroke survivors have few or no deficits one year after their stroke; that is, stroke is not only survivable, but there is life after a stroke.

It is extremely important for patients, families, and health care providers to adopt the "glass is half full" perspective. Patients recover after stroke, and stroke rehabilitation is effective. Examples from history illustrate this point. Woodrow Wilson, Winston Churchill, and Gerald Ford all suffered strokes, recovered, and returned to active public life. More recently, we have seen actors and actresses suffer strokes and then return to work. In some cases, for various television series, the real-life stroke was worked into subsequent scripts!

Predicting which patients will recover from a stroke and which will not is an inexact science. Yet there are data that can guide the clinician in advising the patient and family members. Favorable prognostic factors include younger age, independent prior level of function, small stroke size, and certain locations of the damage within the brain. For example, lacunar infarcts have a very favorable prognosis even though they can initially present with a dense hemiplegia. Intracerebral hemorrhages of less than 30 cc in volume recovery nicely as well. Consultation with a neurologist or physical medicine and rehabilitation (PM&R) (physiatry) specialist can be very important before discussing prognosis with the patient and the family. Some easy-to-remember general statements include:

- The pace of recovery is more week-to-week and month-to-month than day-to-day. It is important to work hard in rehab but also to be patient about the rate of progress.

- Although the pace of recovery can appear to be quickest over the first 90 days after a stroke, it continues for months and months afterwards.

- One rule of thumb is "Where you are after one year is where you're going stay." However, different disabilities after stroke appear to recover over different periods of time. For example, many experts feel that speech and language function continue to improve over several years after stroke, perhaps even for the remainder of the patient's lifetime.

Thus our disappointment in efforts to prevent and emergently treat stroke is fortunately balanced by the continued ability of many of our patients to recover from their deficits. This chapter reviews organized stroke rehabilitation, how stroke patients recover, aspects of medical management, and treatments that may enhance recovery.

The Stroke Continuum of Care

The journey a stroke patient typically travels is one year in duration. It begins the moment he suffers the stroke and continues through the long process of hospitalization, rehabilitation, returning home, and putting a life back together. The patient will pass through many different health care environments and interact with a wide variety of health care providers. This "continuum of care" is somewhat complex and can be distressing, if not anxiety producing, for both patients and their families. It is important for the primary care physician (PCP) to understand this system because he will likely be the only constant element during this journey. The PCP plays a vital role in explaining what has happened and what can be expected, as well as providing reassurance that he will act as guide throughout the journey.

The continuum of care (Figure 8-1) begins in the pre-hospital environment the moment the patient or someone nearby realizes that something is wrong. Somebody calls "911" and the emergency medical system is activated. Pre-hospital providers are now receiving specialized training for stroke throughout the country. In the emergency department, a "Brain

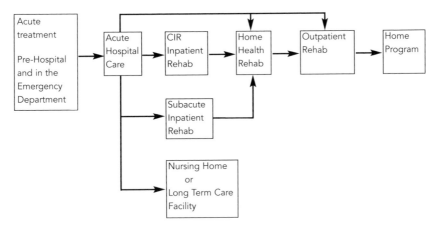

Figure 8-1 Stroke continuum of care.

Attack Team" might swarm over the patient to provide acute treatment. During the subsequent acute hospitalization, the patient will move through many different areas of a hospital for care and diagnostic evaluation. This can be a very disorienting and stressful experience, especially when the patient must spend time in an intensive care unit.

At some point, often toward the later part of the hospitalization, rehabilitation specialists will become involved and agree on a rehabilitation plan. At the time of discharge the patient might move to one of several environments. Comprehensive inpatient rehabilitation (CIR), or acute rehabilitation, is the most intensive. Patients receive at least 3 hours a day of physical, occupational, and speech therapy. They also benefit from an extensive staff of other rehabilitation health care professionals. Subacute inpatient rehabilitation, also known in some areas as TCU (transitional care unit) or SNF (skilled nursing facility), provides a less intense rehabilitation environment. Typically subacute facilities provide up to 1.5 hours of therapy per day, essentially the same amount of therapy that was provided while the patient was hospitalized. Nursing homes or other long-term care facilities can provide therapy sessions once per day up to three times per week; this is similar to what is provided by Home Health agencies. There are complex criteria for what level of rehab a patient qualifies for, not to mention the need for approval by third-party payers. Consultation with a PM&R specialist can be helpful in meeting the challenges of developing a stroke rehabilitation plan that is appropriate for a patient's particular needs and disabilities. Some patients are able to skip this first step of inpatient rehabilitation and go directly to in-home or outpatient rehab.

The outpatient phase of the continuum of care can include a short period of visits from therapists and home health services in the patient's home. However, this typically occurs for only a couple of weeks. Home health therapy ends once a patient has demonstrated the ability to get out of his home and go to appointments. The patient then goes to outpatient therapy appointments, typically three times a week for several weeks. Continuation in outpatient rehab usually is based on patient participation and improvement. When a patient "plateaus," meaning there is no further change in the standard rehabilitation assessment scales, outpatient therapy ends.

Yet, this is not the end of the patient's one-year journey. Often at this point only three months have passed since the stroke. Patients will continue to recover, albeit at a slower pace. Ideally, before the end of therapy, the patient and the family receive a "home program" from the therapists. A home program consists of exercises and activities that the patient can do on his own to continue to promote recovery of function and greater independence.

General Principles

Neurologic Examination vs. Functional Assessment

One important concept to understand when considering stroke rehabilitation is the difference between the neurologic examination and the functional assessment. All physicians are familiar with the neurologic examination: the mental status examination, testing of the cranial nerves, muscle strength and reflexes, sensation, coordination, and gait. However, the neurologic examination does not take into account the environment that the patient is in, or what the patient might be attempting to accomplish. The functional assessment or functional examination, in contrast, analyzes what the patient can actually accomplish with the neurologic deficits he has. For example, the neurologic exam may assess muscle strength or memory, but the functional assessment determines whether a patient can use those abilities to get up from a chair and go to the bathroom. This is an important distinction, as a related concept is that neurologic examination and functional assessment do not necessarily improve in tandem. In fact, they typically diverge. For example, a patient with a dense hemiplegia may experience no significant improvement in voluntary movement of the affected side. Initially, the patient is unable to accomplish the activities of daily living such as going to the bathroom. However, as a result of a comprehensive rehabilitation program, he can learn techniques and the use of special equipment to achieve independence for such as task. The neurologic examination did not change, but the functional examination improved dramatically. Such improvements also can have a profound effect on other vital areas such as patient self-esteem.

Functional activities initially addressed in rehabilitation include the basic activities of daily living: feeding, grooming, bathing, dressing, transfers, mobility, toileting, and continence. As patients improve, higher-level activities are addressed, including homemaking, medication, money management, community socialization, driving, and work retraining. Disability outcome scales have been developed to help measure impairment after a stroke. These outcome scales (such as the Barthel Index, the Rankin Scale, and the Functional Independence Measure [FIM]) have either low sensitivity or difficulty with "floor" or "ceiling" effects. The Stroke Impact Scale, a recently developed scale that includes measurements of quality of life, may better assess stroke survivors, monitor progress during recovery, and evaluate the effectiveness of recovery interventions. Familiarity with scales such as the FIM is important because rehabilitation specialists and third-party payers use them to determine a patient's specific stroke rehabilitation plan (e.g., CIR vs. SNF).

The Rehabilitation Team

Stroke rehabilitation is provided by a coordinated team of health care professionals who work with the stroke patient and their caregiver(s). However, for most physicians stroke rehabilitation is a "black box" (Figure 8-2). Their patients are transferred to this black box after an acute stroke hospitalization, later to re-emerge discharged home and improved in many of their initial impairments. What goes on within that black box is a mystery. The PCP must learn more about what goes on in the black box to dispel the mystery and thus to work effectively with the stroke rehabilitation team members.

The stroke rehabilitation team usually includes physicians, rehabilitation nurses, physical therapists (PTs), occupational therapists (OTs), speech-language pathologists, case managers and/or social workers, dieticians, neuropsychologists, and therapeutic recreation specialists. Each team member concentrates on certain areas of stroke recovery. For example, physical therapists often concentrate on the lower extremities because they

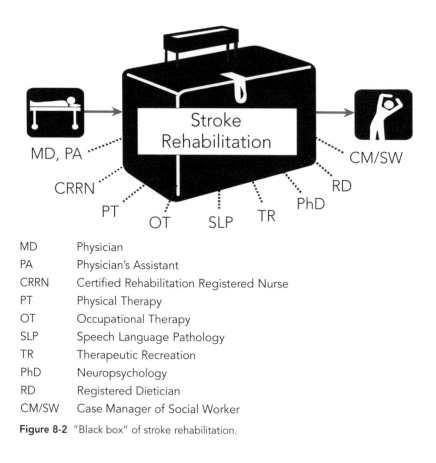

MD	Physician
PA	Physician's Assistant
CRRN	Certified Rehabilitation Registered Nurse
PT	Physical Therapy
OT	Occupational Therapy
SLP	Speech Language Pathology
TR	Therapeutic Recreation
PhD	Neuropsychology
RD	Registered Dietician
CM/SW	Case Manager of Social Worker

Figure 8-2 "Black box" of stroke rehabilitation.

are focusing on mobility issues such as walking. However, their area of expertise also includes bed mobility, transfers to wheelchairs or bedside commodes, and a wide range of equipment to assist patients in improving mobility independence. Occupational therapists might pay attention to upper extremity function and fine motor movements of the hand in order to help improve independence in the activities of daily living. Their area of expertise also includes cognitive function and the variety of equipment they can recommend for patient use.

It is important to understand that there is an enormous overlap of roles and responsibilities among the various therapist disciplines (Figure 8-3). Therapists from different disciplines will often co-treat during a single therapy session because they have complementary expertise in similar areas of rehab. For example, both the PT and OT work on improving transfers from bed to commode or wheelchair. Further, OT and SLP both concentrate on cognitive issues. The rehabilitation team also plays a large role in caregiver and family training.

The goal is to facilitate neurologic return as well as maximize functional recovery and independence. As mentioned above, rehabilitation can be provided in many settings. Traditionally, therapy begins soon after the stroke (while still in acute care hospital) and then continues in an inpatient (acute or subacute rehabilitation unit), in-home, or outpatient setting. "Early Supported Discharge" programs utilizing a home interdisciplinary team allow higher-level patients to be safely discharged home sooner than previously possible.

The Role of the Primary Care Physician

It cannot be emphasized enough that the PCP is a valuable member of the stroke rehabilitation team. He provides advice on treatment strategies for secondary stroke prevention, assists in management of post-stroke complications, and facilitates the patient's transition into the various levels of care

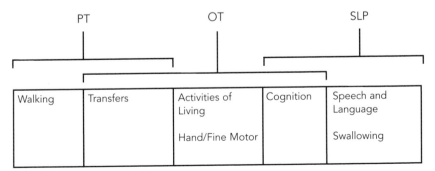

Figure 8-3 Overlapping areas of expertise of physical therapy (PT), occupational therapy (OT), and speech language pathology (SLP).

required during stroke recovery. After hospitalization, orders for therapy and medical equipment are often completed by the PCP, rather than the rehabilitation physician. Also, stroke patients and their families are often emotionally devastated and initially feel hopeless after the sudden impact of stroke. The PCP, well-known to the patient and family, provides comfort, reassurance, support, and hope for recovery. PCPs are perhaps the most important member of the rehabilitation team, providing priceless continuity of care throughout the continuum of stroke care.

Medical Management

General Medical Care

Medical management of patients in stroke rehabilitation includes treating the more common complications seen in recovery and optimizing second-ary prevention of stroke (see Chapter 5). Medical complications occur in up to 75% of stroke patients during inpatient rehabilitation, and 19% of these patients require transfer back to an acute care hospital. The most common reasons for transfer to acute care are thrombolic (deep venous thrombosis or pulmonary embolism), infectious (pneumonia or complicated urinary tract infection), cardiac (ischemic heart disease, heart failure, cardiac arrhythmias), neurologic (recurrent stroke or seizure), and gastrointestinal (upper gastrointestinal bleeding).

One particularly important concern is prevention of deep venous thrombosis and reducing the risk of pulmonary embolism. Asymptomatic and clinically relevant deep venous thrombosis occurs in up to 50% of untreated stroke patients. Cognitive, language, and sensory impairment may delay the diagnosis of thromboembolic disease. Most studies support using low-dose heparin to reduce the risk of developing clinical relevant deep venous thrombosis and pulmonary embolism.

Another important area is nutrition, not only to provide the energy to participate in the rigors of rehabilitation but also to avoid the complications of skin breakdown and the subsequent decubitus ulcers. In many respects, good rehabilitation medicine is actually good internal medicine, with an emphasis on improving health and avoiding complications. One piece of evidence supporting this notion is the fact that aspiration pneumonia dou-bles the morbidity and mortality of stroke patients.

Secondary Prevention

Most stroke patients never had optimal primary prevention, including man-agement of treatable risk factors such as hypertension, hyperlipidemia, dia-betes, and smoking. After a stroke, secondary prevention therefore is of obvious importance.

One area that can be confusing is the management of blood pressure. In the acute setting, current guidelines support allowing blood pressures to rise as high as a systolic pressure of 200 mm Hg. Such "permissive hypertension" is felt to assist in supporting the survival of potential ischemic neurons in the penumbral surrounding the infarct. However, once a patient moves on to the rehabilitation phase, blood pressure will need to be controlled in light of the need for long-term control for secondary prevention. Early in recovery many patients may not need anti-hypertensive medication because they are inactive and resting in bed for long periods of time. If such patients are on anti-hypertensive medication, they can be at greater risk for symptomatic orthostasis when beginning sitting or standing activities from bed or when in therapy. Thus, many patients initially are on little or no medication to start. Exceptions include medications such as clonidine, given the concern for rebound hypertension, as well as cardiac patients in whom beta-blockers are often continued. As recovery continues, and the patient becomes more active, anti-hypertensive medications should be slowly adjusted, emphasizing long-term blood pressure control and medication compliance.

Diabetic management during stroke rehabilitation may be complicated by variability in daily intake (due to dysphagia) and amount of exercise. In addition, patients (and often their caregivers) need re-training for home blood glucose management, including insulin administration, because of new upper extremity impairment. Other aspects of secondary prevention, such as the use of statins and anti-platelet agents, are discussed in Chapter 2.

Pain

Rehabilitation is work and many patients will develop musculoskeletal pain during their recovery. They need to strengthen deconditioned muscles and to learn to move and support their weight using muscles not previously used for such movements. In addition, there is the effect of pre-existing conditions such as osteoarthritis. Neck pain, low back pain, and knee pain are not uncommon. One especially important type of pain that needs special attention is shoulder pain. Shoulder pain is extremely common in hemiplegic stroke patients. Attempts to prevent shoulder pain include positioning the arm properly, wearing shoulder supports, and using prophylactic functional electrical stimulation. One important way to avoid shoulder pain is to ensure that all health care providers, both staff and family caregivers, have been instructed in properly assisting a stroke patient. It is important not to pull or yank on the affected weakened extremity. There are specific techniques to assist with transfers and walking that can be easily learned by any caregiver. Managing shoulder pain depends on the underlying etiology but may include electrical stimulation, local corticosteroid and/or anesthetic injections, and treatment of spasticity. PM&R consultation is often helpful to assist with shoulder pain diagnosis and management. "Shoulder hand syndrome," a form of reflex sympathetic dystrophy, usually presents as shoulder pain combined with a painful and edematous wrist and hand beginning approximately 1-2 months after a stroke. When diagnosed early, shoulder hand syndrome responds to a tapering course of oral corticosteroids. However, it can be very resistant to treatment. The best approach is to prevent its development in the first place, emphasizing the need for proper caregiver training.

Aphasia and Communication

Approximately 25% of stroke patients have language impairment, or aphasia. Aphasia is caused by injury to the dominant hemisphere, typically left hemisphere strokes in most right-handed patients and in almost two thirds of left-handed patients. All patients with aphasia have word-finding problems. Aphasia is further classified based on impairment of fluency, comprehension, and repetition. Stroke patients may also have difficulty with verbal expression due to dysarthria (impaired articulation) or verbal apraxia (impaired voluntary movements for speech). It is important to clarify the diagnosis for type of therapy and for patient and family education. Thus the involvement of a SLP therapist and a neuropsychologist can be invaluable. There is evidence that high-intensity speech therapy improves outcome of aphasia after stroke. Families often need education on effective methods for communication with a patient with aphasia, particularly for patients with impaired verbal comprehension. Special computer aids and pharmacotherapy may be helpful in recovery. Patients have demonstrated benefit from aphasia therapy over a year after a stroke.

Neglect

Hemispatial neglect, which refers to decreased awareness or responsiveness to stimuli on the affected side, occurs more commonly with right hemisphere strokes and is associated with a worse prognosis for recovery. It can be a frustrating problem for both family caregivers and primary care providers. This aspect falls under the purview of OT and SLP, with occasional assistance from neuropsychology. One of the challenges of working with such patients is that successful stroke rehabilitation is totally dependent on a patient's ability to understand what the therapist is trying to teach him. In short, he must be able to learn. Contrary to a common belief among health care providers, patients with aphasia do much better in rehab than patients with a severe neglect. Although they have limited language function, patients with aphasia are often cognitively intact and capable of a great deal of non-verbal learning. In contrast, patients with severe neglect have intact language function but the associated problems with learning and other cognitive dysfunction can make progress in rehab excruciatingly slow. Neglect has been shown to improve with enhanced visual scanning techniques. Other treatments shown to decrease left-sided neglect include prism adaptation (shifting the visual field to the right), electrical stimulation or vibratory stimulation to the left neck, caloric stimulation (cold water to the left ear or warm water to the right ear), and virtual reality.

Dysphagia

Dysphagia can appear particularly vexing early on following a stroke, but actually the prognosis for recovery is typically very good. Stroke patients with dysphagia who suffered damage in areas of the brain above the brain stem do quite well, whereas those involving the brain stem may require specialized care. The importance of early SLP evaluation cannot be overstressed. The presence or absence of a gag reflex is of little importance in the determination of dysphagia and aspiration risk. Many times the SLP therapist cannot determine the safety of eating from the initial bedside swallowing evaluation. In such cases a video fluoroscopy swallow study is required. Some patients may be able to eat and take medicines by mouth by changing the consistency of the food, such as a pureed diet or thickened liquids. Special techniques that the SLP therapist may teach include the "chin tuck" or the "double swallow."

Even with such interventions, however, some patients either are unable to swallow anything safely or they are unable to swallow enough calories or liquid to meet their daily nutritional needs. For such patients the placement of a percutaneous endoscopic gastrostomy (PEG) tube is recommended. PEG tubes themselves will not alleviate aspiration risk, because the patient can still easily develop pneumonia from aspirating their own saliva. However, PEG tubes do allow a patient to no longer need intravenous administration of medications, hydration, and/or nutrition. They are also more comfortable than nasogastric tubes, can be maintained for a long period of time, and can be easily tucked away when not in use to facilitate participation in therapy. Having a PEG tube does not mean the patient cannot take anything by mouth. The patient can eat whatever the SLP therapist feels is safe, and such "recreational eating" is an important symbol of life returning to normal for the patient and the family.

Most patients who require PEG tubes and/or have other complicated dysphagia problems will improve sufficiently over the subsequent weeks or months. There are a variety of surgical procedures that an otolaryngologist with special expertise can offer to dysphagia patients. However, in light of the fact that a great deal of spontaneous recovery does occur, it is often recommended to wait 6 months before referral to such a subspecialist.

Diplopia and Impaired Vision

There are a variety of vision problems that can occur after a stroke. Some of the vision problems involve pre-existing conditions with the eye itself, such as diabetic retinopathy. Other problems, such as diplopia, can result from brainstem infarcts. In addition, injuries to cortical vision areas can impair higher-level visual processing and interpretation. Thus, any injury to the visual system, or a combination of new and pre-existing problems, can challenge the patient during the rehabilitation process.

Two of the most common problems are homonymous hemianopsia and diplopia. Homonymous hemianopsia occurs when the occipital lobe is injured on one side, such as in a unilateral posterior cerebral artery infarction. In the hospital this is usually a minor nuisance, but it can become a more significant issue when a patient attempts to drive or return to work. Each state has specific criteria for the minimal amount of visual field function required in order to drive a car. This topic is discussed in detail in the Driving section below. However, it is important to realize that such laws exist and usually require referral to a neuro-ophthalmologist or other specialist with expertise in this area. From a rehabilitation perspective, there are experimental rehab techniques that may be able to improve the degree of visual field deficit in such cases.

Diplopia is typically the most distressing of the vision problems a stroke patient may experience. Fortunately, like dysphagia, what may initially seem an overwhelming problem can be managed effectively. First, the brain has a remarkable ability to correct diplopia to some degree; for example, infarcts in the lateral medulla (Wallenberg's syndrome) typically produce a diplopia that is initially severe but that can rapidly resolve over days. For patients with persistent diplopia, an eye patch is an easy way to help them achieve more functional independence. However, it is best to advise patients to only use the eye patch when they need it, such as while reading or watching television, because the natural process of brain recovery theoretically will occur faster if the nervous system is confronted with the diplopia as much as possible. Similar to dysphagia, many rehabilitation specialists use the 6-month rule for diplopia. Specifically, it is recommended to wait 6 months to allow the natural recovery process to occur. If diplopia persists at that point, referral to a subspecialist with expertise in this area is indicated. A neuro-ophthalmologist can prescribe special prism glasses to correct the diplopia. In rare cases, using techniques typically used for strabismus, surgery may be recommended.

Bowel and Bladder

Bowel and bladder issues can be the most stressful and humiliating for stroke patients. A variety of mechanisms can lead to urinary incontinence, retention, or a mix of the two. For many patients, the embarrassment of incontinence is their greatest fear. Incontinence can be caused by direct effects of the stroke, such as bladder hyper-reflexia, or indirect effects, such as poor cognition, limited mobility, or limited communication. Other co-morbidities, such as diabetes, can cause "overflow incontinence" secondary to autonomic neuropathy. Lastly, medications such as diuretics can exacerbate incontinence problems due to increased urine output.

One technique that is simple and helpful is "timed voiding." This takes advantage of the post-prandial response, wherein the body is stimulated to void within an hour after a meal. Timed voiding is a regimen where the patient sits on the toilet 30 minutes after each meal and just before bed. He remains there for approximately 15 minutes and tries to void. Thus, although the patient is incontinent, "accidents" are minimized because the patient has the opportunity to use the toilet 4 times per day. Urinary incontinence can also be treated with medications such as oxybutynin. However, discretion is advised before prescribing such medications. They have an anti-cholinergic mechanism of action that can have detrimental side effects on elderly stroke patients, causing cognitive dysfunction or even delirium.

A related problem is urinary retention. This occurs in men more than women, presumably because of concurrent benign prostatic hypertrophy. It is important to remove indwelling Foley catheters as soon as possible, not only to reduce infection risk but to allow greater mobility during therapy sessions. Patients on rehabilitation units with urinary retention are typically on regular bladder catheterization schedules in conjunction with medications such as terazosin, tamsulosin, or doxazosin. These medications will also lower blood pressure. It can often take a few days for them to be effective, so it is best to start at a low dose and slowly titrate for effect.

Spasticity

Spasticity, or increased muscle tone, occurs in almost 40% of patients after a stroke. Occasionally, increased muscle tone may be helpful for the patient's standing or walking. For most patients, however, spasticity leads to worsening functional impairment, contractures, and pain. It is important to rule out treatable causes for increasing tone including infection, pain, urinary retention, constipation, or improper patient positioning. PM&R consultation is often helpful to assist with management of spasticity. Nonpharmacologic treatment includes stretching and positioning programs, splinting, and electrical stimulation. Oral medications, including benzodiazepines, baclofen, dantrolene, and tizanidine, have been tried for generalized tone reduction with variable efficacy. They are often more effective in spasticity because of spinal cord infection. Side effects associated with oral pharmacotherapy include sedation and increasing weakness, so their use should be carefully considered in elderly patients with stroke. Injections of botulinum toxin have been successfully used to locally reduce muscle tone. It takes up to 2 weeks after botulinum toxin injection to demonstrate improvement, and the injections may need to be repeated every 3-6 months. Other options for patients with intractable spasticity include phenol nerve blocks and intrathecal baclofen. Daily active and passive range-of-motion exercises remain an important mainstay of spasticity management. They are easily taught to patients and caregivers. Further, they can help prevent related problems such as frozen shoulder.

Seizures

Seizures are not a common problem in stroke patients. Fewer than 5% of patients will have a seizure at the time of their stroke, more often in situations involving cortical injury or intracerebral hemorrhage. If a stroke patient did not seize at the time of presentation, it is unlikely that he will develop a seizure disorder, and anti-seizure medications are not routinely begun. One common issue is that patients with intracerebral hemorrhage are often routinely placed on anti-seizure medications, whether or not they presented with a seizure. In some situations, such as patients with large lobar hemorrhages with elevated intracranial pressure requiring intensive care, guidelines recommend considering anti-seizure medication for up to 1 month. However, it is also known that anti-seizure medications themselves can cause sedation, cognitive impairment, and impede recovery.

One approach to reconciling these two considerations is that if a patient with an intracerebral hemorrhage has never seized and the hemorrhage itself is small and/or subcortical, then after he has left the ICU and is ready for rehabilitation, the anti-seizure medications can be slowly weaned and discontinued. This plan should be discussed with the patient and family, often in consultation with a neurologist, because there is still a risk of seizures. The rationale is that the seizure medications themselves can impede recovery and the likelihood of having a seizure is low. In most cases they can be safely discontinued over the course of a few days, and only rarely do they need to be restarted should a seizure disorder develop.

Fatigue and Sleep Disorders

Fatigue is a common complaint associated with stroke, as it is for many other chronic neurologic disorders. Assessment and treatment of patients with post-stroke fatigue includes identifying potential contributing factors such as medical co-morbidities, medication and dietary side effects, sleep disorders, and depression. Nonpharmacologic management of post-stroke fatigue usually includes a regular exercise program, scheduling daily rest breaks, and learning stress reduction and relaxation strategies. Medications which may be tried for patients with refractory fatigue include modafanil, amphetamines, ritalin, amantadine, and antidepressants. Proper diagnosis is essential before the initiation of medication.

Sleep disorders associated with stroke include insomnia, hypersomnia, and sleep-disordered breathing. Diagnosing and treating obstructive sleep apnea after a stroke is important for secondary stroke prevention and potentially to improve stroke recovery. Furthermore, obstructive sleep apnea appears to be increasingly common after stroke and is the subject of a great deal of recent research activity. For some patients complaining of cognitive dysfunction or fatigue, the effective treatment is not medication but rather a sleep study followed by use of a CPAP machine at night.

Depression and Mood Disorders

Approximately one third of stroke patients will develop depression or some other form of mood disorder. Depression in particular is associated with worse functional recovery. Depression may be difficult to diagnose when language impairment exists. Treatment of depression not only improves mood but also appears to positively influence stroke recovery. Selective serotonin reuptake inhibitors (SSRIs) and the new "atypical" anti-depressants are often used for depression in stroke patients due to more favorable side-effect profiles. However, these medications have a variety of effects and side effects. For example, some are preferable for geriatric patients (e.g., mirtazapine), some are more stimulating (e.g., sertraline), and still others have better anxiolytic properties (e.g., paroxetine). Further, it is often best to start at a low dose and subsequently titrate for effect.

Often anti-depressant medication can be discontinued 6 to 12 months after the stroke. Tricyclic anti-depressants are often best avoided in stroke patients due to their anti-cholinergic side effects such as sedation and urinary retention. Then again, in some select stroke patients these side effects can be advantageous. For example, a low dose of amitriptyline at bedtime can act as a sleep aid and treat urinary incontinence, as well as provide anti-depressant effects. Consultation with a psychiatrist can be extremely helpful in selecting the best possible anti-depressant medication, dose, and dosing regimen, as well as providing long-term follow-up and counseling to the patient and family.

Other mood disorders include adjustment disorder, anxiety disorder, and emotional lability. Adjustment disorder can be thought of as "a normal response to an abnormal situation." Not unlike grieving the unexpected loss of a loved one, adjustment disorder refers to the intense emotional response that can occur at the time of the initial hospitalization for stroke. This is an extremely stressful time and may be the first major hospitalization for the patient. It also may be the first time the patient has considered his own mortality. Patients often undergo an intense life review. Similar to grieving, this is not typically treated with medication initially, rather with counseling and family support. However, if the patient's depressed or anxious mood becomes dysfunctional or persistent, then alternate diagnoses must be considered, in which case psychiatric evaluation and initiation of medication is advised.

Anxiety disorders also develop in stroke patients. It may be a pre-morbid condition that has been amplified by the situation, often becoming a problem at the time of the initial hospitalization. However, other patients may develop an anxiety disorder weeks or months after their stroke. Psychiatric consultation is often the next best step, because many medications can have cognitive side effects and may impede recovery.

Emotional lability is a common problem for stroke patients and their families. This condition has many other names, including "emotional incontinence" and "post-stroke crying disorder." Patients experience the appropriate emotion for the various circumstances of everyday living, but the intensity of the emotional response is much greater than normal. A wide variety of emotions can be affected. Patients can cry easily, even in seemingly innocuous situations such as television commercials. Similarly they can anger quite easily, developing a "short fuse," which can be very disruptive to family life. Other patients find that they laugh very easily, if not inappropriately, at almost anything or any circumstance. Emotional lability occurs equally in men and women. Most of the time, simply counseling the patient and family that this frequently occurs is sufficient. It is often a transient phenomenon, resolving over the course of several months or even a year. Medication is not typically recommended as initial treatment, unless the emotional lability is causing a problem that is extremely detrimental to the patient's recovery, such as refusing to go outside the home for fear of embarrassment. SSRIs have been shown to be effective (e.g., citalopram for the post-stroke crying syndrome).

Influence of Medications

A concept that has been stressed throughout this chapter is the influence of medications on recovery of function after stroke. Pharmacotherapy to enhance rehabilitation, medications given specifically to improve efficacy of rehabilitation, is a separate topic discussed later in this chapter. The topic of influence of medications is meant to refer to routine medications, prescribed for a variety of other reasons, which may influence stroke rehabilitation. It is not uncommon for physicians to be unaware of this problem. As a general rule, any medication that has a mechanism of action that affects the central nervous system can potentially interfere with a patient's recovery. Anti-seizure medications and sedatives are the more obvious categories. Other, less well-known, potentially "negative" medications include Reglan, often prescribed for gastrointestinal problems, but which has an anti-dopaminergic mechanism of action. Any anti-cholinergic medication can cause problems, such as cognitive dysfunction and delirium in the elderly, as mentioned earlier. Physicians should be careful about their choice of anti-hypertensive medication, avoiding "centrally acting" agents such as clonidine if other choices can be equally effective. There are even case reports suggesting that glaucoma drops have caused delirium in elderly stroke patients. Two studies have suggested that patients receiving centrally acting antihypertensive agents (e.g., clonidine), dopamine receptor antagonists (including neuroleptics), or gamma-aminobutyric acid agonists (e.g., benzodiazepines, certain anticonvulsant agents) had a poorer overall stroke

Table 8-1   Medications That May Affect Stroke Recovery

Positive	Negative
• Amphetamines	• Clonidine
• Levodopa	• Prazosin
• SSRIs	• Phenoxybenzamine
• Bromocriptine	• Haloperidol
• Methylphenidate	• Fluanisone
• Piracetam	• Droperidol
• Cholinergic agents	• Anti-cholinergic agents
• Donezepil	• Metoclopramide
	• Benzodiazepines
	• Phenytoin
	• Barbiturates

outcome. Therefore, when choosing medications for stroke patients, the influence of these medications on potential brain recovery should be considered (Table 8-1).

Other Rehabilitation Issues

Driving

Driving a car, especially to Americans, is often felt to be an inalienable right. However, for stroke patients this issue must be addressed carefully. During the initial phases of stroke rehabilitation, it is best to tell patients that this is one of the last goals to work on. Logically one must learn how to dress, bathe, and walk before one learns to drive again. An appropriate time to move on to driving issues is after the patient has completed outpatient rehabilitation. The next step is for the physician, the patient, and the patient's family to understand that there are specific laws regarding who can and who cannot go back to driving. Because each state has different laws, it is strongly recommended that physicians first contact their state medical board and/or department of motor vehicles before giving advice to patients and families. Further, physicians must admit that it is highly unlikely that they have received any formal driving evaluation training during medical school or residency! Fortunately, in most metropolitan areas, the more sophisticated rehabilitation centers have specialized driving programs, typically run by occupational therapists who have received special training. The physician need only write a prescription for "OT/Driving Evaluation" and then advise the patient to contact the local program for an appointment. Patients receive an office assessment, followed by a driving evaluation. Additional evaluations might be necessary, such as an ophthalmology referral for visual field testing. It is best that all stroke patients have such a formal evaluation, even if the deficits seem minor. The only drawback is that such evaluations are not typically covered by insurance and thus must be paid for out-of-pocket. However, a driving evaluation is one of the best investments the patient can make in terms of safety (the patient's, the family's, and the safety of others) on the road.

Back-to-Work and Community Reintegration

Approximately 25% of stroke patients are under age 65 and thus returning to work is not an uncommon goal for such patients. Further, all patients look forward to returning to their pre-stroke life as much as possible. For some patients, this can be the most challenging part of the stroke rehabilitation journey. In terms of returning to work, consultation with a PM&R physician and a neuropsychologist can be invaluable. The ability to return to work depends on the patient's deficits as well as his occupation. For patients who work in offices and have administrative duties, neuropsychologic evaluation is necessary for a detailed assessment of thinking and memory skills. The patient's relative strengths and weaknesses are determined. In turn, specific recommendations then can be developed for assistive devices and modifications of the work environment and/or schedule. Some comprehensive regional rehabilitation centers have "work hardening" programs that bring together an entire rehab team (PT, OT, SLP, et al.) to help patients get back to work.

It is often best to advise patients not to try to go back to work too soon. The general public still knows very little about stroke and stroke recovery. Going back to work too soon, before recovery is complete, can lead to frustration and disappointment due to problems with fatigue and attention span. Patients who encounter such problems by going back to work too soon can end up having an invisible sign reading "Brain Damaged" hanging around their neck, even long after the fatigue issues have resolved. A gradual approach is best. One way to find out if a patient is ready to go back to work is to try a "simulated work week." The patient gets up at the usual time, then dresses and leaves the house by the usual time as well. However, he doesn't actually go to work. The patient will have planned ahead a day full of activities that will occupy him in a way similar to the usual work environment. Encourage him to have fun but to try to stick to the usual schedule, even, for example, taking an hour for lunch. Many patients who felt they were ready to return to work are stunned by the degree of fatigue they encounter.

As the patient's fatigue problems gradually improve, the next step is a part-time schedule. Certain common trends are usually noticed by stroke patients. One is that they have good days and bad days; another is that they do fine in the morning but fade early in the afternoon. Thus an ideal part-time schedule is not a full-day Monday, Wednesday, and Friday, but instead a weekly schedule consisting of half-days. Overall, returning to work can be accomplished but requires special expertise. The PCP should encourage the patient but, at the same time, obtain appropriate help and consultation for the most efficient rehabilitation methods.

Other aspects of community integration include social events and hobbies and sports. Therapeutic recreation therapists (TRs) are extremely helpful for this aspect of stroke rehabilitation. There is an amazing array of special equipment to help disabled persons participate in the activities they enjoy, from golf to trout fishing to skiing and beyond. Sexuality and interpersonal issues also should be kept in mind. The strain from the hospitalization, low self-esteem, and impaired body image can compound medical problems and mood disorders. Again, consultation is suggested if such issues arise.

The Future: Improving Outcomes

Does Stroke Rehabilitation Work?

Despite our limitations in assessing recovery, studies have demonstrated significant benefit from inpatient stroke rehabilitation programs. In a systematic review of randomized trials, patients receiving rehabilitation had a lower 1-year mortality rate (14% vs. 20%) and were more likely to be living at home independently (41% vs. 35%). Follow-up studies show continued benefit 10 years after rehabilitation. Medicare stroke patients had better outcomes after admission for acute (i.e., CIR) compared with subacute rehabilitation (unlike hip fracture patients in whom there was no difference in outcome between acute and subacute admission). Patients admitted to VA Stroke Programs that follow the Post-Stroke Rehabilitation guidelines had improved outcomes.

Factors predicting improved stroke recovery vary but in general include younger age, higher functional status on admission, small vessel stroke, or diagnosis of hemorrhage rather than infarct. Factors predicting worse recovery include right hemisphere stroke, severe functional impairment at admission, several medical co-morbidities, and lack of a committed caregiver. Although stroke size and severity of impairment are among the strongest predictors of outcome, and thus such severely impaired stroke patients recover less, studies have shown that they actually benefit the most from stroke rehabilitation programs. Less impaired patients will improve a great deal because of natural recovery; however, it is the severely impaired who require the special expertise of intensive rehabilitation. Overall, rehabilitation benefits are seen across all patient populations.

Mechanisms of Recovery

Our understanding of stroke recovery and the influence of cortical reorganization has become clearer over the past two decades. Initial recovery may occur due to improvement in brain activity surrounding the region of infarction, including areas that may have been affected by ischemia, edema, and other metabolic secondary effects from the stroke. Recovery may also occur with resolution of diaschisis, initial changes that occur in other areas of the brain remote to the infarction but still affected due to loss of signals from the damaged region. What excites clinicians and researchers involved in brain recovery is neuroplasticity, the ability of the brain to adapt to the effects of the stroke resulting in cortical reorganization.

Cortical reorganization may occur through recruitment or reinforcement of existing neural pathways (some of which usually lie dormant), as well as through rewiring of the "neural network" with new or enhanced synaptic connections. We now are able to demonstrate cortical reorganization after stroke using functional MRI scanning (fMRI), PET scanning, transcranial magnetic stimulation, and magnetoencephalography. These studies demonstrate the incredible ability of the brain to adapt to the initial insult and to progressively change over time in an attempt to maximize recovery. Primarily from upper extremity motor recovery studies, we have learned that increased activity occurs throughout the brain, involving both ipsilesional and contralesional areas. Most studies have shown increased activation in the primary motor cortex, premotor cortex, supplementary motor areas, and cerebellum. Initially, often a large area of recruitment is seen; patients with limited recovery often demonstrate persistent recruitment in many of these areas. Patients who recover well, however, are often able to focus over time the area of activation toward the ipsilesional network. Studies of language recovery generally suggest that left hemisphere activation is associated with better outcome; however, other studies have shown improvement in patients with right hemisphere activation as well. Transcranial magnetic stimulation has been helpful in determining the significance of the brain activation patterns: its disruption of brain activation helps determine the relative importance of that activation in functional recovery.

Factors Affecting Recovery and Various Techniques

Although it has been demonstrated that the interdisciplinary care of stroke rehabilitation works, current efforts are focusing on trying to determine what types of therapy are the most important for maximal recovery. Important factors include early therapy intervention, increased therapy intensity, adherence to stroke recovery guidelines (but, interestingly, not rigid care pathways), and consistent medical management. Early mobilization and beginning rehabilitation as soon as possible after a stroke appears to be important for maximal recovery. Studies have demonstrated improved functional outcome associated with greater intensity and frequency of therapy. Patients receiving daily additional sensorimotor stimulation of the arm for 6 weeks post-stroke demonstrated improved outcomes still noticeable 5 years after treatment. Bimanual activities may be helpful in stroke recovery. For example, one study demonstrated increased activation in the affected hemisphere initially when both arms were used in an activity. Later, as the patient improved, this increased activity was no longer seen. Other promising techniques being studied for motor recovery include mirror therapy, biofeedback, virtual reality, and mental practice.

Task-Specific Therapy

Task-specific therapies refer to rehabilitation techniques derived from studies of motor learning in humans. Importantly, the methods through which humans learn a new motor task, such as playing the piano or hitting a baseball, are goal-oriented and non-transferable. *Goal-oriented* refers to the need for a specific goal such as reaching for a glass in order to drink. Meaningless repetition without a goal is far less effective. *Non-transferable* refers to the phenomenon that in order to improve a specific task you must practice that specific task. For example, if a patient wants to improve walking, they must practice walking; spending a great deal of time on a stationary bicycle will be far less effective. Repetitive exercises can build gross strength and endurance, but the issue is more one of improving coordination and accuracy of a movement. Task-specific therapies have been demonstrated to be helpful for the more severely impaired patient and can even help patients after they were determined to have completed conventional rehabilitation programs.

Treadmill Training

An example of task-specific therapy is body-weight-support treadmill training. If a patient's goal is to improve walking, his initial deficits could be too significant to even begin therapy. In order to address this problem, the patient is supported by a harness while walking on a treadmill with therapists assisting advancement of the leg as well as support of the pelvis. One difficulty with body-weight-support treadmill training is the need for two therapists to assist each patient. Newer robotic technologies can now fully support the patient and also move the legs as necessary with a motorized exoskeleton. In addition, robotic technology is being studied to provide active-assistance, task-specific therapy to promote upper extremity recovery function. Benefits have been demonstrated for both acute and chronic stroke patients, as well as for mild and severely impaired patients.

Electrical Stimulation

Electrical stimulation is being evaluated as an additional treatment for stroke recovery. Electrical stimulation is likely helpful for treatment, and perhaps prevention, of post-stroke shoulder pain. Using electrical stimulation to increase ankle dorsiflexion is helpful in combination with physical therapy for successful gait training. Electrical stimulation of the upper extremities is being studied, including evaluation of EMG-triggered devices and exoskeletal-stimulating wrist splints. Cutaneous electrical stimulation (below sensory thresholds) used in combination with therapy may additionally improve upper extremity function. Electrical stimulation is also being used to improve recovery for stroke patients with swallowing impairment.

Constraint-Induced Movement Therapy

Constraint-induced movement therapy (CIMT) has expanded our knowledge of brain recovery and so far has shown very promising results. The theory behind CIMT is that persistent weakness seen in stroke patients is a result of learned non-use or suppression of movement that occurred early on post stroke. Patients will often stop using the "bad arm" because it can be frustrating, and develop the habit of only using their "good arm." By restricting movement of the unaffected upper extremity (usually placing in a sling) in combination with a progressive training program ("shaping") of the affected extremity, patients as long as 17 years post-stroke have demonstrated upper extremity recovery. CIMT involves restricting movement for 90% of the day for 2-3 weeks in combination with a "shaping" program with a therapist for 6 hours daily. A multicenter trial is underway to determine whether CIMT will be helpful for patients 3-6 months post-stroke. Increased areas of activation have been seen after CIMT in the contralateral motor and premotor areas of recovered patients. Alternative approaches to classic CIMT are being studied, including modifying intensity and using an automated workstation in an attempt to decrease the need for direct therapy supervision. Constraint-induced studies are also being done for aphasia, lower extremity movement, brain injury, hip fracture, spinal cord injury, and focal hand dystonia.

Pharmacotherapy

Medications have been used alone or in combination with therapy in an attempt to improve stroke outcome. Pharmacotherapy has often been based on known influences of neurotransmitters on brain recovery. Stroke outcome may depend on medication timing; for example, GABA agonists drugs may be helpful (due to neuroprotection) initially after a stroke, whereas later use of these same medications may inhibit brain recovery. Amphetamines increase brain norepinephrine, dopamine, and serotonin.

When administered 30 minutes before therapy sessions they appear to improve outcomes in motor and language recovery. Levodopa, also when combined with therapy, has been shown to improve motor recovery. Hemiparetic patients demonstrated increased brain activation and improved motor performance after a single dose of the seritonergic medication fluoxetine. Other medications that may be helpful in stroke recovery include cholinesterase inhibitors, methylphenidate, and piracetam. This area of stroke rehabilitation research is very promising.

Conclusions

Not only have there been advances in the prevention and treatment of stroke but it is now realized that stroke is an event from which recovery is often possible. The brain has natural recovery processes that occur after stroke. Stroke rehabilitation takes advantage of these processes and is effective at improving outcomes. Although the journey of a stroke patient through the process of recovery is long and challenging for both patients and caregivers, the end results can be remarkable. The primary care physician has an invaluable role in this process of healing.

SUGGESTED READING

PUBLICATIONS, TEXTS AND JOURNAL ARTICLES

Clinical Practice Guidelines Number 16: Post-Stroke Rehabilitation. AHCPR Publication 95-0662. Washington, DC: Department of Health and Human Services; May 1995.

Dobkin BH. The Contemporary Science of Neurologic Rehabilitation. New York: Oxford University Press; 2003.

Dobkin BH. Rehabilitation after stroke. N Engl J Med. 2005;352:1677-84.

Losseff N, Thompson AJ. Neurological Rehabilitation of Stroke. The Queen Square Neurological Rehabilitation Series. London: Taylor and Francis; 2004.

WEB SITES FOR PATIENTS, FAMILIES, AND HEALTH CARE PROVIDERS

American Stroke Association: www.strokeassociation.org
National Stroke Association: www.stroke.org

Chapter 9

Carotid Artery Disease

JUDY HUANG, MD

Key Points

- Atherosclerosis is the most common cause of cerebral ischemia and infarction.
- Diagnostic evaluation of carotid stenosis includes a thorough neurological examination, carotid Duplex ultrasonography, brain magnetic resonance imaging and angiography, and frequently digital subtraction angiography.
- Nearly all symptomatic and many asymptomatic patients with carotid stenosis may benefit from carotid endarterectomy.
- Evaluation for carotid endarterectomy in patients with symptoms of anterior circulation ischemia should proceed urgently after presentation.
- The major morbidity of carotid endarterectomy is perioperative stroke.

A s the most common cause of cerebral ischemia and infarction, atherosclerosis affects primarily the large intracranial and extracranial arteries. The most frequent location of flow-limiting arterial stenosis caused by occlusive atherosclerotic plaques is the origin of the proximal internal carotid artery at the bifurcation of the common carotid artery in the neck. Fortunately, timely identification of individuals who are at risk for stroke due to atherosclerosis at this extracranial location allows for the institution of preventive measures. A number of preventive measures, both medical and surgical, are possible. All patients derive benefit from medical therapy for stroke prevention. Control of risk factors by treatment of hypertension, diabetes mellitus, and hyperlipidemia is a mainstay of prevention. Smoking cessation and anti-platelet therapy with aspirin are also essential.

Carotid endarterectomy is an integral part of a comprehensive approach that diminishes the devastating morbidity and mortality associated with stroke in patients who are at risk.

In 1952, Fisher described the causal relationship between atherosclerotic disease of the cervical carotid artery and increased risk of cerebral ischemia (1). Soon thereafter, Eastcott and associates reported the successful use of carotid endarterectomy in treating a patient with intermittent hemiplegia (2). The pathophysiological basis of this procedure centers on the removal of the atheromatous plaque as a source of emboli while restoring blood flow through the previously narrowed internal carotid artery.

Carotid endarterectomy rapidly became a widely utilized procedure after its introduction as a surgical means to achieve stroke prophylaxis. Early on, risk-benefit analysis was unavoidably incomplete due to poor definitions of clinical indications and acceptable procedure-related risks. However, since the 1980s, several large-scale trials comparing patients randomized to surgical or medical treatment have critically assessed the utility of this procedure in the prevention of stroke in patients with atherosclerotic disease of the carotid artery. It is clear from several prospective, randomized trials that carotid endarterectomy is effective in reducing the risk of stroke in carefully selected patients.

Indications for Surgery

There are three critical factors that shape the risk-benefit analysis for each patient undergoing consideration for carotid endarterectomy: 1) whether the patient is symptomatic or asymptomatic, 2) the degree of internal carotid artery stenosis, and 3) the risk of perioperative complications of stroke or death. There is strong evidence to suggest that nearly all symptomatic patients have great potential to benefit from carotid endarterectomy, while the procedure may benefit most asymptomatic patients with carotid stenosis.

Although recent innovations in the clinical armamentarium include percutaneous carotid angioplasty and stenting, these experimental techniques have not yet been subjected to rigorous randomized studies with long-term follow-up. At present, carotid stenting is best reserved for the subset of patients with a relative contraindication to surgery, such as prior endarterectomy or history of neck irradiation (3). In the absence of these risk factors, patients should only receive carotid stenting when enrolled in a prospective, randomized trial (4). The results of multicenter studies such as Carotid Revascularization Endarterectomy versus Stenting Trial (CREST) are eagerly anticipated (5). Examination of data on in-stent restenosis rates is also necessary (6).

Review of the data from several prospective, randomized trials enables a critical assessment of the existing evidence on the benefits of carotid endarterectomy. The risk-benefit considerations that guide the clinical decision-making algorithm for symptomatic and asymptomatic patient populations are so different that they must be considered separately.

Symptomatic Carotid Stenosis Trials

The European Carotid Surgery Trial (ECST) included 3024 patients in 97 centers with at least one transient or mild ischemic vascular event referable to the carotid circulation within 6 months of enrollment. Patients underwent angiography and were subsequently randomized to surgery plus best medical care (60%) or to best medical treatment only (40%) (7). Best medical care consisted of antiplatelet medications and control of hypertension. Approximately one third of the enrolled patients in both the surgical and medical groups had either severe stenosis (70%-99%) or moderate stenosis (50%-69%). Outcome events were major strokes and death.

The major finding of the final results of the ECST reported in 1998 is that the frequency of a major stroke or death at 3 years is reduced from 26.5% in the control group to 14.9% in the surgical group, with the absolute risk reduction offered by surgery equaling 11.6%. Stated differently, for 1000 symptomatic patients treated with carotid endarterectomy, 116 major strokes or deaths might be avoided at 3 years. When stenosis was greater than 80%, the long-term risk of stroke without surgery outweighed the risk of surgery (7).

The North American Symptomatic Carotid Endarterectomy Trial (NASCET) enrolled 2885 patients beginning in 1987. Randomization of symptomatic patients with severe stenosis (greater than 70%) was terminated prematurely in 1991 (after 659 patients) due to the finding of an overwhelming reduction in stroke risk among the surgically treated group. The risk of ipsilateral stroke at 2 years was reduced from 26% in the nonsurgical group to 9% in the surgical cohort, yielding an absolute risk reduction of 17% by carotid endarterectomy (Figure 9-1) (8). Thus, compared with medical therapy alone, the number needed to treat in order to prevent one additional ipsilateral stroke in the 2-year period following endarterectomy is 6. The durability of carotid endarterectomy has also been recently established. Compared with a 2.1% rate of disabling ipsilateral stroke at 30 days for patients with severe symptomatic stenosis who underwent endarterectomy, by 5 years the rate was only 5.1% and at 8 years it had increased to 6.7% (9).

The NASCET results for the subgroup of patients with moderate (50%-69%) stenosis have been recently reported. The rate of any ipsilateral stroke with best medical care was 22.2% compared with 15.7% with endarterectomy at 5 years of follow-up. Therefore 15 patients with symptomatic moderate stenosis would require endarterectomy to prevent one ipsilateral stroke during 5 years (9).

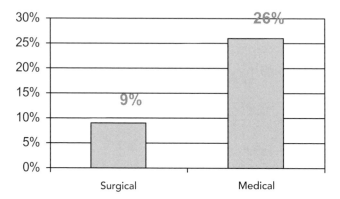

Figure 9-1 Medical versus carotid endarterectomy in symptomatic carotid disease. Ipsilateral stroke risk at two years in patients treated with surgical or medical therapy.

Asymptomatic Carotid Artery Stenosis

In 1995, the Asymptomatic Carotid Atherosclerosis Study (ACAS) supported the hypothesis that carotid endarterectomy reduces the risk of stroke in certain patients with asymptomatic carotid stenosis. This prospective trial randomized 1662 patients with greater than 60% stenosis in 39 centers in North America. All patients received daily aspirin and risk factor management while those randomized to the surgical arm received carotid endarterectomy. The 5-year aggregate risk of ipsilateral stroke and any perioperative stroke or death was reduced from 11% in the medical group to 5.1% for patients receiving prophylactic carotid endarterectomy. This benefit is realized only if carotid endarterectomy is performed by a surgeon with a less than 3% rate of perioperative morbidity and mortality. For this study, complications of diagnostic angiography contributed to perioperative stroke risk. In light of recent technical improvements in MRA and its supplanting of catheter angiography, surgical risks are even further diminished. The ACAS trial reaffirmed the success of carotid endarterectomy as an integral part of stroke prevention in the management of carefully selected patients with asymptomatic atherosclerotic carotid stenosis. The benefits of carotid endarterectomy appear greater for symptomatic carotid stenosis than asymptomatic stenosis (Figure 9-2). This is supported by recommendations from the American Heart Association and National Stroke Council (10,11).

Preoperative Evaluation

Diagnostic evaluation of carotid stenosis includes a thorough neurological examination, carotid Duplex ultrasonography, brain magnetic resonance

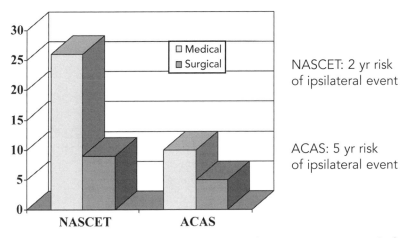

Figure 9-2 Carotid surgery benefits for symptomatic disease (NASCET: 2-year risk of ipsilateral event) versus asymptomatic disease (ACAS: 5-year risk of ipsilateral event).

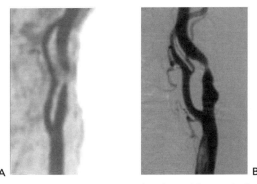

Figure 9-3 **A**, Magnetic resonance angiography of carotid stenosis. **B**, Digital subtraction angiography of carotid stenosis.

imaging and angiography (MRI/MRA) (Figure 9-3, *A*), and, frequently, digital subtraction angiography (DSA) (Figure 9-3, *B*). See Case Study 9-1.

A complete history and examination is central in the diagnostic evaluation of potential candidates for carotid endarterectomy. In addition to assessment of the nature and time course of the neurological event, consideration of potential stroke and cardiac risk factors is essential. Classification of the neurological event into transient ischemic attack or completed stroke is useful in guiding the timing of surgical intervention, which is relatively more urgent in patients with transischemic attacks (TIAs). Preoperative assessment of perioperative risk is warranted, with a thorough medical and cardiac evaluation, including echocardiography. Optimal control of medical conditions such as hypertension and diabetes mellitus should be achieved before surgery (Case Study 9-2).

The initial diagnostic test in the evaluation of carotid artery stenosis is based on ultrasound. Duplex ultrasound combines Doppler analysis of blood flow together with B-mode ultrasound of vessel wall morphology. Because accuracy of ultrasound evaluation of carotid artery stenosis may be variable across operators and laboratories, consideration of accreditation and independent verification of reproducibility is necessary. In order to diminish the risk of misclassification of degree of stenosis, Duplex ultrasound should be combined with MRA of the neck in order to increase the sensitivity and specificity of these noninvasive diagnostic modalities (12,13).

Digital subtraction angiography is currently the gold standard of diagnostic studies for the evaluation of carotid stenosis, with a low risk of adverse neurological complications ranging from 0.45% to 2.6% (14). Although some clinicians obtain a cerebral angiogram routinely as part of the diagnostic evaluation, others proceed to angiography only if there is a discrepancy in the results of the noninvasive studies. However, MRA utilizing 3D contrast-enhanced techniques are rapidly improving and gaining acceptance as a substitute for conventional angiography (14,15). Furthermore, as computed tomography (CT) angiography is increasingly developed, its potential utility as a diagnostic tool will be further analyzed (16).

The degree of stenosis by NASCET criteria is calculated by measuring the diameter of the internal carotid artery at its most narrowed point (N), divided by the diameter of the normal internal carotid artery distal to the stenosis (D) and converting to a percentage (Figure 9-4). This is represented as a formula:

$$\% \text{ stenosis} = (1 - N/D) \times 100$$

For instance, if the lumen of the internal carotid artery measures 5 mm at its narrowest point, and the diameter of the normal internal carotid artery beyond the plaque is 17 mm, the percent stenosis is calculated as:

$$(1 - 5/17) \times 100 = 70\% \text{ stenosis}$$

Timing of Carotid Endarterectomy for Cerebral Ischemia

Acute Stroke

Because the risk for subsequent stroke is highest in the first 30 days after the presenting ischemic symptoms, evaluation for carotid endarterectomy in patients with symptoms of anterior circulation ischemia should proceed urgently after presentation. This allows endarterectomy to be performed in a timely fashion if indicated, based upon the patient's clinical scenario (17,18). Patients with crescendo TIAs or unstable neurological symptoms

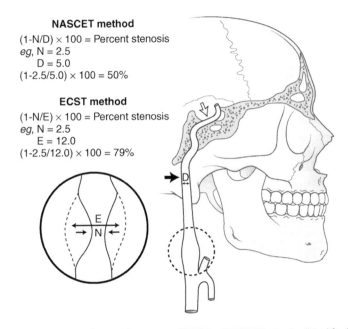

NASCET method
$(1-N/D) \times 100$ = Percent stenosis
eg, N = 2.5
    D = 5.0
$(1-2.5/5.0) \times 100 = 50\%$

ECST method
$(1-N/E) \times 100$ = Percent stenosis
eg, N = 2.5
    E = 12.0
$(1-2.5/12.0) \times 100 = 79\%$

Figure 9-4 Measurement of carotid stenosis of DSA by NASCET criteria. (Modified from Rothwell PM, Eliasziw M, Gutnikov SA, et al. Analysis of pooled data from the randomized controlled trials of endarterectomy for symptomatic carotid stenosis. Lancet. 2003;361:107-16; with permission.)

should be considered for endarterectomy on an emergency basis. In contrast, patients with depressed levels of consciousness, a major fixed neurological deficit, or evidence of cerebral edema or hemorrhage on radiographic studies are not considered immediate surgical candidates. In such patients, carotid endarterectomy is commonly performed after an empiric delay of 3 to 6 weeks (19).

Concurrent Carotid and Coronary Artery Disease

In patients who are candidates for coronary revascularization procedures who are found to have an asymptomatic carotid artery stenosis of greater than 60%, consideration of carotid endarterectomy before coronary artery bypass grafting is supported by ACAS. Similarly, staged carotid endarterectomy followed by coronary revascularization is appropriate for individuals with symptomatic cerebral ischemia and a surgical coronary lesion. The performance of combined cerebral and coronary revascularization during the same operative event and general anesthesia in patients with either asymptomatic or symptomatic carotid stenosis remains controversial, with groups reporting either no increased or slightly higher risk of perioperative complications with combined procedures (20-22). These divergent outcomes are likely the result of differences in patient selection.

Complications of Endarterectomy

The major morbidity of carotid endarterectomy is perioperative stroke, which may occur as a result of diminished cerebral perfusion during intraoperative carotid clamping or distal embolization of plaque during dissection. Strategies to minimize this risk include routine intraoperative monitoring with EEG or transcranial Doppler, as well as performing the operation under local anesthesia. Another strategy is the routine or selective use of shunting as an operative adjunct. Differences in surgical techniques include primary closure, patch grafting, or eversion arteriotomy. Although there are no significant differences in outcome between neurosurgeons and vascular surgeons as a whole, it is well established that improved outcome is directly correlated with increasing individual surgeon volume (23). Regardless of the specific surgical procedure employed, careful attention to technical detail is essential to complication avoidance in carotid endarterectomy.

Cranial nerve injuries are usually transient and completely avoidable with meticulous surgical technique. Hypoglossal nerve injury results in unilateral tongue weakness and dysarthria. Injury to the vagus nerve is usually manifest by dysphagia or hoarseness. A potentially disfiguring facial weakness may occur after injury to the marginal mandibular branch of the facial nerve.

Due to the high incidence of concurrent atherosclerotic disease of the carotid and coronary arteries, myocardial infarction is a major source of potential perioperative morbidity and mortality and has a significant impact on overall outcome at 5 years (24).

During the immediate post-operative period, fluctuations in blood pressure are common, necessitating close neurological and hemodynamic monitoring, preferably in an intensive care unit setting. Close monitoring enables rapid recognition, evaluation, and treatment of new neurological or cardiac events. Patients are typically discharged home on the first or second postoperative day (25).

After carotid endarterectomy, nearly all patients have asymptomatic increases in ipsilateral cerebral blood flow, ranging from 20% to 40% above preoperative baseline, which usually persist for several hours. In a small subset of patients with presumed defective vascular autoregulation, hyperemia of greater magnitude and duration may occur. Cerebral blood flow may be more than doubled compared with baseline and remain elevated for several days to weeks. Patients with cerebral hyperperfusion syndrome usually present with headache, and a small number may progress to develop seizures, hemorrhage, or focal neurological deficits. The incidence of cerebral hyperperfusion syndrome as a devastating complication of endarterectomy is approximately 1%.

Predisposing factors for post-endarterectomy hyperperfusion syndrome include severe carotid stenosis (>70%), a large pressure gradient across the stenosis, contralateral carotid occlusion, poor collateral circulation, and pre- and post-operative hypertension. Establishing the presence of increased cerebreal blood flow is central to confirming a clinical suspicion of cerebral hyperperfusion syndrome. It is typically impossible to distinguish on clinical grounds alone whether neurological deficits occurring after endarterectomy originate from thromboembolism or cerebral hyperperfusion. Various modalities have been employed, including transcranial Doppler ultrasonography, xenon-CT, and SPECT. Intraoperative transcranial Doppler monitoring has been recently employed to predict those patients at higher risk for post-endarterectomy cerebral hyperperfusion in order to identify patients that require more stringent post-operative blood pressure management (26).

Cerebral hyperperfusion leading to intracranial hemorrhage, ipsilateral hemispheric edema, and neurological deficits has also been described to occur after percutaneous transluminal carotid stenting and angioplasty (27).

Follow-Up Care

Aspirin is resumed immediately after surgery and is continued indefinitely. Because atherosclerotic disease is an ongoing process, interval surveillance of restenosis is routinely performed. Patients enrolled in the ACAS study were followed prospectively with Doppler ultrasound to determine restenosis rates. The incidence of early restenosis occurring within 3 to 18 months is 7.6%, while that of late restenosis occurring from 18 to 60 months is 1.9%. The natural history of restenosis is often benign and does not necessarily warrant intervention in all instances (28). Pursuit of medical management, carotid artery stenting, or reoperative carotid endarterectomy is tailored to the individual.

Other Causes of Extracranial Occlusive Carotid Disease

Fibromuscular Dysplasia

As the second most common cause of extracranial carotid artery stenosis, fibromuscular dysplasia is a nonatherosclerotic disease of small-to-medium-sized arteries, which more frequently affects young individuals and women. The most common vascular bed affected is the renal arteries, followed by the cervicocranial carotid arteries, often bilaterally. Three main subtypes have been identified, based upon the arterial wall layer primarily involved. Medial dysplasia comprises the majority of all cases, with its angiographic appearance typically described as a "string of beads." Histologically, these lesions are characterized by regions of thinned media alternating with thickened fibromuscular collagen ridges. In contrast to atherosclerotic carotid disease that is found at the carotid bifurcation, fibromuscular dysplasia usually occurs several centimeters distal to the bifurcation at the C1 and C2 levels.

The etiology of fibromuscular dysplasia is incompletely understood. An inheritance pattern of autosomal dominance with variable penetrance has been suggested, but a number of cases are due to sporadic mutations. Associations have included cigarette smoking, alpha-1-antitypsin deficiency, use of ergotamine preparations, and other diseases such as intracranial aneurysms, neurofibromatosis, pheochromocytoma, Ehlers-Danlos syndrome type IV, Alport's syndrome, and coarctation of the aorta. As a noninflammatory process, fibromuscular dysplasia should be distinguished from vasculitis

When neurologically symptomatic, cervicocranial fibromuscular dysplasia often presents with transient ischemic attack, cerebral infarction, or subarachnoid hemorrhage. Nonspecific symptoms include headache, altered mental status, vertigo, tinnitus, and neck pain. The diagnosis can be established by noninvasive techniques such as carotid Duplex ultrasound and magnetic resonance angiography, but cerebral angiography remains the gold standard.

Treatment is tailored to the presence or absence of symptoms. Antiplatelet agents are recommended for patients without symptoms. Associated intracranial aneurysms should be surgically treated to prevent the risk of rupture. Percutaneous transluminal angioplasty is the treatment of choice in most patients who are symptomatic, although a number of surgical bypass grafting procedures have been effectively employed (29).

Carotid Dissection

Spontaneous or traumatic carotid artery dissection occurs rarely, with an estimated annual incidence of approximately 3 per 100,000. Although these cases account for less than 2% of all ischemic strokes, they account for up to 25% of strokes affecting the young and middle-aged population, with peak incidence occurring during the fourth decade.

Dissections with traumatic origin are thought to arise from contact with bony structures such as the cervical vertebrae, transverse process of C2, or the styloid process. Spontaneous dissections can be associated with atherosclerosis or fibromuscular dysplasia and are also frequently linked to minor trauma. A history of minor trauma with neck rotation or hyperextension as a precipitating event is often elicited. The inciting event is an intimal tear, leading to entry of blood into the tunica media to form an intramural hematoma, or the false lumen. If the dissection is subintimal, the arterial lumen becomes stenotic; however, if the dissection is subadventitial, a pseudoaneurysm may form.

Presentation is typically with pain on one side of the face, head, or neck, with Horner's syndrome, and subsequent ipsilateral cerebral ischemia. Other clinical manifestations include lower cranial nerve palsies and pulsatile tinnitus. From one half to nearly all patients with spontaneous carotid artery dissection report cerebral or retinal ischemic symptoms.

Cerebral angiography is the diagnostic test of choice. However, MRA and CT angiography is becoming increasingly developed to produce high-resolution images. The classic appearance of carotid artery dissection is irregular stenosis beginning centimeters distal to the carotid bifurcation and extending for various lengths into the cervical internal carotid artery but not beyond the entry of the internal carotid artery into the skull base. Arterial occlusion is visualized as having a tapered, flame-like appearance. Approximately one third of patients have fusiform aneurysmal dilatations.

The clinical course of carotid dissection is usually shaped by the severity of the initial ischemic insult. Nearly all carotid stenoses resolve, the majority of occlusions become recanalized, and some aneurysmal dilatations diminish in size within the first 2 to 3 months after the dissection. Because the cerebral infarcts arising from carotid dissections are thromboembolic rather than due to hemodynamic flow failure, treatment consists of anticoagulation with intravenous heparin followed by oral warfarin for 3-6 months, with a target international normalized ratio of 2.0 to 3.0. There is a very limited role for surgical or endovascular treatment if ischemic symptoms persist despite therapeutic anticoagulation (30).

Conclusion

Recent advances in therapeutic interventions for stroke have occurred in the form of thrombolysis and the ongoing development of neuroprotective pharmacological agents. However, stroke remains the third leading cause of morbidity and mortality in the United States, with an enormous economic and social burden. Prevention remains the cornerstone of management of this difficult medical condition. Medical managment can make an impact on modifiable risk factors. Carotid stenting requires more scrupulous study with long-term follow-up before direct comparisons to carotid endarterectomy are valid. In the majority of cases, carotid endarterectomy is an enduring prophylactic procedure with well-proven efficacy that is a crucial part of the comprehensive management of patients at risk for stroke.

Referral to an experienced neurosurgeon or vascular surgeon is recommended for most patients with symptomatic high-grade carotid artery stenosis. For other patients with carotid artery disease who are high-risk or have less clear-cut indications for intervention, consultation with a neurologist in addition to a surgeon or interventional neuroradiologist is recommended.

Given the controversial nature of carotid endarterectomy, it is necessary for physicians to remain up-to-date on the relevant literature. Reference 31 provides a recent evidence-based review.

Case Study 9-1

A 65-year-old man with hypertension and diabetes mellitus presents complaining of right arm numbness and weakness lasting 30 minutes. On neurological examination in the ER, he is completely intact. He is admitted for work-up of a TIA. Head CT demonstrates no abnormalities. Carotid duplex Dopplers reveal severe, 80%-99% left internal carotid artery stenosis. Brain MRI demonstrates diffusion-weighted changes in the middle cerebral artery distribution. Severe, 90% narrowing of the distal portion of the internal carotid artery is present on the neck MRA (Figure 9-3, *A*). Cerebral angiogram reveals 70% stenosis of the left internal carotid artery (Figure 9-3, *B*). Carotid endarterectomy is indicated for severe, symptomatic carotid artery stenosis. Postoperatively, the patient is monitored in the ICU; he is discharged home on the following day with instructions to continue daily aspirin. He is counseled to have regular monitoring of his blood pressure and serum glucose levels in order to reduce his risk factors for subsequent stroke.

Case Study 9-2

A 70-year-old woman with hypertension and cigarette smoking is found to have a carotid bruit during a routine office visit. She denies any prior episodes of visual changes, paresthesias, weakness, or difficulty speaking. She is referred for screening carotid Doppler ultrasound, which reveals 80%-99% stenosis of the right internal carotid artery. This is subsequently confirmed with a neck MRA that demonstrates 80% stenosis. Brain MRI findings include only periventricular white matter changes. Prophylactic carotid endarterectomy is recommended for asymptomatic carotid stenosis. Based upon ACAS data, her risk of stroke over the next 5 years will be diminished from 11% to 5%, provided that her procedure is performed by an experienced surgeon with a perioperative complication rate of less than 3%. The patient is advised to take daily aspirin, continue regular check-ups for blood pressure monitoring, and be once again counseled on smoking cessation.

REFERENCES

1. **Fisher CM**. Transient monocular blindness associated with hemiplegia. Arch Ophthalmol. 1952;47:167-203.
2. **Eastcott HG, Pickering GW, Rob CG**. Reconstruction of internal carotid artery in a patient with intermittent attacks of hemiplegia. Lancet. 1954;2:994-8.
3. **Gasparis AP, Ricotta L, Cuadra SA, et al**. High-risk carotid endarterectomy: fact or fiction? J Vasc Surg. 2003;37:40-6.
4. **Chaturvedi S, Fessler R**. Angioplasty and stenting for stroke prevention: good questions that need answers. Neurology. 2002;59:664-8.
5. **Hobson RW**. Update on the Carotid Revascularization Endarterectomy versus Stent Trial (CREST) protocol. J Am Coll Surg. 2002;194:S9-14.
6. **Schillinger M, Exner M, Mlekusch W, et al**. Acute-phase response after stent implantation in the carotid artery: association with 6-month in-stent restenosis. Radiology. 2003;227:516-21.
7. Randomised trial of endarterectomy for recently symptomatic carotid stenosis: final results of the MRC European Carotid Surgery Trial (ECST). Lancet. 1998;351:1379-87.
8. **North American Symptomatic Carotid Endarterectomy Trial Collaborators**. Beneficial effect of carotid endarterectomy in symptomatic patients with high-grade carotid stenosis. N Engl J Med. 1991;325:445-53.
9. **Barnett HJ, Taylor DW, Eliasziw M, et al**. Benefit of carotid endarterectomy in patients with symptomatic moderate or severe stenosis. North American Symptomatic Carotid Endarterectomy Trial Collaborators. N Engl J Med. 1998;339:1415-25.
10. **Biller J, Feinberg WM, Castaldo JE, et al**. Guidelines for carotid endarterectomy: a statement for healthcare professionals from a special writing group of the Stroke Council, American Heart Association. Circulation. 1998;97:501-9.
11. **Biller J, Feinberg WM, Castaldo JE, et al**. Guidelines for carotid endarterectomy: a statement for healthcare professionals from a special writing group of the Stroke Council, American Heart Association. Stroke. 1998;29:554-62.
12. **Nederkoorn PJ, Mali WP, Eikelboom BC, et al**. Preoperative diagnosis of carotid artery stenosis: accuracy of noninvasive testing. Stroke. 2002;33:2003-8.
13. **Johnston DCC, Goldstein LB**. Clinical carotid endarterectomy decision making: noninvasive vascular imaging versus angiography. Neurology. 2001;56:1009-15.
14. **Remonda L, Senn P, Barth A, et al**. Contrast-enhanced 3D MR angiography of the carotid artery: comparison with conventional digital subtraction angiography. Am J Neuroradiol. 2002;23:213-9.
15. **Sundgren PC, Sunden P, Lindgren A, et al**. Carotid artery stenosis: contrast-enhanced MR angiography with two different scan times compared with digital subtraction angiography. Neuroradiology. 2002;44:592-9.
16. **Randoux B, Marro B, Koskas F, et al**. Carotid artery stenosis: prospective comparison of CT, three-dimensional gadolinium-enhanced MR, and conventional angiography. Radiology. 2001;220:179-85.
17. **Blaser T, Hofmann K, Buerger T, et al**. Risk of stroke, transient ischemic attack, and vessel occlusion before endarterectomy in patients with symptomatic severe carotid stenosis. Stroke. 2002;33:1057-62.
18. **Eckstein HH, Ringleb P, Dorfler A, et al**. The carotid surgery for ischemic stroke trial: a prospective observational study on carotid endarterectomy in the early period after ischemic stroke. J Vasc Surg. 2002;36:997-1004.
19. **Loftus CM, Quest DO**. Technical issues in carotid artery surgery, 1995. Neurosurgery. 1995;36:629-47.
20. **Farooq MM, Reil TD, Gelabert HA, et al**. Combined carotid endarterectomy and coronary bypass: a decade's experience at UCLA. Cardiovasc Surg. 2001;9:339-44.
21. **Brown KR, Kresowik TF, Chin MH, et al**. Multistate population-based outcomes of combined carotid endarterectomy and coronary artery bypass. J Vasc Surg. 2003;37:32-9.

22. Estes JM, Khabbaz KR, Barnatan M, et al. Outcome after combined carotid endarterectomy and coronary artery bypass is related to patient selection. J Vasc Surg. 2001;33:1179-84.

23. Cowan JA Jr., Dimick JB, et al. Surgeon volume as an indicator of outcomes after carotid endarterectomy. an effect independent of specialty practice and hospital volume. J Am Coll Surg. 2002;195:814-21.

24. Gates PC, Eliasziw M, Algra A, et al. Identifying patients with symptomatic carotid artery disease at high and low risk of severe myocardial infarction and cardiac death. Stroke. 2002;33:2413-6.

25. Angevine PD, Choudhri TF, Huang J, et al. Significant reductions in length of stay after carotid endarterectomy can be safely accomplished without modifying either anesthetic technique or postoperative ICU monitoring. Stroke. 1999;30:2341-6.

26. Baker CJ, Mayer SA, Prestigiacomo CJ, et al. Diagnosis and monitoring of cerebral hyper-fusion after carotid endarterectomy with single photon emission computed tomography: case report. Neurosurgery. 1998;43:157-60; discussion 160-1.

27. Meyers PM, Higashida RT, Phatouros CC, et al. Cerebral hyperperfusion syndrome after percutaneous transluminal stenting of the craniocervical arteries. Neurosurgery. 2000;47:335-43; discussion 343-5.

28. Moore WS, Kempczinski RF, Nelson JJ, et al. Recurrent carotid stenosis: results of the asymptomatic carotid atherosclerosis study. Stroke. 1998;29:2018-25.

29. Begelman SM, Olin JW. Fibromuscular dysplasia. Curr Opin Rheumatol. 2000;12:41-7.

30. Schievink WI. Spontaneous dissection of the carotid and vertebral arteries. N Engl J Med. 2001;344:898-906.

31. Chaturvedi S, Bruno A, Feasby T, et al. Carotid endarterectomy: an evidence-based review. Report of the Therapeutics and Technology Assessment Subcommittee of the American Association of Neurologists. Neurology. 2005;65:794-801. See also: www.aan.com/professionals/practice/index/cfm.

Chapter 10

Cardioembolic Stroke

ADRIAN GOLDSZMIDT, MD

Key Points

- Cardioembolic stroke can be definitively diagnosed in patients with a clear cardiac source in the absence of significant cerebrovascular disease.
- Clinical presentations that result in diagnosis of cardiac embolism likely include history of cardiac disease, palpitations or chest pain, or stroke in a young patient without risk factors for atherosclerosis.
- Patients with atrial fibrillation due to rheumatic heart disease have a 17- to 18-fold increased risk of stroke. These patients should in almost all instances receive anticoagulation with warfarin.
- Acute management within the first 6 hours of symptom onset is similar to the management of other ischemic stroke.
- Patients with a cardioembolic stroke who can be treated within 3 hours of symptom onset are candidates for thrombolytic therapy with t-PA.
- Intra-arterial thrombolysis within 6 hours of symptom onset should be considered for patients who cannot receive IV t-PA within 3 hours.
- Heparin should be reserved for patients who are at higher than average risk for recurrent stroke from a clear cardiac source and at low risk for hemorrhagic transformation.

Emboli arising from the heart account for 15%-20% of ischemic strokes. While the cardioembolic stroke may be suggested on the basis of the patient's history and presentation, few features by themselves are sensitive or specific enough to firmly make the diagnosis, which makes appropriate testing crucial. Patients may have more than one potential cause for stroke, and many patients have atherosclerotic cerebrovascular disease in addition to a potential cardiac source of stroke. Cardioembolic stroke can be definitively diagnosed in the presence of a clear cardiac source (by history and/or testing) in the absence of significant cerebrovascular disease. Often, a complete work-up reveals that patients with embolic stroke have multiple potential sources but no single clear cause. In the Stroke Prevention in Atrial Fibrillation trial, only 52% of all strokes in patients with known atrial fibrillation were classified as "probably cardioembolic"; 24% were noncardioembolic and 24% were classified as uncertain cause (1). Clinical judgment is therefore required to determine the cause of the stroke. Patients with embolic strokes are more likely to undergo hemorrhagic transformation; this occurs 20% of the time. Large areas of hemorrhage deep in the infarct, thought secondary to reperfusion after the embolism clears, are more specific to cardiogenic embolism. Petechial hemorrhage may also occur.

In 20%-30% of patients, no source of stroke is found even after extensive workup; in those cases, all diagnosed potential causes should be appropriately treated. It is likely that many of these patients with "cryptogenic stroke" have cardiac emboli, and adequate cardiac testing is vital in these patients. Understanding the potential role of the heart in ischemic stroke is necessary for the prevention of stroke in at-risk patients and in working up patients with suspected cardioembolic stroke.

Diagnosis

The diagnosis of cardioembolic stroke can only be made in the appropriate clinical setting with supportive diagnostic evidence (electrocardiography, rhythm monitoring, echocardiography). Distinguishing cardioembolic embolism from other sources of embolism can be difficult. Clues come from the patient's history and presentation, as well as initial testing. A final diagnosis of cardiac embolism depends on finding a cardiac source in the absence of other potential causes. Evidence of non-lacunar infarction in multiple territories and evidence of systemic emboli are clues to a likely cardiac source. Aortic arch plaque can, however, present similarly. About one third of ischemic stroke patients will have a potential cardiac source of embolism suggested by history or examination; in turn, one third of patients with a potential cardiac source will have concomitant cerebrovascular atherosclerosis and potential artery-to-artery emboli. Proximal atherosclerotic embolic sources (carotid artery stenosis, vertebral and/or basilar disease, and aortic arch plaque) should be worked up concurrently even if cardiogenic embolism is strongly suspected.

Clinical Presentation

No clinical presentation is sufficiently specific to diagnose cardiac embolism. Nonetheless, there are several features that make cardiogenic embolism more likely: a history of cardiac disease (myocardial infarction, valvular disease, or atrial fibrillation); palpitations or chest pain; and stroke in a young patient without risk factors for atherosclerosis. Most cardiac emboli lodge in the middle cerebral artery (MCA) stem or branches, the distal basilar artery, or the posterior cerebral arteries. Cerebral emboli can also lodge at branch points, or proximally in the cervical vessels, especially in the presence of pre-existing stenosis. Less commonly, large subcortical infarcts (>1.5 cm), suggesting obstruction of more than one penetrating artery, may be due to cardiac emboli. Last, even small deep infarcts typically attributed to hypertension can be caused by cardiogenic emboli. The lack of the typical "lacunar" risk factors (older age, hypertension, diabetes) is usually a clue in these cases that extensive cardiac investigation is warranted.

The specific clinical symptoms are referable to the function of the brain served by the affected artery. Certain clinical syndromes—Wernicke's aphasia without hemiparesis (from a dominant hemisphere inferior division MCA lesion) and homonymous hemianopia (from the PCA)—are overrepresented in patients with cardioembolic stroke. Symptoms most commonly occur during activity. Symptoms are maximal at onset in about 80% of patients with cardiac embolism. A minority of patients will have symptoms that progress after onset; this is thought to be due to an embolism which initially lodges proximally (without disrupting collateral flow to the more distal regions) and then moves more distally.

Compared with non-cardiac origin strokes, cardioembolic strokes are more likely abrupt in onset, are more likely large, and are more often associated with hemorrhagic transformation. Infarcts in multiple territories are also suggestive of a central or cardiac source. Transient ischemic attacks, especially in the same vascular territory, are far less common in patients with cardioembolic stroke than in patients with large artery stenosis as the cause of their stroke. However, patients with cardioembolic stroke are more likely to have a history of strokes in other vascular territories. Cardiac embolism is also a more common stroke type in younger patients.

Diagnostic Testing

Review of electrocardiograms obtained by emergency medical services on the scene may help diagnose a paroxysmal rhythm disorder. Because >20% of non-fatal acute myocardial infarctions (MIs) may be silent, it is important to rule out acute MI in all patients who present with stroke. Specific questions about angina and anginal equivalents should be asked. An EKG should be ordered in all cases, and cardiac enzymes ordered if indicated.

In addition to changes suggestive of acute MI, EKG may show arrhythmia, left atrial enlargement, left ventricular hypertrophy, or anterior Q waves suggestive of prior anterior MI with a hypokinetic or akinetic segment. Crochetage (an M-shaped bifid notch on the ascent or peak of the R wave in inferior EKG leads) is sometimes seen in patients with patent foramen ovale (PFO).

Prolonged cardiac rhythm monitoring (in-hospital telemetry or Holter monitoring) may reveal dysrhythmias in patients with stroke. Whether to perform cardiac rhythm monitoring in all patients with ischemic stroke remains controversial. While the yield of routine cardiac rhythm monitoring is relatively low, the evidence favoring anticoagulation of patients with atrial fibrillation with warfarin is strong enough to warrant monitoring in almost all patients. At many institutions, stroke patients are admitted to a stroke unit with cardiac telemetry for the first few days. The literature suggests a yield of 2%-4% unsuspected arrhythmia rate (atrial fibrillation, sick sinus syndrome) in stroke patients.

Imaging can suggest cardiac embolism as well. Cardiac embolism should be suspected in the presence of a wedge-shaped infarct on CT or MRI, abutting the cortical surface. This is especially true in the absence of coexisting atherosclerotic disease (which can result in artery-to-artery emboli, which would have a similar radiographic appearance). The CT scan can be normal in the first 6-24 hours, but there are subtle findings that can suggest ischemia. One is the hyper-dense MCA sign; it is associated with poor patient outcome (see Chapter 4). This is a density seen on CT in the area of the MCA. There can be loss of grey/white differentiation, loss of clear delineation of the lentiform nucleus, and subtle hypodensity seen in the area of ischemia early on. These signs are difficult to see often and require a trained neurologist or neuroradiologist to evaluate.

Conventional angiography is rarely performed in acute stroke unless the patient is a candidate for intra-arterial thrombolysis or there are abnormalities on noninvasive vascular imaging that need further delineation. Cerebral angiography can show the presence of occlusions in the absence of atherosclerotic disease, highly suggestive of cardiac embolism; or the presence of "vanishing occlusions," filling defects that vanish on a follow-up study. Transcranial ultrasonography (transcranial doppler [TCD]) can also show lack of flow in an affected vessel, for example an MCA, with subsequent recanalization, which is diagnostic of an embolic infarct.

Management

Acute management of cardioembolic stroke patients within the first 6 hours of symptom onset is similar to the management of other ischemic stroke patients. Patients with a cardioembolic stroke who can be treated within 3 hours of symptom onset are candidates for thrombolytic therapy with t-PA.

Patients with cardioembolic stroke treated with t-PA in the NINDS t-PA trial improved about 25% more often than those receiving placebo, with a similar complication rate. Patients who should not be considered for t-PA include those who are on warfarin with a PT > 15 (or INR > 1.7); those with minor deficits who are not likely to benefit from treatment; and those whose deficits are rapidly improving at the time therapy is being considered (see Table 7-1 in Chapter 7 for more contraindications). In some cases, intravenous t-PA may be considered for patients beyond 3 hours after symptom onset who show a large perfusion deficit on MRI with a small lesion on diffusion MRI imaging. Intravenous t-PA, however, is not FDA approved beyond 3 hours after a stroke.

Intra-arterial thrombolysis (with t-PA or prourokinase) within 6 hours of symptom onset may also be considered, at experienced treatment centers, for patients who cannot get intravenous t-PA within 3 hours. In a randomized clinical trial, patients with MCA syndromes and appropriate angiographic findings had a 15% better chance of a good outcome if treated with intra-arterial thrombolysis. This treatment is not yet widely available and does not have FDA approval.

For patients in whom thrombolytic therapy is not an option, the goal of treatment should be to maximize cerebral perfusion (to improve outcome from the current stroke) while preventing further emboli. The role of heparin in this circumstance remains controversial. While heparin has never conclusively been shown to prevent recurrent cardiac emboli, small studies of cardiac emboli in the 1980s showed a trend toward fewer recurrent strokes in patients treated with heparin. More recent data, however, have cast doubt on the efficacy of heparin (2). Although many neurologists taking care of stroke patients continue to use heparin, its role even in cardiogenic emboli has been increasingly questioned. A joint committee of the American Academy of Neurology and the American Stroke Association issued a report in 2002 summarizing the existing data on the use of heparin in all strokes (3). The committee reached the following conclusion: "IV, unfractionated heparin or high-dose LMW heparin/heparinoids are not recommended for any specific subgroup of patients with acute ischemic stroke that is based on any presumed stroke mechanism or location (e.g., cardioembolic)."

In a post-stroke setting, the role of anticoagulation is secondary prevention. The potential benefit of heparin should be understood in light of the patient's risk for recurrent stroke and heparin's ability to prevent recurrence. The risk of recurrent emboli has varied widely in the literature. Some estimates are as high as 5% within 48 hours, with an additional 12% over 2 weeks. Some recent large prospective studies have given a substantially lower risk of stroke in the setting of atrial fibrillation. In the International Stroke Trial of nearly 20,000 patients (of whom 3169 had atrial fibrillation), the risk of recurrent stroke for patients with atrial fibrillation not receiving either heparin or aspirin was 2.5% at 1 week (4). Even if heparin were 100%

effective at preventing recurrence, and risk free, the benefit would not be large in this setting. The risk of hemorrhage in this trial using high-dose subcutaneous heparin was close to 1% greater than that seen in placebo-treated patients. This study did report a high risk of early death within 14 days after stroke in patients with atrial fibrillation. However, this risk was not because of recurrent stroke, but neurological damage from the initial strokes, due to edema and other complications. The patients with atrial fibrillation were also older than other patients in the trial. There was no effect of heparin on death rate.

Even without the use of heparin, hemorrhagic transformation occurs over 30% of the time in cardioembolic stroke. Usually, this is asymptomatic; it is associated with clinical worsening in only 5% of patients. The risk of hemorrhagic transformation increases with increasing infarct size, and increases further with anticoagulant therapy (especially supratherapeutic dosing or with an initial bolus) or uncontrolled hypertension. Hemorrhagic transformation usually occurs within the first 48 hours. To minimize risk of intracranial bleeding, it is common practice to withhold initiation of anticoagulation for 48 hours or so after intracranial hemorrhage or large stroke. If necessary, it can be withheld for up to a few weeks (see Chapter 5).

In practice, heparin, if used at all, should be reserved for patients who are at higher than average risk for recurrent stroke from a clear cardiac source (rheumatic heart disease, prosthetic valves, acute MI, cardiomyopathy, or thrombi visualized on echocardiography) and at low risk of hemorrhagic transformation. A large infarct suggested by examination (for example lethargy, gaze preference, dense hemiplegia and aphasia, indicative of a large MCA infarction) or on initial CT (>3 cm, or more than 33% of the MCA territory) is a contraindication to immediate anticoagulation with heparin. Anticoagulation should be used with extreme caution in patients with uncontrolled hypertension. If begun, heparin should be started at up to 1000 units/hour, without a bolus, and adjusted to achieve an aPTT of 1.5-2.5 times control.

For patients with cardioembolic stroke not anticoagulated with heparin (the vast majority), aspirin 160-325 mg per day has been shown to safely reduce recurrence, although the effect is not large. This should be begun as soon as possible after initial evaluation.

The data for long-term use of warfarin are much stronger (as reviewed below). Warfarin should be begun as soon as possible in all patients with suspected atrial fibrillation, left atrial thrombus, or cardiomyopathy. After 48 hours, the risk of hemorrhagic transformation declines, and warfarin can be started safely for secondary prevention at that point.

Identification and Management of Specific Sources of Cardiogenic Embolism

Numerous cardiac lesions are associated with embolism; some of these conditions confer a high risk, while in others, emboli are rare. In some cases, such as in the presence of atrial fibrillation, the finding is significant enough to warrant treatment (although other potential causes of stroke should still be sought). In other cases, the cardiac abnormality may or may not have an association with the stroke, depending on the clinical circumstance. For example, PFO is often seen in normal patients and should not routinely be considered the cause of stroke unless the patient has a DVT or is at high risk for one.

Atrial Fibrillation

Atrial fibrillation is an arrhythmia in which there is an electrical and mechanical change in heart function, resulting in stasis of blood in the atria and subsequent thrombus formation. Non-valvular atrial fibrillation is the source of 45% of cardioembolic strokes. If cardiac emboli account for 15%-20% of all ischemic strokes, then 7%-10% of all strokes are due to non-valvular atrial fibrillation. Among all patients with atrial fibrillation, 70% have non-valvular atrial fibrillation. In 20% of cases, atrial fibrillation is due to rheumatic heart disease with mitral stenosis. The remaining 10% of patients have no obvious heart disease ("lone atrial fibrillation").

Compared with the population as a whole, those with atrial fibrillation due to rheumatic heart disease have a 17-to-18-fold increased risk of stroke. Patients with non-valvular atrial fibrillation have a risk of stroke that is five times that of the population as a whole. While some studies have reported a lower risk of embolism for patients with paroxysmal atrial fibrillation compared with chronic atrial fibrillation, other studies have shown that both paroxysmal and chronic atrial fibrillation confer similar thromboembolic risk.

Lone atrial fibrillation is defined as atrial fibrillation unassociated with clinical, EKG, or other evidence of heart disease, and without prior history of embolic events; it occurs predominantly in younger patients, mainly men. The risk of stroke in these patients is quite low, about 0.5% annually for those under 60 years old. However, older patients (above age 60) and patients with hypertension even in the absence of overt heart disease or valvular abnormalities may be at higher risk of stroke.

The prevalence of atrial fibrillation is <2% of the adult population in the United States, but is much more common in elderly Americans. The prevalence is less than 1% in patients aged 40-65, but rises to >5% in those over age 75. One in three patients with atrial fibrillation will have an ischemic stroke in their lifetime. Overall, the annual risk of stroke with atrial fibrillation is 5% per year. The Stroke Prevention in Atrial Fibrillation III investigators (5) stratified patients with atrial fibrillation into several risk groups:

1. Patients below 65, without risk factors associated with increased stroke rates (hypertension, diabetes, prior stroke or TIA, coronary arterial disease or congestive heart failure) (Table 10-1). These patients have an annual stroke risk of 1%.

2. Patients with hypertension but no other risk factors who had an annual stroke risk of 3.5% per year.

3. Patients with systolic blood pressure greater than 160 mm Hg, left ventricular dysfunction, and women over 75. These factors increased the risk of stroke somewhat, to 6% per year.

4. Patients with a history of prior stroke or TIA. In these patients, annual stroke risk was 12%.

Transesophageal echocardiography (TEE) can offer meaningful information in the management of patients with atrial fibrillation by demonstrating left atrial thrombus, spontaneous echo contrast ("smoke"), or aortic plaque. These factors increase the likelihood of cardioembolic stroke. However, the benefit for warfarin in patients with atrial fibrillation is well enough established that patients with stroke and atrial fibrillation should in

---

Table 10-1 Independent Predictors of Stroke in Nonvalvular Atrial Fibrillation

Consistent Predictors
- Advancing age
- Hypertension
- Previous stroke/TIA
- Left ventricular dysfunction

Possible Predictor
- Diabetes
- Systolic blood pressure >160 mm Hg
- Hormone replacement therapy, women >75 years old
- Coronary artery disease/prior myocardial infarction
- TEE appendage thrombi

Not Predictive
- Left atrial diameter
- Intermittency of atrial fibrillation

From Hart RG, Halperin JL. Atrial fibrillation and stroke: concepts and controversies. Stroke. 2001;32:803-8; with permission.

almost all instances be anticoagulated with warfarin, even if another cause of their infarct is suspected.

Valvular Heart Disease

While cardioembolism from rheumatic heart disease usually occurs in the setting of atrial fibrillation, 20% of emboli in patients with rheumatic heart disease occur in sinus rhythm. Often, a systemic embolus is the presenting sign of mitral stenosis. Patients with rheumatic mitral stenosis and systemic embolism should be anticoagulated with warfarin. Patients with left atrial size greater than 5.5 cm are also considered to be at high risk for emboli. Recurrent systemic emboli despite adequate anticoagulation may be an indication for mitral valve surgery or commissurotomy.

Left Atrial Thrombus

Left atrial thrombus is most commonly seen in the setting of atrial fibrillation but may also be present in the setting of an enlarged left atrium or with mitral stenosis. The majority of left atrial thrombi occur in the left atrial appendage. These are far better seen by TEE, rarely by TTE. Left atrial thrombus may be seen in patients with unsuspected paroxysmal atrial fibrillation who are in sinus rhythm at the time of presentation; the left atrium should be explored fully in patients with embolic stroke with no source.

Prosthetic Valves

Systemic emboli occur in the setting of prosthetic heart valves at a rate of 1%-4% per year. Mitral valves have a higher rate of embolism than do aortic valves. The risk is highest in patients with atrial fibrillation. The risk of emboli also depends on the valve type: bioprosthetic valves have a lower risk than mechanical valves. Caged-ball and tilting disc valves are associated with increased risk of embolism, whereas bileaflet valves are associated with lower risk.

Mitral Valve Prolapse

The association with cardioembolic stroke with mitral valve prolapse (MVP) is controversial. Reports of the incidence of mitral valve prolapse (MVP) in the population are as high as 35%, with most studies in the 5%-15% range. MVP has also been shown to occur with increased frequency (as high as 30%) in young patients with ischemic stroke. Mitral valve prolapse is also associated with an increased risk of bacterial endocarditis.

Part of the variability in the literature comes from echocardiographic criteria for MVP. Early M-mode and 2-dimensional echocardiography tended to overestimate the prevalence. More recent studies with strict echocardiographic criteria incorporating three-dimensional analysis of valve shape report a population prevalence of less than 3% (6). In this study, only one of 84 patients with MVP had cerebrovascular disease. A recent case-control study of patients older than 45 with ischemic stroke or TIA, again using strict echocardiographic criteria, found an incidence of MVP of 1.9%, lower than that in the control subjects (7). MVP was present in 2.8% of patients with cryptogenic stroke, nearly identical to the incidence in the control group. In another study, most patients with stroke and MVP had other risk factors for stroke, and the mechanism of the stroke was not likely a cardiac embolism.

MVP should be viewed as a spectrum, with patients who have marked myxomatous proliferation of the valves, with elongation of the chordae at one end, and patients with normal-appearing valve leaflets with some bulging into the atrium at the other end. Patients with normal-appearing valve leaflets likely are not at elevated risk for stroke.

Overall, the risk of embolic complications for patients with MVP is low, and the presence of MVP alone does not place the patient at high risk for recurrent stroke. However, older patients with redundant leaflets and thickened valves may be at higher risk for stroke. There are no published data on antiplatelet therapy or anticoagulation for patients with MVP and stroke or TIA. Aspirin or other antiplatelet agents are most often recommended.

Bacterial and Nonbacterial Endocarditis

Bacterial endocarditis accounts for less than 1% of all embolic strokes. However, the clinical incidence of systemic embolism is high in patients with bacterial endocarditis, occurring 11%-43% of the time. Stroke occurs in up to 20%. Pathologically, up to 65% of patients have evidence of embolism at autopsy. Vegetations larger than 10 mm, and those attached to the mitral valve, especially the anterior leaflet, are at highest risk of embolizing. Patients may develop ischemic stroke, hemorrhage, abscess, or encephalopathy, presumably from cerebritis. Most strokes occur within 48 hours of diagnosis. The risk of stroke is 6% per day before the initiation of appropriate antibiotics. After the infection is controlled, the risk of stroke is low, and treatment should be directed at appropriate control of the underlying infection. The most common species of bacteria are viridans streptococci, enterococci, and coagulase-positive or negative staphylococci. Fungal infections can be seen in immunocompromised patients, such as those with HIV or malignancy. The mainstays of diagnosis are blood cultures and echocardiography. Transesophageal echocardiography has proven more sensitive than transthoracic echocardiography (TTE) in detecting small vegetations, especially on the mitral valve.

Fever is the most common presenting sign, although it may be minimal or absent in elderly or debilitated patients. Splinter hemorrhages, petechiae, and Osler's nodes may be seen but are often absent. The diagnosis should be considered in any patient who presents with a stroke and fever, a stroke and a new cardiac murmur, or multiple systemic emboli.

Populations at risk for bacterial endocarditis include patients with pre-existing valvular abnormalities, especially mitral valve prolapse, which accounts for up to 30% of native valve endocarditis not related to drug abuse or nosocomial infection. The risk of developing endocarditis with MVP is three to eight times that in the population as a whole. Also at risk are patients with HIV, and intravenous drug abusers, who most commonly have *Staphylocccus* species and more commonly have right-sided endo-carditis. Patients with prosthetic valves are at increased risk as well.

There is no proven role for anticoagulation for patients with native valve endocarditis. *For patients with prosthetic valve endocarditis, anticoagulation therapy should be continued.* If anticoagulation in this setting is discontinued, the risk of subsequent embolism is high (42%); with continuing anticoagu-lation, the risk is 12%. If embolism does occur, CT scan should be per-formed to rule out hemorrhage, and anticoagulation should be discontinued for several days because of the increased risk of hemorrhage in this setting.

Intracerebral hemorrhage due to mycotic aneurysm, arteritis, or hemor-rhage into an infarct, occurs 5% of the time in bacterial endocarditis. Subarachnoid hemorrhage can also occur. Mycotic aneurysms occur at branch points, generally distally over the cerebral cortex, usually in branches of the MCA. Patients may present with unremitting headache or other signs of meningeal irritation. Cerebral angiography is required for evaluation. Ruptured aneurysms should be repaired surgically if feasible; unruptured aneurysms that are found during the course of antimicrobial therapy may resolve without intervention but should be followed (with conventional, magnetic resonance, or CT angiography). A growing lesion, however, should be treated surgically.

Most patients respond well to antibiotic therapy; embolic events are rare beyond 48 hours after initiation of appropriate antibiotic therapy. Surgery (valve replacement) should be reserved for patients who continue to embolize or who have significant valve dysfunction. Some authors recommend early surgery for patients with endocarditis caused by *Staphylo-coccus aureus* and vegetations that are visible by transthoracic echo-cardiography because of increased risk for arterial emboli with *S. aureus* and large vegetations.

Non-bacterial thrombotic endocarditis most often occurs in malignancy (most commonly in lung adenocarcinoma), disseminated intravascular coagulation, in the setting of connective tissue disorders such as systemic lupus erythematosis, and with other illnesses including acquired immuno-deficiency syndrome. It is a common cause of stroke in these conditions, although diagnosis can be difficult. Murmurs may or may not be present, and there are no specific clinical signs; sometimes the underlying disorder is not initially apparent. Echocardiography is the most useful diagnostic modality, and the vegetations must be distinguished from bacterial endocarditis. Vegetations composed of fibrin and platelets form on an uninfected valve leaflet. In autopsy series, the rate of embolism (to renal and cerebral arteries) is 40%; in an ante-mortem surgical series, 33% of patients had proven or suspected emboli.

Patients with antiphospholipid antibody syndrome have abnormalities of cardiac valves about 1/3 of the time. Half of these patients have primary antiphospholipid antibody syndrome, the other half have antiphospholipid antibodies in the setting of systemic lupus erythematosis. Patients with lupus and antiphospholipid antibodies are much more likely than those without antibodies to have valvular abnormalities. The term "Libman-Sacks endocarditis" is sometimes used for this entity; the findings in Libman-Sacks range from lesions on the valvular and mural endocardium, with vegetations on the ventricular aspect of the posterior mitral leaflet, to thickened, functionally impaired cardiac valves. Some authors consider Libman-Sacks to be a subset of nonbacterial thrombotic endocarditis (NBTE); others consider it a distinct entity.

NBTE should be considered in patients with known malignancy, diffuse intravascular coagulation (DIC), HIV, or connective tissue disease. Echocardiography is the most sensitive diagnostic test; because of the frequency of mitral valve pathology in NBTE, TEE (which provides a better look at the mitral valve) should be more sensitive than TTE to detect the lesions. NBTE should also be considered in patients with culture-negative vegetations. An underlying systemic illness (malignancy, connective tissue disease, HIV, DIC) should be ruled out.

Other Cardiac Valvular Lesions

Mitral regurgitation may result in left atrial enlargement. By producing stasis in the left atrium, mitral regurgitation may lead to cardiac embolism. If a patient has a systolic murmur suggestive of mitral regurgitation, or if transthoracic echocardiography shows mitral regurgitation, transesophageal echocardiography should be undertaken to ensure that there is no thrombus in the left atrial appendage. Many patients with mitral regurgitation and left atrial enlargement will have atrial fibrillation as well.

Valvular strands are small processes often seen on the mitral and aortic valves. They are often multiple and measure 1.5 by 10 mm in size. These strands are highly mobile and consist of fibrin deposits over damaged endocardial valvular surfaces. While several studies have shown an increased risk of systemic embolism and stroke, other studies have not shown an increased risk of strands in patients with cryptogenic stroke. The association between strands and stroke is not yet definite, and isolated small strands should not be considered a source of stroke unless there are other abnormalities. Treatment studies have not been done.

Patent Foramen Ovale

PFO is found in as many as 35% of all autopsies. While common as an incidental finding, there is also an increased incidence of PFO in patients without another identifiable cause for stroke. Issues concerning diagnosis and management of stroke patients with PFO are covered in Chapter 13.

Ischemic Heart Disease and Acute Myocardial Infarction

Data from the Framingham Heart Study show that coronary artery disease, either angina or prior MI, increases the risk of stroke threefold. Stroke complicates up to 5% of MI, although this risk is reduced to less than 1% in patients treated with anticoagulation. Even with small MIs, changes in contractility can lead to stasis and predispose to embolism formation. Endothelial damage can also occur, which can lead to platelet-thrombin deposits and subsequent thrombus formation. Patients with transmural MIs have a greater risk of embolic stroke.

Hypokinetic or akinetic segments or ventricular aneurysms predispose to mural thrombus formation and subsequent embolic stroke. These will often be seen with echocardiography, but thrombi often form and dislodge, so cardiac embolism should be considered in patients with akinetic segments even without mural thrombi seen on echocardiography. Mural thrombi can be seen in 11% of patients with anterior wall MI. They occur in >10% of patients with MI and ejection fractions <40%. Nearly one in three strokes associated with MI occur simultaneously with the MI, and the vast majority occur within the first month after the MI. The following factors place patients at higher risk for stroke in the setting of MI: increasing age; prior history of stroke; history of atrial fibrillation; anterior or apical location of MI; larger MIs by enzymes; and history of congestive heart failure.

Cardiomyopathy

Cardiomyopathy refers to a group of diseases of the myocardium that impair cardiac performance. The etiology may be ischemia or infarction from coronary artery disease, or non-ischemic. Ischemic cardiomyopathy is common in patients with atherosclerosis; nonischemic cardiomyopathy is often caused by a virus or toxins (especially alcohol). While stroke in this population is common, the most common cause of death in patients with cardiomyopathy is due to left ventricular dysfunction or sudden cardiac death due to MI or ventricular tachyarrhythmia.

Congestive heart failure increases stroke risk by two to three times. While this is less than the increased risk from atrial fibrillation (a fivefold increased risk), there are twice as many patients with congestive heart failure than with atrial fibrillation. Heart failure is therefore an important risk factor for stroke. In addition, the prevalence of heart failure is increasing as the population ages. However, younger patients with heart failure are at higher relative risk of stroke than are older patients; this may be due to increasing stroke risk from other causes among older patients without heart failure.

The risk of stroke is inversely proportional to ejection fraction, that is, patients with lower ejection fractions are at higher risk for stroke. In the Survival and Ventricular Enlargement (SAVE) study, there was an 18% increase in stroke risk for every 5% fall in ejection fraction (8). Other comorbidities—patient age, prior stroke, hypertension, and diabetes—increase the risk of stroke in patients with cardiomyopathy. Stroke rates appear similar between patients with ischemic and nonischemic cardiomyopathy. The rates of embolic events with cardiomyopathy are 1.7%-3.5% per year.

However, there has been limited study of stroke subypes in patients with cardiomyopathy. While most strokes in patients with nonischemic cardiomyopathy (and therefore little intrinsic atherosclerotic disease) are likely cardioembolic, the same cannot be said of patients with ischemic cardiomyopathy, who usually have systemic and cerebral atherosclerosis as well as atherosclerotic coronary artery disease. As with other potential cardioembolic strokes, exclusion of other potential causes is appropriate.

Coronary Artery Bypass Surgery

Nearly 1 million patients throughout the world annually undergo myocardial revascularization procedures. There is an increased risk of stroke during CABG, from atherosclerosis, hemodynamic fluctuations, and embolism of atherosclerotic plaque, as well as air or fat. In one prospective, multicenter study, 3.1% of >2100 patients who underwent CABG had neurological complications: death due to cerebral injury, non-fatal stroke, TIA, or persistent stupor (9). Over 20% of patients who had stroke died. An additional 3% had deterioration in intellectual function or seizures without focal findings on exam or imaging.

Proximal aortic atherosclerosis increased the risk of stroke, death, or stupor by 4-fold compared with patients without this risk factor. Older age (>70), history of neurological disease, pulmonary disease, and perioperative hypotension also increased the risk of adverse neurological outcome.

Intracardiac Mass Lesions

Primary tumors of the heart occur in less than 2 per 1000 patients. Most are benign; half of these are myxomas. Lipomas, papillary fibroelastomas, and rhabdomyomas are also seen. Rhabdomyomas are the most common tumors in children, but myxomas are most common in adults. Malignant cardiac tumors, like angiosarcoma and rhabdomyosarcoma, occur in the myocardium. Cardiac metastases are 20-40 times more common than primary tumors and result from lymphatic or hematogenous spread, or direct extension. However, these tumors are almost always in the pericardium, sometimes in the myocardium, rarely in the endocardium; they therefore are unlikely to be the source of cardiogenic emboli.

Myxomas are endocardial neoplasms, usually projecting from the endocardium into the atrium. The cells giving rise to the tumor are multipotential mesenchymal cells. The clinical features are determined by their location, size, and mobility. Patients can present with embolism, intracardiac obstruction, and constitutional symptoms. Embolism occurs 30%-40% of the time, most commonly to the brain or retinal arteries. Symptoms can mimic bacterial endocarditis, with constitutional symptoms such as fever, fatigue, arthralgia, and myalgia, as well as an elevated sedimentation rate and serum C-reactive protein. Myxomas can become infected, with increased risk of systemic embolism. In the pre-echocardiography era, the diagnosis of a cardiac myxoma was almost always post-mortem; the first pre-mortem diagnosis was made by angiocardiography in 1951. Transesophageal echocardiography is superior to transthoracic echocardiography in detecting myxomas, especially in the left atrium.

The treatment of choice is surgical. The root of the pedicle and the full thickness of the adjacent interatrial septum should be excised. All chambers of the heart should be inspected to rule out a multifocal tumor. Recurrences have been reported.

Primary and Secondary Prevention

The best data for warfarin anticoagulation as primary or secondary prevention for stroke are in the case of atrial fibrillation. However, both the source and composition of emboli is variable and not all of these will respond to warfarin. Emboli can be predominantly platelets (as in nonbacterial thrombotic endocarditis), fibrin-rich thrombi which arise from ventricular clot, calcific material from valvular disease, tumor in the case of a myxoma, or infective material in bacterial endocarditis. Treatment that is effective for one type of embolism should not be assumed to be effective for another. For many sources of cardiac embolism, more data are needed before definitive statements on appropriate therapy can be made.

Atrial Fibrillation

There is clear evidence to support the use of warfarin for most patients with atrial fibrillation, even without a history of stroke (primary prevention). The complications of warfarin therapy are skin necrosis, which is uncommon, as well as drug interactions and bleeding, both of which are more common. Five major clinical trials have shown that warfarin reduces the subsequent risk of stroke in patients with non-valvular atrial fibrillation. A meta-analysis of these trials showed that treatment with warfarin results in a 68% risk reduction compared to placebo. However, there were patients in the studies in whom the risk was significantly lower: patients with lone atrial fibrillation who were younger than age 60 had no increased risk of stroke. Conversely, patients with congestive heart failure and coronary artery disease had a stroke rate three times higher than those without these risk factors. Stroke risk increased as age increased, but so did the rate of hemorrhage for those patients placed on warfarin.

What is the optimum international normalized ratio (INR) for patients receiving warfarin for atrial fibrillation? The INR goals in the major studies varied somewhat, ranging from a low of 1.7 to a high of 4.6. Anticoagulation at the higher intensities increases bleeding risk, and subtherapeutic INRs are associated with increased risk of cardioembolic stroke. The upper and lower limits of "therapeutic anticoagulation" remain under some debate. In two studies, Hylek et al determined that the optimal intensity of anticoagulation is an INR of 2.0-3.0 (10,11). In a case-control study, she found a steep increase in cardioembolic stroke risk as INR fell below 2.0. At an INR of 1.7, the risk was double compared with an INR of 2.0; at an INR of 1.5 the risk was triple; and at an INR of 1.3 the risk was sixfold. The same investigators also found that the risk of ischemic stroke did not go down significantly at INRs greater than 2.0, remaining similar up to an INR of 7.0. In a separate study, a substantially increased risk of intracranial hemorrhage was found as the INR increased above 4.0. In another trial, an unacceptably high incidence of major bleeding complications was seen with an INR range of 3.0-4.5. Because there is no increased benefit for an INR over 3.0, the recommendation is an INR of 2.0-3.0.

However, in a Japanese population, Yasaka et al demonstrated efficacy with a somewhat less intensive anticoagulation (12). In that study, an INR of 1.6-2.6 was associated with reduced risk of stroke with low hemorrhage rates. Hemorrhage rate increased as INR increased above 2.6. The hemorrhage rate was higher in patients older than 75. Because hemorrhage rates are higher in Japan than they are in the United States, it is not clear that these data are applicable to an American population. Most authors recommend an INR of 2.0-3.0 for primary prevention of stroke in patients with atrial fibrillation, but an upper limit of 2.5 for older patients seems reasonable. In a meta-analysis of the five large warfarin atrial fibrillation trials, the risk of intracranial or systemic hemorrhage requiring hospitalization or transfusion was 1.3% per year in the warfarin-treated group; it was 1% in the placebo group, for a difference of only 0.3%. These complications are more likely to occur with an elevated INR.

Despite the efficacy and safety data, there continues to be evidence that warfarin anticoagulation is underutilized in patients with atrial fibrillation. It is estimated that increased use of warfarin for patients in atrial fibrillation could reduce stroke in the United States annually by 20,000 to 30,000. For the physician seeing a patient with atrial fibrillation who is on the fence about anticoagulation, careful history and examination, supplemented by neuroimaging, can reveal evidence for previously unrecognized stroke. Silent strokes may be seen 15% of the time by CT in patients with atrial fibrillation and without a clinical history of stroke or TIA or abnormalities on examination. The presence of these infarcts places the patient in a higher-risk category and may tilt the clinician's judgment toward the use of warfarin. The incidence of potential complications can be reduced with vigilant follow-up and patient and family education about the importance of compliance with warfarin therapy and side effects. Other potential contraindications to anticoagulation with warfarin include dementia or gait disturbance, which may predispose the patient to falls and brain hemorrhages (Table 10-2). These should be assessed in each patient before initiating therapy. In certain instances, home safety evaluations may be useful to identify patients at risk for falls; safety modifications can sometimes allow a patient to safely start or continue warfarin. Because the incidence of cerebral amyloid angiopathy (which predisposes to intracerebral hemorrhage) increases with patient age, in some patients a gradient echo MRI scan (which is sensitive for old hemorrhages that would not be seen on CT) may help reassure the physician that the patient is not at undue risk from warfarin.

For patients who have a contraindication to warfarin, aspirin is warranted. Aspirin has been shown to reduce risk of stroke by 21% in patients with atrial fibrillation. Existing data warrant the use of at least 325 mg/day of aspirin for patients with atrial fibrillation who are not on warfarin. The only patients who do not not clearly benefit from warfarin are those who are younger than age 60 and have lone atrial fibrillation without any other risk factors: these patients should be on aspirin (as myocardial infarction prophylaxis) or no therapy. Patients aged 60-75 with no other stroke risk factors have a higher risk of stroke than do their counterparts below age 60, making their risk of stroke and hemorrhage comparable. However, in these patients, any additional factors that increase the risk for stroke (abnormalities on echocardiography, hypertension, or diabetes) would tilt the balance in favor of warfarin.

Table 10-2 Relative Contraindications to Warfarin

• Arteriovenous malformation of the brain	• Bleeding disorder
• Brain tumor	• Pregnancy
• Previous hemorrhagic stroke	• Allergic to warfarin
• Systolic blood pressure at discharge > 200 mm Hg	• Frequent falls
• Active peptic ulcer disease with bleeding	• Alcoholism
• Major trauma/surgery < 2 months previous	• Hepatic disease
• Bacterial endocarditis	

The role of aspirin for patients on warfarin is somewhat controversial. Among patients treated with warfarin with hypertension, aspirin significantly further reduces stroke risk. This is likely due to the increased chance of atherosclerosis in these patients, which leads to other types of stroke. Patients on warfarin for atrial fibrillation remain at risk for stroke from carotid stenosis or other causes that do not respond to warfarin. These patients are also at increased risk for MI. A baby aspirin should therefore be considered in these patients.

Prosthetic Valves

There is high risk of stroke in patients with prosthetic valves, and primary prevention is therefore warranted. For all patients with a mechanical prosthetic valve, anticoagulation with warfarin is recommended, with INR goals of 3.0 (for bileaflet valves) to 4.0-4.9 (for caged-ball and tilting disc valves). For patients with recurrent emboli despite adequate anticoagulation, low-dose aspirin (81-162 mg/day), dipyridamole (75-400 mg/day), or clopidogrel (75 mg/day) may be added as secondary prevention. For patients with bioprosthetic valves in the aortic position, empiric aspirin 325 mg/day is recommended as primary prevention. For patients with mitral bioprosthetic valves, warfarin (INR goal 2.0-3.0) is usually prescribed initially for 3 months, followed by lifelong aspirin. If a patient with a bioprosthetic valve develops a cardiac embolism, warfarin therapy with an INR of 2.0-3.0 should be inititated.

Myocardial Infarction

Intravenous heparin (initial weight-based dose of approximately 1000 U/hour with an IV bolus of 2500-5000 U, adjusted to maintain aPTT at 1.5-2.5 times control) is recommended after anterior MIs, MIs complicated by congestive heart failure or atrial fibrillation, and when mural thrombi are seen by echocardiography. After severe left ventricular dysfunction, congestive heart failure, mural thrombus, or Q-wave anterior infarctions, patients should be anticoagulated with warfarin, with a target INR of 2.0-3.0 for 3-6 months. There are not sufficient data to recommend anticoagulation in other post-MI situations; antiplatelet therapy and risk-factor management are warranted.

Cardiomyopathy

Retrospective data suggest that anticoagulation with warfarin as primary prevention may decrease stroke risk in patients with depressed left ventricular ejection fraction and normal coronary arteries (idiopathic dilated cardiomyopathy). However, no randomized prospective studies exist, and the available data are confounded by the severity of the cardiomyopathy in the patients treated with warfarin compared with those who were not anticoagulated. For patients with ischemic cardiomyopathy, warfarin should be considered when there is increased risk of emboli—for example, in patients with large, protruding, or mobile ventricular thrombi. Aspirin has been shown to reduce thromboembolism in cardiomyopathy, as well. Oral anticoagulation with warfarin should be considered in all patients with cardiomyopathy and embolic stroke, regardless of whether thrombus is seen on echocardiography.

Conclusion

Cardiac embolization accounts for approximately 20% of strokes. The cardiac evaluation is a vital part of the stroke workup. Evaluation of the cardiac status is important because there are interventions that have been proven to reduce the recurrence of strokes if addressed specifically. Significant risks exist when a patient has had a stroke and either atrial fibrillation or paroxysmal atrial fibrillation is found. Both states are clear indications for anticoagulation with warfarin as long as the risks of fall or head injury are not too great. Although evidence that low left ejection fraction, post-MI, and mobile plaque within the arch of the aorta may indicate warfarin use, the issues have not been studied completely. There is significant debate about patent formaen ovale leading to strokes. There appear to be reasonable data to suggest that patent formaen ovale with atrial septal defects increase the changes of recurrent stroke. Trials are underway to determine how best to treat these patients.

Lastly, it is vital to remember that a stroke or TIA suggests a risk of future myocardial infarction as well as recurrent stroke. Evaluation of cardiac status, rhythm, and anatomy is vital for the overall health and well-being of the patient. A stroke or TIA should be considered an opportunity to address hypertension, hypercholesterolemia, smoking, and obesity, which are all risk factors for cardiac and cerebrovascular disease.

REFERENCES

1. Hart RG, Pearce LA, Miller VT, et al. Cardioembolic vs. noncardioembolic strokes in atrial fibrillation: frequency and effect of antithrombotic agents in the Stroke Prevention in Atrial Fibrillation Studies. Cerebrovasc Dis. 2000;10:39-43.
2. Swanson RA. Intravenous heparin for acute stroke: what can we learn from the mega-trials? Neurology. 1999;52:1746-50.
3. Coull BM, William LS, Goldstein LB. Anticoagulants and antiplatelet agents in acute ischemic stroke. Neurology. 2002;59:13-22.
4. Saxena R, Lewis S, Berge E, et al. Risk of early death and recurrent stroke and effect of heparin in 3169 patients with acute ischemic stroke and atrial fibrillation in the International Stroke Trial. Stroke. 2001;32:2333-7.
5. The SPAF III Writing Committee for the Stroke Prevention in Atrial Fibrillation Investigators. Patients with nonvalvular atrial fibrillation at low risk of stroke during treatment with aspirin: stroke prevention in Atrial Fibrillation III Study. JAMA. 1998;279:1273-7.

6. Freed LA, Levy D, Levine RA, et al. Prevalence and clinical outcome of mitral-valve prolapse. N Engl J Med. 1999;341:1-7.

7. Gilon D, Buonanno FS, et al. Lack of evidence of an association between mitral-valve prolapse and stroke in young patients. N Engl J Med. 1999;341:8-13.

8. Pullicino PM, Halperin JL, Thompson JL. Stroke in patients with heart failure and reduced left ventricular ejection fraction. Neurology. 2000;54:288-94.

9. Roach GW, Kanchuger M, Mangana CM, et al. Adverse cerebral outcomes after coronary bypass surgery. N Engl J Med. 1996;335:1857-63.

10. Hylek EM, Skates SJ, Sheehan MA, Singer DE. An analysis of the lowest effective intensity of prophylactic anticoagulation for patients with nonrheumatic atrial fibrillation. N Engl J Med. 1996;335:540-6.

11. Hylek EM, Singer DE. Risk factors for intracranial hemorrhage in outpatients taking warfarin. Ann Intern Med. 1994;120:897-902.

12. Yasaka M, Minematsu K, Yamaguchi T. Optimal intensity of international normalized ratio in warfarin therapy for secondary prevention of stroke in patients with non-valvular atrial fibrillation. Intern Med. 2001;40:1183-8.

Chapter 11

Lacunar Stroke

DOROTHY S. CHUNG, MD, PhD

Key Points

- Lacunar stroke may be defined as a stroke that has small vessel disease as its pathogenesis. However, 15%-36% of patients with small strokes may have associated large vessel or embolic disease.
- Lacunar strokes may present with sudden hemiplegia, hemi-anesthesia, ataxia, clumsiness of a limb, or dysarthria.
- The prognosis for recovery from lacunar infarcts is very good, and the risk of recurrent stroke or death immediately following a lacunar infarct is low.
- Treatment includes antiplatelet therapy and reducing cerebro-vascular risk factors.

Approximately 15%-28% of all ischemic strokes are lacunar strokes (1–5). Lacunar infarcts can be described pathologically, radiographically, or, less precisely, by clinical syndromes. The etymology of *lacune* (from the French word for "lake") can be traced back to Durand-Fardel, who in 1843 first used the term to describe the pathologic appearance of small infarcts which appeared as small "holes" in the brain, particularly in subcortical regions (6). Lacunar strokes were long recognized as a potentially significant sub-category of stroke, differing from non-lacunar strokes in pathogenesis and prognosis. When C. Miller Fisher published his seminal paper on the pathologic description of lacunes in 1965, it was part of a larger effort to categorize and identify underlying stroke processes to better stratify treatment and prevention (7).

Lacunes, as defined by Fisher, are ischemic infarcts of limited size (0.5-15 mm diameter) in deeper parts of the brain, excluding the cerebral and cerebellar hemispheres. These lesions are associated with cerebral atherosclerosis and arterial hypertension and result from occlusion of penetrating arteries or "small vessels" from either anterior or posterior circulation arteries. Pathologically, the most frequent sites of involvement in descending order are the putamen, caudate, thalamus, pons, internal capsule, and subcortical white matter (7,8).

Microscopically, a typical lacune appears as an irregular cavity containing a few strands of fine fibrillar connective tissue and occasional fatty macrophages, some enclosing a tiny artery or vein. A dense fibroglial matting with many astrocytes surround the walls. Lacunes are traditionally thought to result from lipohyalinosis or microatheroma formation within small penetrating vessels; they are less likely to result from embolism.

Definition of Terms

The terms *lacune, lacunar syndrome, lacunar stroke or infarct,* and *small vessel stroke* often generate confusion, even within the stroke literature. A *lacune* is a pathologic and radiographic description of a small ischemic lesion less than 15 mm in diameter occurring in the subcortical and deep structures of the brain. *Lacunar syndrome* refers to a constellation of clinical features that may be associated with, though not invariably, a radiographic or pathologic lacune (4,9). Broadly speaking, even small hemorrhages and large ischemic infarcts may produce *lacunar clinical syndromes* (9). Lacunar strokes, however, have come to imply a stroke which has small vessel disease as its pathogenesis (4). Lacunar stroke is more appropriately used to designate a mechanism of stroke, much as large vessel stroke or cardioembolic stroke is used to designate alternative mechanisms of stroke. Lacunar strokes imply small vessel stroke and can be used interchangeably with this term. Thus *lacunar stroke* can be strictly defined as a stroke usually presenting with a typical clinical syndrome supported by radiographic findings of a small (<15 mm diameter) deep ischemic infarct or lacune, with no evidence of large artery stenosis and no source of cardiac embolism or rare etiologies, such as arterial dissection, vasculitis, or hematologic disorders (Fig. 11-1).

Lacunar Syndromes

While lacunar infarcts may be described pathologically and radiographically, over 20 different clinical syndromes have been associated with lacunes (8). The most recognizable of these are pure motor hemiparesis, pure sensory stroke, ataxic hemiparesis, sensorimotor stroke, and dysarthria-clumsy hand syndrome. It is important to remember that these clinical syndromes may be associated with ischemic infarcts as well as discrete hemorrhages and other non-ischemic etiologies (10,11).

Pure motor hemiparesis is characterized by a unilateral motor deficit involving the face, arm, and leg with no associated sensory loss. This usually affects the limbs equally but may affect one extremity more than the other (12). While classically pure motor hemiparesis involves the face, arm, and leg, some have broadened the syndrome to include patients presenting with a pure motor stroke involving at least one limb. However, broadening the definition decreases the positive predictive value that the syndrome represents a lacunar stroke. Some even suggest that pure motor monoparesis is rarely caused by a deep infarct (11). Pure motor hemiparesis may be associated mild dysarthria, but this is of no localizing value. Importantly, because there is no involvement of higher cortical structures, aphasia, apraxia, neglect, visual loss, and disturbance of other higher cortical functions are absent. This syndrome may result from a lesion anywhere along the motor tract: in the contralateral posterior limb of the internal capsule, corona radiata, cerebral peduncle, basis pontis, or the medullary pyramid (13,14). Although rare, an ischemic cortical lesion may cause a pure motor hemiparesis (10).

Pure sensory stroke (pure hemisensory or paresthetic stroke) is characterized by unilateral numbness, paresthesias, and a hemisensory deficit typically involving the face, arm, trunk, and leg. Lacunes in the thalamus or pons (localized to the medial leminiscus) may present with this syndrome (15). However, ischemic infarctions in the corona radiata or in the parietal cortex may cause pure sensory stroke (10,14). An important complication of pure sensory stroke is delayed central pain syndrome, where patients complain of continuous burning on one side of the body or unpleasant sensations to minor stimuli such as brushing of clothes or cold water.

Ataxic hemiparesis (homolateral ataxia and crural paresis) is characterized by a combination of cerebellar and motor symptoms on the same side of the body (Case Study 11-1). Unilateral weakness more prominent in the lower extremity is associated with unilateral arm and leg ataxia. Dysarthria and involvement of the face is uncommon. Generally, lesions in the contralateral posterior limb of the internal capsule, basis pontis, or thalamocapsular region cause this syndrome (10,14,16,17). Although less frequently, lesions in other regions such as corona radiata, lentiform nucleus, red nucleus, lateral medulla, cerebellum, and even frontal cortex are reported (11,14,18).

The dysarthria-clumsy hand syndrome is characterized by unilateral hand weakness and dysarthria. There is often supranuclear facial weakness, tongue deviation, dysphagia, dysarthria (many times severe), impaired fine motor control of the hand, and an extensor plantar response. There is no sensory deficit. Lacunar strokes in the basis pontis, or in the genu of the internal capsule may cause this syndrome (10,14).

Strokes in patients with sensory and motor impairment generally involve large territories in the cortex. However, in those patients with a clear sensorium and no other deficits, a lacunar infarct may be the etiology of the symptoms. Huang et al suggested that sensorimotor stroke as a lacunar syndrome may be restricted to those with only mild-to-moderate hemiparesis and sensory impairment in both upper and lower limbs (19). Lacunes located in the thalamocapsular region or corona radiata may give rise to this syndrome (4,19).

Clinical Features

Lacunar strokes may present with sudden hemiplegia, hemianesthesia, ataxia, clumsiness of a limb, or dysarthria, as described above. Many are also silent (20). In a study of 246 neurologically normal adults, Kobayashi et al found that 13% of these subjects had silent lacunar infarcts defined by MRI imaging (21). While the prognosis is generally good for recovery, and mortality of this stroke subtype is low compared with other stroke types (22), multiple bilateral lacunes can lead to pseudobulbar palsy or dementing states. Pseudobulbar palsy refers to the condition where bilateral lacunes result in spasticity of the brainstem functions (the "bulb"), causing spastic dysarthria, swallowing difficulties and the curious disorder of "emotional incontinence" where uncontrolled expressions such as laughing or crying are provoked by minor stimuli. A disorder known as CADASIL (Cerebral Autosomal Dominant Arteriopathy Subcortical Infarcts and Leukoencephalopathy), involving the early onset of lacunar strokes, subcortical dementia, psychiatric disturbances, and migraine, results from mutations in the Notch 3 gene; however, this mutation is rare and routine screening is not indicated (23).

The reported positive predictive value of a lacunar syndrome varies widely and depends on the stroke subtype studied. For example, the positive predictive value of pure motor hemiparesis is reported from 58% to 79% (4,24). In one study, the positive predictive values of pure sensory syndrome, ataxic-hemiparesis, sensorimotor syndrome, and pure motor hemiparesis in predicting a radiographic lacune were 100%, 95%, 87%, and 79% respectively (4). However, nearly 25% of patients who presented with a lacunar syndrome confirmed radiologically were eventually diagnosed as having a nonlacunar mechanism of infarction, either atherosclerosis of a large vessel, cardioembolism, or other potential source of stroke (Case Studies 11-2 and 11-3). On the other hand, of patients who presented with a non-lacunar syndrome but had a radiographic lacune, only 26% of cases were deemed due to a lacunar mechanism.

Lacunar strokes tend to occur in patients with chronic hypertension (21,25), hyperlipidemia (26), and smoking habit (20,27,28). Lacunar strokes are less often associated with diabetes (27), though diabetic patients compared with those without diabetes are more likely to present with lacunar strokes (29). The proportion of lacunar strokes is also significantly higher in blacks and Hispanics compared with whites (4), and lacunar stroke has increasing incidence with age and male sex (28). Furthermore, frequent physical exercise is associated with significantly decreased risk of lacunar stroke (27). It is estimated that, while the vast majority of lacunar syndromes result from small vessel disease, as many as 15% to 36% of these patients are found to have large vessel disease, cardioembolic, or other sources which may explain their infarct (4,12,24,25,30,31). Although these findings may be associative rather than causative, patients presenting with a lacunar syndrome must be evaluated for other potential preventable causes of stroke.

The risk of hemorrhagic transformation or edema in patients with lacunar stroke is rare. However, many patients can clinically fluctuate or "worsen" in the first few days without imaging correlates, possibly representing "completion" of the original stroke.

The prognosis for recovery from lacunar infarcts is generally very good. There is general acknowledgement of the low risk of recurrent stroke and death immediately following a lacunar infarct (32,33). A recent report examined the long-term follow-up of 180 patients with pure motor hemiparesis (34). In the first 5 years after stroke, the survival rates were similar to the general population, but beyond this time death rates were increased. During the 10-year follow-up, 60% of the patients died, most commonly as a result of coronary heart disease. Recurrent strokes occurred at an annual rate of 2.4%, and hypertension and diabetes were independent risk factors. Thus the emphasis in patients who present with a lacunar infarct should be on reduction of risk factors and secondary prevention of future strokes and cardiovascular complications (35). Stroke recovery is also improved in patients participating in rehabilitation (36,37).

In general, patients with lacunar stroke have a more benign clinical evolution, do not share the same pathogenetic mechanisms, and require different clinical management than patients who do not have a lacunar stroke.

Mechanism of Infarction

The current concept of categorizing strokes based on underlying mechanisms of infarct has led to tailoring specific stroke management and treatment to specific stroke subtypes.

A cerebral embolism results from a clot that forms in another portion of the body, such as the heart (in the case of atrial fibrillation), is carried through the bloodstream, and becomes lodged in an artery that supplies blood to the brain, blocking the flow of blood. On the other hand, atherosclerotic cerebrovascular disease, or so-called large vessel disease, results in stroke when there is an impediment to normal blood flow as a result of severe arterial stenosis or occlusion due to atherosclerosis in large and medium vessels and coexisting thrombosis. In this case, a stroke is thought to occur much in the same way that has been described for acute coronary syndromes. Typically, this is caused by rupture or erosion of an atherosclerotic plaque followed by formation of a platelet-rich thrombus, which proceeds to cause an acute stroke. This thrombus can either completely occlude the artery or break off and travel downstream to lodge in smaller vessels.

Lacunar infarcts have been described to result from microatheroma or lipohyalinosis of the small penetrating arteries of the brain. Lipohyalinosis is characterized by arterial wall disorganization, resulting in thickening of the small-vessel wall accompanied by luminal narrowing, and in the acute stage demonstrates fibrinoid necrosis. While some suggest that lacunar infarcts result from a mechanism of atherosclerosis and microthrombus formation, others suggest that breakdown of the blood-brain barrier and leakage of plasma contents into the vessel wall and surrounding brain tissue may be the etiology (38).

Thus, while anticoagulation with warfarin may prevent clot formation within the heart, it may not be the ideal way to prevent the platelet aggregation that occurs during the rupture of a thrombus or the lipohyalinosis that occurs during a lacunar infarct. Many clinical trials have begun to answer these questions, and a conceptual framework for the management of different stroke types has recently taken shape.

Diagnosis

As discussed above, although a lacunar stroke generally implies small vessel stroke, as many as 15%-36% of patients presenting with a lacunar syndrome may have associated large vessel or embolic disease that may be the etiology of the stroke. Thus all patients presenting with a suspected lacunar infarct should receive a full workup to determine the etiology of the infarct (Figure 11-1). These patients should receive a carotid duplex to study the carotid artery for lesions amenable to surgery or stenting. In addition, studies to evaluate the intracranial vasculature, including MRI and MR angiography, CT angiography, or transcranial Doppler, should be performed. Finally, patients should receive a transesophageal echocardiogram (TEE) to rule out cardioembolic sources to complete the workup. (Treatment of these patients based on positive results of these studies is discussed in other chapters.) Furthermore, depending upon the clinical scenario, other potential rare etiologies of stroke, such as dissection, vasculitis, fibromuscular dysplasia, or hematologic abnormalities, should be excluded. If these studies are negative, the presumed etiology of the lacune is a small vessel stroke, likely secondary to small vessel changes and possible microthrombosis that occur with chronic hypertension, diabetes, and/or hyperlipidemia. A search for modifiable risk factors, such as hypertension, hypercholesterolemia, diabetes mellitus, and smoking, should be undertaken and treated accordingly.

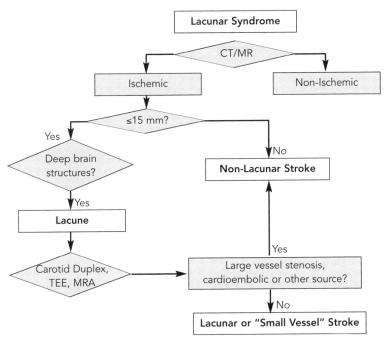

Figure 11-1 Diagnosis of lacunar stroke.

Treatment

Reduction of Risk Factors

Treatment of lacunar strokes should include reduction of cerebrovascular and cardiovascular risk factors and the institution of antiplatelet therapy. Furthermore, early involvement of physical therapy and occupational therapy promotes faster recovery and earlier time to independence (37). While there have been no specific clinical trials looking at risk factor reduction in specific stroke subtypes, there have been clear benefits in reducing the risk of all strokes with reduction of blood pressure and hyperlipidemia and with smoking cessation. Non-modifiable risk factors for stroke include age, sex, race/ethnicity, and heredity, whereas potentially modifiable risk factors for lacunar strokes include hypertension, diabetes, hypercholesterolemia, cigarette smoking, and physical inactivity. Thus, in patients with lacunar strokes, aggressive management of hypertension, diabetes, hypercholesterolemia, as well as positive lifestyle modifications should be strongly encouraged.

Antiplatelet Therapy

While many patients presenting with an acute lacunar stroke likely do not meet NIH stroke scale criteria for thrombolysis, those that do within the 3-hour allotted window should receive intravenous tissue plasminogen activator (see Chapter 7). While there has been no systematic clinical trial specifically studying acute lacunar strokes and thrombolytics, these patients were included in the original thrombolytic trials (39,40) and no interaction was found between type of stroke at baseline and responses following treatment (39). Furthermore, the positive predictive value of pure motor hemiparesis or sensorimotor stroke was found to be poor in a retrospective analysis of the ECASS trial for predicting acute lacunar infarcts, thus making separation of this group for future prospective analysis in acute stroke trials difficult (41). Interestingly, there has even been a recent case report of reversal of the MRI deficits of a lacunar infarct with thrombolytics (42). Thus, excluding patients for thrombolytic therapy based upon suspicion of a small vessel stroke may be inappropriate.

Anticoagulation versus Antiplatelet Therapy

While warfarin is clearly the anticoagulant of choice in patients with a cardioembolic source of stroke, this is not necessarily the case in patients with strokes of other etiologies. In a recent multi-center, randomized, double-blind study of 1103 patients with strokes of non-cardioembolic origin (the Warfarin–Aspirin Recurrent Stroke Study [WARSS]), there was no significant difference between aspirin and warfarin in the prevention of recurrent strokes or death in two years of follow-up (43). Furthermore, there were no significant differences in treatment outcome between patients who presented with lacunar strokes, cryptogenic strokes, or strokes of large vessel origin. Thus there is no role for warfarin therapy in patients with non-cardioembolic strokes, including lacunar infarcts, because antiplatelet therapy is similarly effective with fewer potential hemorrhagic complications.

Summary of Lacunar Stroke Treatment

A patient presenting with a lacunar syndrome should have a full workup to determine the etiology of the stroke. If a lacune is found on imaging studies but no other etiology, then a small vessel stroke is assumed. A search for modifiable risk factors should then be undertaken. Hypertension, hypercholesterolemia, and diabetes management should be optimized and lifestyle changes, such as smoking cessation, weight loss, diet, and physical activity, should be encouraged. Patients should then be placed on antiplatelet therapy for optimal secondary prevention of future strokes. Patients who meet NIH stroke scale criteria for thrombolysis should receive t-PA.

Conclusion

Lacunar infarcts have been described pathologically as well as clinically, and the extent to which these correlate is great, but imperfect. Lacunar strokes tend to occur in specific patient populations, with hypertension, hyperlipidemia, diabetes, and smoking the major risk factors for their development. Furthermore, pathological examinations of small subcortical infarcts reveal varying degrees of atherosclerotic changes in the small vessels. Thus it is assumed that the primary pathology in most lacunar infarcts is within the small vessels. However, up to 15%-36% of these infarcts may actually have a large vessel stenosis, atheroemboli, cardioembolic, or other source as an etiology.

The prognosis, clinical course, and response to treatment of lacunar strokes are distinct from non-lacunar strokes and therefore have survived clinical stratification. However, because these definitions are imperfect, lacunar syndromes may also, in some cases, be attributed to larger vessel disease or even embolic disease. Thus, while the vast majority of patients presenting clinically with a lacunar syndrome have indeed a stroke caused by small vessel disease, they are also at risk for large vessel or embolic strokes, and a search to exclude these possibilities must be included as part of the stroke workup. With a negative workup, it is possible to assure the patient and family of a fairly good prognosis as well as a relatively low risk of recurrence, particularly with aggressive secondary prevention.

Secondary prevention of stroke lies in the active management and reduction of known risk factors for cerebrovascular and cardiovascular disease, particularly hypertension, hyperlipidemia, diabetes, and smoking. Encouragement of positive lifestyle modifications, such as diet, weight-loss, and physical activity, helps to lower these risk factors as well. There does not appear to be a role for heparin or warfarin in the treatment of lacunar strokes, because neither is more efficacious than antiplatelet therapy alone in preventing recurrence. The choice of antiplatelet therapy at this point is a matter of personal preference and choosing the appropriate side-effect profile, although clinical trials now underway will clarify this issue.

Case Study 11-1

A 58-year-old male with a history of hypertension, tobacco use, and myocardial infarction reports that he awoke with "numbness" of the index and middle fingers of his right hand and weakness and unsteadiness of his right lower extremity. On admission, his blood pressure was 182/122; his higher cognitive functions and his cranial nerves were intact. He had mild weakness of his right upper and lower extremities accompanied by hyper-reflexia. Sensory loss was restricted to a stocking glove distribution bilaterally. The patient had dysmetria in his upper and lower extremities out of proportion to his weakness. He was determined to have ataxic-hemiparesis by clinical examination.

MRI revealed a new corona radiata infarction on the left. There was also evidence of old lacunes in his basal ganglia bilaterally and in his left corona radiata (Figure 11-2). Carotid duplex and MRA revealed no

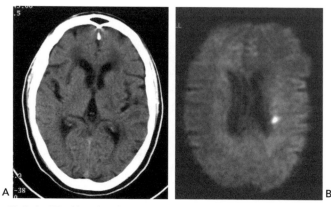

Figure 11-2 A, CT of head without contrast, revealing previous lacunes in the putamen and thalamus on the left. **B,** MRI diffusion-weighted image showing a small acute infarct in the corona radiata on the left.

evidence of hemodynamically significant stenosis in large arteries. TEE was negative for cardioembolic source. During hospitalization, the patient was found to have hypercholesterolemia and was started on a statin agent. There was no evidence of glucose intolerance. The patient was counseled to quit smoking. He had been on 1 aspirin per day and was discharged from the hospital on clopidrogel.

Discussion and Follow-Up

This patient presented with a typical lacunar syndrome, ataxic-hemiparesis. Diffusion-weighted imaging by MRI revealed an acute lacunar infarct in appropriate region. Workup revealed no other source of embolic or large vessel disease. Given a history of chronic hypertension and tobacco use, as well as evidence of previous lacunes on head CT, the likely etiology of his stroke is small vessel disease. Thus antiplatelets and aggressive risk factor modification is indicated for secondary prevention of future strokes. Given that he had been on aspirin at the time of this stroke, he was considered an aspirin "failure" and clopidrogel was added to his regimen. Aggressive blood pressure management, cholesterol modification, and smoking cessation were encouraged.

One year later, the patient returned to the hospital with similar symptoms. Another lacunar stroke was found in the same region. The patient reported being non-compliant with his medications because he felt they were interfering with his sexual function. He was encouraged to at least take an aspirin a day and follow up with his primary care physician. Again, aggressive management of risk factors was encouraged.

Case Study 11-2

A 77-year-old female with a history of tobacco use awoke to find that she had a "funny" and "heavy" sensation in her right hand, particularly in her last three fingers. She felt that her right hand was "cramped." Her daughter noticed an hour later that the patient's right hand appeared to be clumsy and that her mother was unable to butter the toast. These symptoms began to resolve when she arrived at the emergency department. There was no suggestion of any mental status changes. On admission her blood pressure was 186/66. Examination was normal except for mild pronator drift of the right upper extremity and poor rapid alternating movements and finger taps on the right compared with the left. There was no noticeable dysarthria, aphasia, or neglect. An MRI of the head revealed a small infarct in the left hemisphere centrum semiovale. Carotid duplex revealed less than 40% stenosis bilaterally, and transesophageal echocardiogram revealed a large (7 by 1.5 cm) thrombus with a mobile component in the aortic arch (Figure 11-3). The patient was immediately started on IV heparin and converted to warfarin therapy before returning home.

Discussion and Follow-Up

Although this patient presented with monoparesis and slight clumsiness of the hand, she did not have dysarthria or pure motor hemiparesis. While up to 80% of those presenting with pure motor hemiparesis involving the face, arm, and leg and a history of hypertension have a deep infarct, pure motor monoparesis is less common and is rarely caused by a deep infarct (12). The patient's

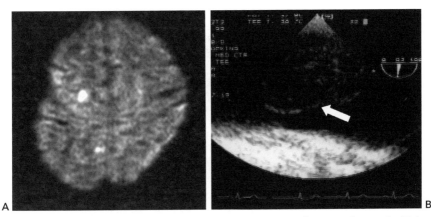

Figure 11-3 A, MRI diffusion-weighted image revealing a small acute infarct in the high white matter at right. **B,** TEE showing a large mobile plaque (*arrow*) in the aortic arch.

presenting symptoms, though minor, were not typical for a lacunar infarct, and her lack of history of hypertension also suggests another etiology. Indeed, although her infarct was small, it was located superficially and was likely caused by an embolic source. She was therefore treated with warfarin. The patient has done well in several years of follow-up.

Case Study 11-3

A 51-year-old morbidly obese male with a history of chronic hypertension, obstructive sleep apnea, and hypercholesterolemia presented with the sudden onset of right-hand numbness and tingling. This progressed to involve his right arm and right leg. He had been taking one aspirin per day. On admission his blood pressure was 195/102 and he was alert and oriented. Neurological examination was normal except for a slight right pronator drift and mild right-sided weakness. There was no evidence of dysarthria, aphasia, or neglect. On sensory examination he had decreased light touch to his right lower face and hand, but hyperesthesia to pin prick and cold sensation of his right face, arm, and leg. Later, he reported dysesthesias to pain and light touch to his right upper and lower extremity. The patient was felt to have a sensorimotor syndrome and a thalamocapsular infarct by clinical findings.

Head CT was initially negative but later revealed a small CVA at the posterior limb of the internal capsule, extending into the thalamus (Figure 11-4). He could not undergo MRI due to his obesity. Carotid duplex was negative for significant stenosis, and TEE revealed no cardioembolic stroke. Transcranial Dopplers were performed due to

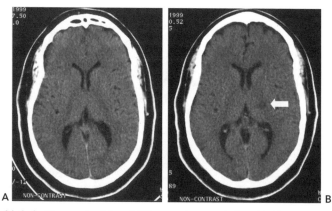

Figure 11-4 A, Non-contrast head CT scan at presentation. **B,** Non-contrast head CT scan 3 days later revealing new left thalamocapsular stroke (*arrow*).

the inability to perform MRI; they revealed possible stenosis of one segment of his left MCA. CT angiography revealed evidence of a severely stenotic lesion in the M1 segment of his left MCA.

It was recommended that the patient be started on clopidrogel instead of aspirin in combination with aggressive reduction of cerebrovascular risk factors. There was no evidence of diabetes mellitus. Warfarin was considered, but the patient was non-compliant in the past with follow-up visits and, upon discussion, the patient declined the intervention. Lifestyle changes including diet, weight-loss, and physical activity were encouraged.

Discussion and Follow-Up

This patient presented with a sensorimotor stroke suggestive of a lacunar syndrome. Furthermore, given his history of hypertension and hypercholesterolemia, the suspicion for small vessel disease was high. However, further evaluation revealed a large vessel stenosis as the likely etiology of his stroke, emphasizing that a potential large-vessel arterial or cardiac source of embolism should not be overlooked in patients presenting with suspected lacunar stroke. While in this case the eventual treatment was unchanged, patients with intracranial large vessel stenosis may be candidates for stenting; future clinical trials should clarify this issue. Patients with carotid stenosis or a cardio-embolic source may be candidates for carotid endarterectomy or anticoagulation, respectively. The patient in this case remained compliant with his medications and had no further strokes in several years of follow-up.

REFERENCES

1. Bamford J, Sandercock P, Jones L, Warlow C. The natural history of lacunar infarction. The Oxfordshire Community Stroke Project. Stroke. 1987;18:545-51.
2. Petty GW, Brown RD Jr., Whisnant JP, et al. Ischemic stroke subtypes: a population-based study of incidence and risk factors. Stroke. 1999;30:2513-6.
3. Mohr JP, Caplan LR, Melski JW, et al. The Harvard Cooperative Stroke Registry: a prospective registry. Neurology. 1978;28:754-62.
4. Gan R, Sacco RL, Kargman DE, et al. Testing the validity of the lacunar hypothesis. The Northern Manhattan Stroke Study experience. Neurology. 1997;48:1204-11.
5. Giroud M, Milan C, Beuriat P, et al. Incidence and survival rates during a two-year period of intracerebral and subarachnoid haemorrhages, cortical infarcts, lacunes and transient ischaemic attacks. The Stroke Registry of Dijon: 1985-1989. Int J Epidemiol. 1991;20:892-9.
6. Durand-Fardel M. Traite du ramollissement du cerveau. Paris: Bailliere; 1843.
7. Fisher CM. Lacunes: Small, deep cerebral infarcts. Neurology. 1965;15:774-84.
8. Fisher CM. Lacunar strokes and infarcts: a review. Neurology. 1982;32:871-6.
9. Millikan C, Futrell N. The fallacy of the lacune hypothesis. Stroke. 1990;21:1251-7.
10. Kappelle LJ, van Gijn J. Lacunar infarcts. Clin Neurol Neurosurg. 1986;88:3-17.
11. Moulin T, Bogousslavsky J, Chopard JL, et al. Vascular ataxic hemiparesis: a re-evaluation. J Neurol Neurosurg Psychiatry. 1995;58:422-7.

12. Melo TP, Bogousslavsky J, van Melle G, Regli F. Pure motor stroke: a reappraisal. Neurology. 1992;42:789-95.

13. Chokroverty S, Rubino FA, Haller C. Pure motor hemiplegia due to pyramidal infarction. Arch Neurol. 1975;32:647-8.

14. Brazis PW. Localization in Clinical Neurology, 3rd ed. New York: Little, Brown; 1996.

15. Hommel M, Besson G, Pollak P, et al. Pure sensory stroke due to a pontine lacune. Stroke. 1989;20:406-8.

16. Helweg-Larsen S, Larsson H, Henriksen O, Sorensen PS. Ataxic hemiparesis: three different locations of lesions studied by MRI. Neurology. 1988;38:1322-4.

17. Gorman MJ, Dafer R, Levine SR. Ataxic hemiparesis: critical appraisal of a lacunar syndrome. Stroke. 1998;29:2549-55.

18. Schonewille WJ, Tuhrim S, Singer MB, Atlas SW. Diffusion-weighted MRI in acute lacunar syndromes: a clinical-radiological correlation study. Stroke. 1999;30:2066-9.

19. Huang CY, Woo E, Yu YL, Chan FL. When is sensorimotor stroke a lacunar syndrome? J Neurol Neurosurg Psychiatry. 1987;50:720-6.

20. Herderschee D, Hijdra A, Algra A, et al. Silent stroke in patients with transient ischemic attack or minor ischemic stroke. The Dutch TIA Trial Study Group. Stroke 1992; 23:1220-4.

21. Kobayashi S, Okada K, Yamashita K. Incidence of silent lacunar lesion in normal adults and its relation to cerebral blood flow and risk factors. Stroke. 1991;22:1379-83.

22. de Jong G, van Raak L, Kessels F, Lodder J. Stroke subtype and mortality. a follow-up study in 998 patients with a first cerebral infarct. J Clin Epidemiol. 2003;56:262-8.

23. Dong Y, Hassan A, Zhang Z, et al. Yield of screening for CADASIL mutations in lacunar stroke and leukoaraiosis. Stroke. 2003;34:203-5.

24. Toni D, Del Duca R, Fiorelli M, et al. Pure motor hemiparesis and sensorimotor stroke. Accuracy of very early clinical diagnosis of lacunar strokes. Stroke. 1994;25:92-6.

25. Horowitz DR, Tuhrim S, Weinberger JM, Rudolph SH. Mechanisms in lacunar infarction. Stroke. 1992;23:325-7.

26. Inzitari D, Eliasziw M, Sharpe BL, et al. Risk factors and outcome of patients with carotid artery stenosis presenting with lacunar stroke. North American Symptomatic Carotid Endarterectomy Trial Group. Neurology. 2000;54:660-6.

27. You R, McNeil JJ, O'Malley HM, et al. Risk factors for lacunar infarction syndromes. Neurology. 1995;45:1483-7.

28. Longstreth WT Jr., Bernick C, Manolio TA, et al. Lacunar infarcts defined by magnetic resonance imaging of 3660 elderly people: the Cardiovascular Health Study. Arch Neurol. 1998;55:1217-25.

29. Megherbi SE, Milan C, Minier D, et al. Association between diabetes and stroke subtype on survival and functional outcome 3 months after stroke: data from the European BIOMED Stroke Project. Stroke. 2003;34:688-94.

30. Pullicino P, Nelson RF, Kendall BE, Marshall J. Small deep infarcts diagnosed on computed tomography. Neurology. 1980;30:1090-6.

31. Baumgartner RW, Sidler C, Mosso M, Georgiadis D. Ischemic lacunar stroke in patients with and without potential mechanism other than small-artery disease. Stroke. 2003;34:653-9.

32. Samuelsson M, Soderfeldt B, Olsson GB. Functional outcome in patients with lacunar infarction. Stroke. 1996;27:842-6.

33. Clavier I, Hommel M, Besson G, et al. Long-term prognosis of symptomatic lacunar infarcts: a hospital-based study. Stroke. 1994;25:2005-9.

34. Staaf G, Lindgren A, Norrving B. Pure motor stroke from presumed lacunar infarct: long-term prognosis for survival and risk of recurrent stroke. Stroke. 2001;32:2592-6.

35. Albers GW, Hart RG, Lutsep HL, et al. AHA Scientific Statement. Supplement to the guidelines for the management of transient ischemic attacks: a statement from the Ad Hoc

Committee on Guidelines for the Management of Transient Ischemic Attacks, Stroke Council, American Heart Association. Stroke. 1999;30:2502-11.

36. Teasell R. Stroke recovery and rehabilitation. Stroke. 2003;34:365-6.

37. Musicco M, Emberti L, Nappi G, Caltagirone C. Early and long-term outcome of rehabilitation in stroke patients: the role of patient characteristics, time of initiation, and duration of interventions. Arch Phys Med Rehabil. 2003;84:551-8.

38. Wardlaw JM, Sandercock PA, Dennis MS, Starr J. Is breakdown of the blood-brain barrier responsible for lacunar stroke, leukoaraiosis, and dementia? Stroke. 2003;34:806-12.

39. Kwiatkowski TG, Libman RB, Frankel M, et al. Effects of tissue plasminogen activator for acute ischemic stroke at one year. National Institute of Neurological Disorders and Stroke Recombinant Tissue Plasminogen Activator Stroke Study Group. N Engl J Med. 1999;340:1781-7.

40. Hacke W, Kaste M, Fieschi C, et al. Intravenous thrombolysis with recombinant tissue plasminogen activator for acute hemispheric stroke. The European Cooperative Acute Stroke Study (ECASS). JAMA. 1995;274:1017-25.

41. Toni D, Iweins F, von Kummer R, et al. Identification of lacunar infarcts before thrombolysis in the ECASS I study. Neurology. 2000;54:684-8.

42. Chalela JA, Ezzeddine M, Latour L, Warach S. Reversal of perfusion and diffusion abnormalities after intravenous thrombolysis for a lacunar infarction. J Neuroimaging. 2003;13:152-4.

43. Mohr JP, Thompson JL, Lazar RM, et al. A comparison of warfarin and aspirin for the prevention of recurrent ischemic stroke. N Engl J Med. 2001;345:1444-51.

Chapter 12

Posterior Circulation Stroke

ISHTIAQ AHMAD, MD, PhD
ROBERT J. WITYK, MD

Key Points

- Diagnostic evaluation and treatment of posterior circulation stroke is similar to that of anterior circulation disease.
- Common but vague symptoms such as dizziness or impaired balance in an elderly patient may be the only warning sign of posterior circulation stroke.
- The vertebral artery is a common site of atherosclerosis. The vertebral artery dissection can result from neck injury.
- Patients with stroke resulting from vertebral artery disease have vertigo and ataxia as their primary symptoms.
- Motor or oculomotor signs are the characteristic symptoms of stroke from basilar artery disease.
- The most important abnormalities in patients with posterior cerebral artery disease infarcts relate to vision, memory, sensation, higher cortical function, and behavior.

Vertebrobasilar (posterior circulation) occlusive disease differs from anterior circulation ischemic disease in clinical presentation and prognosis. Its diagnosis and management are challenging because the structures supplied by the posterior circulation are complex, and the patient may present with a wide spectrum of signs and symptoms during ischemia. One should be careful when evaluating common but vague symptoms such as dizziness or impaired balance in an elderly patient because they may be the only warning signs of a potentially devastating posterior circulation stroke.

New technological advances have improved our ability to detect lesions in vertebrobasilar circulation and now include several reliable noninvasive means. Magnetic resonance imaging (MRI) clearly delineates cerebellar strokes and is able to detect many small brain stem lesions. Doppler ultrasound and transcranial Doppler (TCD) allow dynamic and repeatable measurement of blood flow velocity in the cervical and intracranial portions of the posterior circulation. Magnetic resonance angiography (MRA) and computed tomographic angiography (CTA) now promise a noninvasive means of imaging the arteries of the posterior circulation and providing important anatomical data. With these improved diagnostic capabilities, we can evaluate more closely our current therapies for vertebrobasilar ischemia, including the use of anticoagulation, thrombolytic agents, angioplasty, stenting, and arterial reconstructive surgery. This chapter discusses the anatomy of the posterior circulation and the clinical presentation of its various lesions.

Anatomy of the Posterior Brain and Vasculature

The vertebral artery (VA) rises at an acute angle as the first branch of the subclavian arteries (Figure 12-1). Its course is divided into four segments: the first part from the origin at the subclavian artery to its entrance into the foramen transversarium at C6; the second part within the foramen transversarium from C6 to C2; the third part starting at C2 and winding around the atlas; and the fourth part from where it pierces the dura at the foramen magnum to the junction with the other vertebral artery to the basilar artery (BA) at the pontomedullary junction. The VA is relatively fixed at its origin, its second and intracranial segment. The third segment is more loosely anchored and vulnerable to trauma during neck motion. The extracranial vertebral artery gives off a number of deep muscular branches; its rich collateral circulation comes from the ascending cervical and transverse cervical branches of the thyrocervical trunk, the occipital branches of the external carotid arteries, and the contralateral branches of the subclavian and external carotid arteries, which come from the other vertebral artery.

The intracranial vertebral artery supplies the medulla and the inferior surfaces of the cerebellum. Its two most important branches are the posteroinferior cerebellar artery (PICA), which emerges laterally from segment four of the VA, and a branch which runs medially from this segment to merge with its contralateral branch and form the anterior spinal artery. The BA runs along the base of the pons on the clivus and terminates at the level of the midbrain, where it divides into the two posterior cerebral arteries (PCAs). The BA supplies the pons and has two major circumferential branches: the anteroinferior cerebellar artery (AICA), which supplies the lateral pontine tegmentum and the inferior rostral cerebellum, and the superior cerebellar artery (SCA), which supplies the superior surface of the cerebellum.

Numerous smaller branches arising from the dorsal and lateral portions of the basilar artery penetrate the brainstem and supply the bulk of the

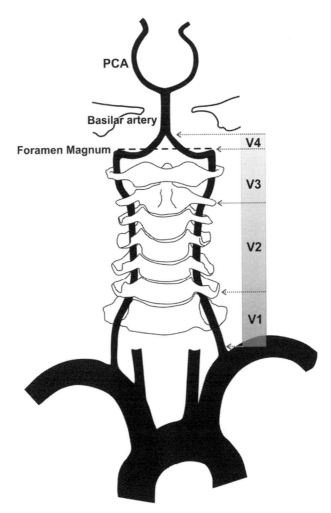

Figure 12-1 Diagram showing the four segments of the vertebral artery. *V1 segment:* Origin from subclavian artery to foramen transversarium of C6. *V2 segment:* C6 to C2 foramen transversarium. *V3 segment:* C2 to the vessel pierced dura. *V4 segment:* Intradural vertebral artery until it joins the other vertebral artery to form the basilar artery.

pons. Other small penetrating arteries that arise from the distal basilar artery supply parts of the midbrain and medial thalamus. The two PCAs communicate with the internal carotid arteries via the posterior communicating arteries as part of the circle of Willis. The PCAs then course around the midbrain, giving off a group of small thalamogeniculate branches to the lateral thalami. The major branches of the PCA supply the medial temporal lobes and the occipital lobes, including the striate visual cortex on the banks of the calcarine fissure.

Clinical Features

Different portions of the vertebrobasilar arterial system supply specific anatomic loci. Described below are the diseases related to the vertebral, basilar, and posterior cerebral arteries, respectively.

Vertebral Artery Diseases

The VA, from its penetration of the dura to its junction with the BA, is a common site of atherosclerosis. In a normal VA, there are three sites of physiological narrowing: 1) just after it pierces the dura; 2) proximal to the origin of the PICA; and 3) just before the junction with the basilar artery. Emboli can lodge at these locations and may produce symptoms. Whether the patient will be symptomatic depends on the adequacy of blood flow through the other VA.

Subclavian Steal Syndrome

Disease of the subclavian artery proximal to the vertebral artery origin may cause posterior circulation ischemia due to hypoperfusion (Figure 12-2). When both VAs are patent, blood may sometimes flow antegrade up one VA, and then flow retrograde down the VA associated with the subclavian stenosis to supply the ischemic arm, resulting in the subclavian steal syndrome. Limb symptoms associated with this syndrome are fatigue, claudication upon exercise, paresthesia, sensitivity to cold, and heaviness or coolness of the affected arm. Neurologic symptoms of subclavian steal syndrome include dizziness or vertigo, visual blurring, inability to fixate (probably due to vestibular dysfunction), and nystagmus. Perioral or limb numbness and unilateral or bilateral weakness occur infrequently.

On examination, brachial blood pressure is at least 20 mm Hg lower on the involved side. The radial pulse is invariably small, absent, or difficult to palpate in the involved side. A bruit is sometimes audible in the supraclavicular fossa. Vertebral bruits can be bilateral because of the increased flow in both the VAs. Another helpful sign is arm or cerebral ischemia when exercising the arm with the diminished pulse.

The most common cause of subclavian artery disease is atherosclerosis. Congenital lesions such as preductal coarctation of the aorta associated with patent ductus arteriosus, atresia of the left subclavian artery, or pseudocoarctation of the aorta with kinked left subclavian artery occasionally cause this syndrome (1). Sometimes subclavian steal syndrome can be caused by surgery for the repair of tetrology of Fallot, Takayasu disease, and temporal arteritis (2).

Despite the well-known description of subclavian steal syndrome, it is surprising to find that many patients with subclavian stenosis and angiographic subclavian steal are asymptomatic and that, among patients with

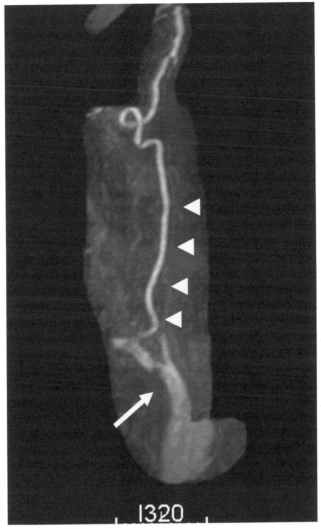

Figure 12-2 Subclavian artery stenosis. Magnetic resonance angiography of the neck and chest showing stenosis (*arrow*) at proximal right subclavian artery just after the origin of right common carotid artery. The vertebral artery (*arrowheads*) arises from the subclavian artery and shows a normal lumen.

symptoms, transischemic attacks (TIAs) may be common but actual stroke is not.

Vertebral Artery Dissection
The VA can be injured during sudden neck rotation or movement or after direct neck injury (e.g., whiplash injury or chiropractic manipulation of the neck). The most common location of the injury is the third segment of

the VA near the C1 and C2 vertebrae before it pierces the dura (Figure 12-3). Injury to the vascular intima of the vertebral artery results in development of a mural hematoma, which can narrow or even occlude the arterial lumen. In addition, the dissection and intimal disruption activates the clotting mechanism, so that a thrombus can form in the distal VA and embolize to the distal BA or PCAs. Formation of a dissecting pseudoaneurysm and perforation of the artery can also occur.

In most patients with traumatic dissection of the distal extracranial VA, the syndrome is unilateral and the ischemia is limited to the lateral medulla,

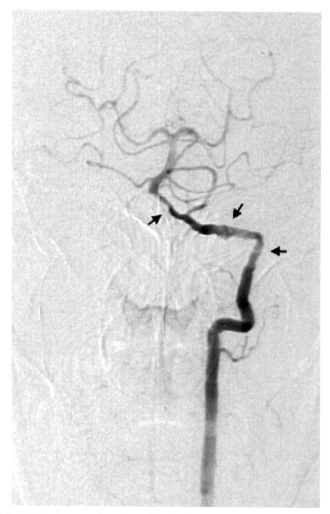

Figure 12-3 Vertebral artery dissection. Cerebral angiogram (AP view of left vertebral artery injection) shows marked irregularity of the distal left vertebral artery dissection involving the V3 and V4 segments, consistent with vertebral artery dissection.

pons, and ipsilateral cerebellum. When initial findings indicate bilateral brainstem ischemia, the course is often progressive and fatal. Bilateral spontaneous dissections of the VAs are not uncommon and suggest an underlying process in the artery predisposing to dissection. The nature of this underlying process is not known at this time, but subtle inflammatory or connective tissue disorders have been hypothesized.

Spontaneous dissection of the intracranial VA has been reported, but it is much less common. Acute-onset headache is the earliest symptom, often accompanied by posterior neck pain, and may be noted hours to days before the onset of neurologic symptoms. The dissection can progress to the basilar artery, resulting in quadriparesis and coma, or remain limited to the unilateral VA, with symptoms related to unilateral medullary or lower pontine ischemia. Subarachnoid hemorrhage is a common complication of dissection of the intracranial VA (3).

Cerebellar Stroke

Cardiogenic embolism and the atherosclerotic occlusion of arteries supplying the cerebellum (PICA, AICA, and SCA) are frequent causes of cerebellar stroke. Commonly, an embolus lodged in the intracranial VA produces an ipsilateral PICA territory infarct. The typical clinical presentation is sudden onset of gait ataxia, dizziness, and vomiting. Sometimes it is associated with prominent nystagmus, dysarthria, ipsilateral limb ataxia, and occipital headache. Some infarcts affecting the cerebellar vermis (the medial branch of the PICA) present solely with vestibular symptoms that may have a positional character and be mistaken for acute labyrinthitis. Potential swelling of the infarct and brainstem compression make this a treacherous diagnosis to miss. Patients with labyrinthitis typically have horizontal and rotatory nystagmus in one direction that is contralateral to the affected ear. Vertical nystagmus or nystagmus that changes direction depending on the gaze is indicative of brainstem or cerebellar lesions. With cerebellar infarct, the nystagmus tends to be more prominent with gaze toward the lesion. With both cerebellar and labyrinthine lesions, patients tend to veer toward the lesion when walking, but severe ataxia, particularly out of proportion to the degree of dizziness, suggests a cerebellar lesion. A patient with normal tandem gait is unlikely to have an acute large PICA infarct.

Large infarcts can swell and lead to new neurologic deficits 2-3 days after stroke. The edematous hemisphere compresses the ipsilateral brainstem, initially producing ipsilateral sixth nerve palsy or gaze palsy and sometimes an associated facial weakness and Horner's syndrome. The eyes deviate away from the lesion and, unlike hemispheric gaze deviation, they cannot be brought across the midline with either caloric stimulation or head rotation. Hydrocephalus may develop from the compression of the fourth ventricle (Figure 12-4), leading to confusion, agitation, and rapid progression to coma. This deterioration can occur in a matter of hours. One then sees pinpoint pupils and decerebrate quadriparesis from pontine

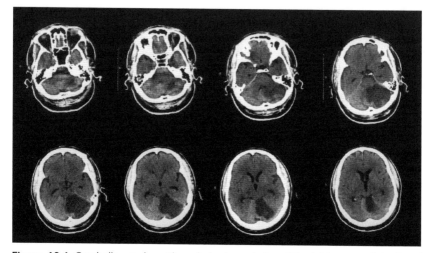

Figure 12-4 Cerebellar stroke with early hydrocephalus. CT axial images of the head showing left inferior cerebellar infarct (PICA territory) seen as a low-density (*dark*) area. There is swelling with compression of fourth ventricle and subtle enlargement of frontal and temporal horns of lateral ventricle, indicating early obstructive hydrocephalus.

compression. Ataxic respiration and later apnea signify medullary compression from tonsillar herniation shortly before death. For this reason, patients with cerebellar strokes should be closely monitored for the first 48 hours after admission, and patients with large cerebellar strokes should be admitted to an intensive care unit.

CT may not show the cerebellar infarct in the first 24-48 hours, and bone artifact may make interpretation of structures in the posterior fossa difficult. Special attention should be paid to the detection of early hydrocephalus as indicated by dilatation of the temporal horns and any compression or change in position of the fourth ventricle (see Figure 12-4). Often the cerebellopontine angle and the ambient cisterns are compressed. MRI can show an infarct within hours. Surgical decompression before progression to coma is the treatment of choice, but ventricular drainage alone for hydrocephalus may be an option in selected patients. Hyperventilation and osmotic agents such as mannitol or hypertonic saline may be beneficial while definitive treatment is pursued.

AICA distribution infarcts are less common and present with ipsilateral facial palsy (cranial nerve VII), deafness and tinnitus (cochlear nucleus), facial sensory loss (trigeminal nucleus), appendicular ataxia (anterior cerebellum), and crossed sensory loss (spinothalamic tract). The typical presenting symptoms include vertigo, nausea, and vomiting from the involvement of flocculus and vestibular nuclei.

Infarction in the SCA territory classically produces dizziness, ipsilateral limb ataxia, Horner's syndrome, and contralateral loss of pain and temperature. There may also be sixth nerve palsy and choreiform, restless

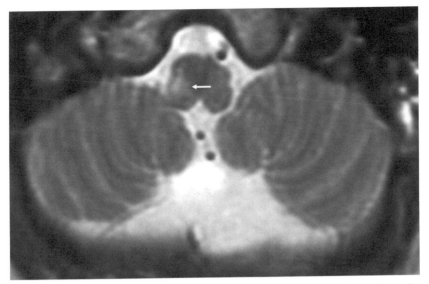

Figure 12-5 Lateral medullary infarct. T_2-weighted MRI shows high signal intensity in the right medulla (*arrow*) consistent with a stroke causing the lateral medullary syndrome.

movements of the ipsilateral limbs, for a day or two after the onset of symptoms. Strokes involving the SCA territory can occasionally develop enough edema to compress the brain stem.

Lateral Medullary Syndrome
A direct branch from VA or PICA usually supplies the lateral medulla. Infarction of this area is variable because of the potential collaterals to this region (Figure 12-5). Patients typically present with headache, dizziness, nausea, vomiting, visual difficulty, and staggering gait. The symptoms may develop suddenly, but a stepwise progression over 24-48 hours is also common. Half the patients will have had transient spells of dizziness, diplopia, and staggering gait prior to stroke. The headache is often steady pain in the ipsilateral occiput, retroauricular or frontal. About 50% of patients have facial pain, usually in the ipsilateral periorbital area and often described as stinging, burning or pricking. This suggests lateral medullary ischemia involving the spinal nucleus of the descending tract of the trigeminal nerve. Dizziness can range from severe vertigo with nausea and vomiting to a slight sense of impaired balance toward the side of the lesion. The ipsilateral ataxia of the arm and leg is due to infarction of the restiform body, the spinocerebellar tract, or the ipsilateral cerebellum. Nystagmus is almost always present with rotatory and horizontal components.

Another hallmark of lateral medullary syndrome is crossed sensory signs, with loss of pain and temperature sensations involving the ipsilateral face and contralateral arm and leg. Involvement of the nucleus ambiguus in the medulla produces dysphonia, dysphagia, hiccups, and vomiting. The ipsilateral vocal cord can be paralyzed, producing a hoarse voice. On examination of the pharynx, the ipsilateral palate fails to elevate so that the uvula pulls toward the intact side. Inadequate attention to swallowing difficulties can lead to aspiration pneumonia, a common cause of morbidity. Dysautonomia with tachycardia, labile blood pressure, and occasionally the failure of automatic respiration can occur from medullary ischemia. Finally, one typically sees a Horner's syndrome on the side of the stroke, due to the interruption of sympathetic fibers from the hypothalamus descending in the lateral medullary tegmentum.

In most patients, the prognosis is good with gradual resolution of symptoms and recovery of bulbar function. The sensory loss and impaired balance during walking often persist. Poor outcome may be related to the propagation of a clot distally or the involvement of other intracranial arteries. An associated large cerebellar (PICA) infarct may swell from edema, producing obstructive hydrocephalus or brainstem compression. Severe headache, decreased alertness, and head tilt are signs of cerebellar involvement. CT scan may miss the infarct due to artifact from bone, but MRI depicts the region well. Angiography or MRA may be needed to diagnose VA occlusion (Figure 12-6).

Basilar Artery Disease

Clinical features of BA disease are variable and depend on the size of the lesion and its etiology. Patients tend to develop more motor or oculomotor signs in BA disease, whereas in VA disease patients primarily have vertigo and ataxia. Focal atherosclerotic stenosis is most commonly seen in the proximal and midbasilar artery, at the level of the AICA (Figure 12-7). Emboli to the basilar artery usually lodge in the distal segment as it becomes smaller rostrally. A lesion in this region produces a characteristic set of findings referred to as the "top-of-the-basilar" syndrome, discussed below.

Basilar Artery Stenosis/Thrombosis

The signs and symptoms of acute stroke depend on the extent of thrombosis of the BA and the acuteness of the onset. With slowly progressive stenosis, TIAs are common starting weeks to months prior to occlusion. Dizziness, blurred vision, dysarthria, diplopia, crossed motor, or sensory symptoms are common. Although basilar stenosis should be part of the differential diagnosis of near syncope, a sudden and transient loss of consciousness without premonitory symptoms or other history of vertebrobasilar TIAs is rarely due to basilar stenosis.

Some degree of motor weakness from ischemia of the corticospinal tracts in the basis pontis is seen in almost all cases of basilar occlusion. Some patients present initially with hemiparesis mimicking MCA stroke, but careful exam shows bilateral motor involvement, with perhaps only hyperreflexia or

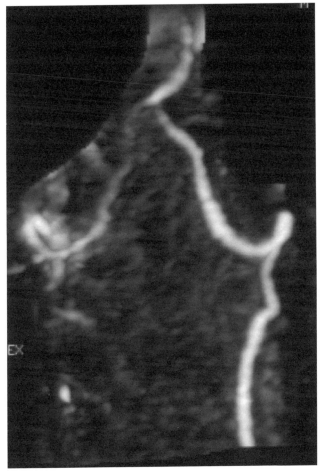

Figure 12-6 Magnetic resonance angiography of the upper neck and head shows a diseased right vertebral artery with probable proximal occlusion and a small amount of residual flow into the V4 segment. The left vertebral artery is normal and fills the basilar artery at the top of the figure.

a Babinski sign on the intact side. Injury to the corticobulbar fibers and the lower cranial nerves cause facial weakness, dysarthria, and dysphagia with pooling of secretion and hyperactive jaw jerk. Pontine infarction classically produces pinpoint pupils that do react to light, though it is difficult to see without magnification. Ptosis can occur from the interruption of the descending sympathetic fibers, and some degree of nystagmus and skew deviation is common, depending on the location of the infarction.

The extreme form of motor weakness is the "locked in" state, in which there is paralysis of all limbs and impairment of the lower cranial nerves. The patient has no motor movement and is unable to communicate, appearing to be in a coma while actually alert and awake. Consciousness

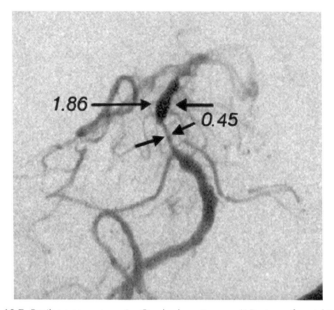

Figure 12-7 Basilar artery stenosis. Cerebral angiogram (AP view of a right vertebral artery injection) shows a high-grade proximal basilar artery stenosis of more than 70% stenosis (*arrows*).

is retained, because the collateral circulation spares the reticular formation of the pontine tegmentum. The midbrain structures are often spared, with the patient retaining control of blinking and vertical eye movement, which can be used for communication.

Because of the potentially severe outcome, patients with suspected basilar thrombosis should be monitored carefully, ideally in an intensive care unit. As brainstem ischemia progresses, the patient is often at risk for bulbar dysfunction, leading to aspiration and sometimes cessation of adequate respiration.

MRI may show abnormal signal in the basis pontis; MRA, CTA, TCD, or angiography will reveal the BA stenosis of occlusion (Figure 12-8).

Disease of the Perforators from the Basilar Artery
Atheromatous plaque on the wall of the BA can occlude the orifice of perforating and the short circumferential branch arteries, leading to hypoperfusion of a small portion of the pons. Usually, the MRI shows a small pontine lesion with a patent BA (Figure 12-9). Fisher described microscopic changes of lipohyalinosis in the small penetrating vessels of hypertensive patients, which may progress to occlusion and produce small, deep lacunar infarcts (4). Pontine lesions can cause three types of lacunar syndrome.

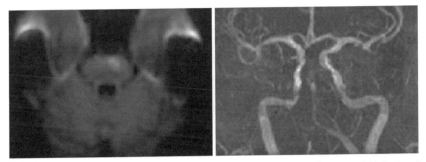

Figure 12-8 Pontine stroke. Diffusion-weighted MRI shows a small region of high signal intensity in left pons consistent with an acute infarct (*left*). Magnetic resonance angiography shows normal flow in both carotid arteries inside the head but poor flow in the vertebral arteries and suggestion of multifocal stenosis of the basilar artery (*right*).

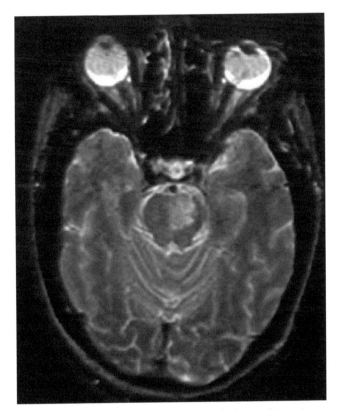

Figure 12-9 Pontine stroke. T$_2$-weighted MRI shows a high signal intensity representing a left pontine lesion primarily in the left pons consistent with infarct. Magnetic resonance angiography (not shown) revealed good flow in the vertebrobasilar system, which indicated that the pontine infarct was likely related to occlusion of a paramedian perforator from the basilar trunk.

Pure motor hemiparesis can occur with a paramedian pontine infarct involving corticospinal fiber on one side, causing a contralateral hemiparesis often sparing the face. Pure motor hemiparesis can also occur in the internal capsule-corona radiata lacunar infarct, the area supplied by the lenticulostriate branch of the MCA. A lacunar lesion at the contralateral basis pontis can produce the dysarthria, clumsy hand syndrome, which consists of moderate to severe dysarthria, corticobulbar weakness of the lower face and tongue, and slowness of fine movement of the hand. Ataxic hemiparesis is the third lacunar syndrome, consisting of mild hemiparesis with cerebellar-type ataxia in the affected limb out of proportion to the degree of weakness. The autopsy of the first reported such case found a lesion in the rostral pons, but now MRI shows that lesions at the posterior limb of the internal capsule can also cause this syndrome.

Top-of-the-Basilar Syndrome

The vessels arising from the rostral BA include the SCA, PCA, and small perforating arteries that supply the medial midbrain and paramedian diencephalic structures. Occlusive lesions that extend into the PCA can involve small branches to the midbrain, the thalamogeniculate artery, and the distal PCA territory in the medial temporal and occipital lobes.

Prominent behavioral changes and subtle oculomotor deficit are the major findings in patients with an embolus at the top of the basilar artery. The patient may present with agitated delirium and cognitive deficits, prompting a workup for metabolic encephalopathy. It is easy to overlook the vascular nature of the disease, but subtle abnormalities of the eye movements are usually the best clues to the diagnosis.

A patient may have a loss of voluntary vertical gaze, papillary abnormalities, and difficulty with convergence. A center for vertical gaze is located in the pretectal region and affected by this stroke syndrome. Rostral basilar ischemia causes alteration of consciousness and hypersomnolence, because of the involvement of midbrain perforators supplying the medial mesencephalon and diencephalon that contain the rostral portion of the reticular formation. Anterograde and retrograde amnesia occur due to the involvement of medial thalamic structures, which have extensive connections with the medial temporal and frontal lobes.

Patients with the top-of-the-basilar syndrome are often difficult to diagnose because their somnolence or cognitive impairments limit detailed neurologic examination. Some patients have a visual field deficit due to associated PCA stroke. Other patients are discovered when MRI is performed as part of the evaluation of persistent cognitive change (Figure 12-10). Remarkably, small infarcts in the medial thalamus may produce profound behavioral changes. Because of the midline nature of the vascular supply, many patients have simultaneous bilateral medial thalamic strokes, which may result in long-term memory deficits.

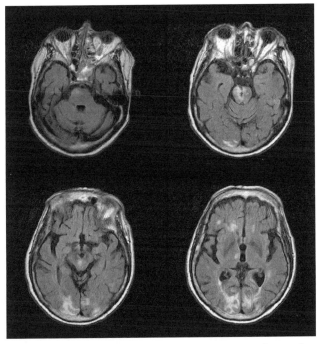

Figure 12-10 Top-of-the-basilar stroke. Brain MRI (FLAIR images) shows infarcts involving the pons, upper midbrain, and both occipital lobes due to an embolus lodged in the distal basilar artery and blocking both posterior cerebral arteries.

Posterior Cerebral Artery Disease

The PCA territory includes the occipital lobe, the inferior and medial portions of the temporal lobe, and the posterolateral part of the thalamus. Occlusion of PCA branches is most often embolic, but intrinsic disease of the PCA does occur; angiography helps make this distinction. The most important abnormalities in patients with PCA infarcts relate to vision, memory, sensation, higher cortical function, and behavior.

Thalamic Infarct

Infarct in the thalamus can be caused by occlusion of small perforating vessels from the PCA by lipohyalinosis or atherosclerosis (Figure 12-11). Clinical findings of thalamogeniculate infarcts include hemibody numbness and paresthesias. The contralateral limbs have a cerebellar-type dysmetria due to loss of sensory feedback. Weeks or months after the infarct, the patient may present with neuropathic pain in the paresthetic limbs, the so-called "thalamic pain syndrome." While many patients spontaneously improve over months to a year, some patients remain with a distressing central pain syndrome lasting years. Traditional treatments have included

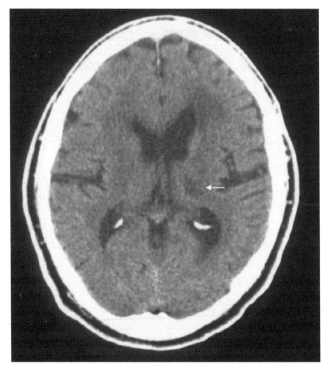

Figure 12-11 Thalamic lacune. Computed tomography of the head shows a left thalamic lacune (*arrow*).

tricyclic antidepressants (e.g., amitriptyline) and anticonvulsant agents, with gabapentin having the best results and least side effects.

Smaller lacunes in the somatosensory nuclei of the thalamus (ventral posterolateral and ventral posteromedial) produce the lacunar syndrome of "pure sensory stroke." Patients complain of tingling, prickling, and a numb feeling on one side of the body with slightly diminished pinprick sense in the affected region. Involvement of the half of the body, including the chest and abdomen, is characteristic of a thalamic lesion and is not generally seen in MCA strokes involving the sensory cortex.

Hemianopia

Infarction of the striate cortex of the occipital lobe causes a homonymous hemianopia of the contralateral visual field. The patient is usually aware of the deficit and describes it as darkness to one side sparing the macular zone. It is remarkable that many patients with hemianopia describe this as loss of vision in one eye, rather than loss of vision in both eyes in the same hemifield. (This is different than hemianopia from MCA stroke, which often involves the parietal lobe and causes neglect as well as hemianopia—the patient cannot see to one side, but is not aware of the deficit.) At times, the visual defect is partial. If it affects only color recognition, the deficit is called hemiachromatopsia, which can be discovered by testing the visual fields with confrontation using a colored pin.

Infarcts in other areas of the occipital and temporal lobes can result in unusual visual and linguistic abnormalities. For example, interruption of connections of the visual cortex with the temporal lobe result in spared vision, but difficulty with interpretation of vision. Some patients, for example, have loss of face recognition, even though they can see and even describe the face. Another classical disconnection syndrome is alexia without agraphia, where the patient can write words but cannot read them. Patients typically have right hemianopia and involvement of the corpus callosum: visual information fed into the right occipital lobe is disconnected from the left hemisphere, where the language systems for reading are located.

Fortunately, many patients with visual loss from occipital infarction have some degree of recovery over time. Presumably, adjacent areas of visual cortex can take over function. In addition, most usable vision involves the macular region in the very center of vision, and if this is spared, reading may be intact. Peripheral visual field defects, however, may limit the patient's mobility and ability to drive a motor vehicle.

Diagnosis and Treatment

In most respects, diagnostic evaluation and treatment of stroke or atherosclerosis involving the posterior circulation is similar to the anterior circulation disease, as described in other chapters of this book. Many years ago, a clinical diagnosis of "vertebrobasilar insufficiency" was felt to be sufficient, but with modern diagnostic techniques full evaluation of vertebrobasilar stroke is warranted.

Several points concerning evaluation and treatment bear mention. The symptoms of vertebrobasilar disease may be relatively non-specific, with complaints of lightheadedness or "dizziness" possibly due to a variety of other disorders. Patients with dizziness who have vascular risk factors should be referred to a neurologist for consultation, particularly to consider vertebrobasilar disease. A careful history of the symptoms and clinical suspicion of vascular disease may lead one to evaluate for cerebrovascular disease. Treatment options for vertebral and basilar artery lesions are increasingly studied and utilized, particularly with the advent of stenting and angioplasty of cerebral vessels (5). While this field is not as advanced as the treatment of carotid disease, the techniques of vertebral artery stenting are not much different. Finally, the severe deficits and poor prognosis for basilar artery thrombosis have led many to pursue very aggressive treatment for progressing brainstem infarction (Case Study 12-1) (6). Some patients have dramatic improvement with intra-arterial thrombolysis of basilar artery clot, although the uncommon nature of this disease has not led to any randomized clinical trials at this time.

Conclusion

Vertebrobasilar ischemia remains a challenge in terms of diagnosis and treatment for both general practitioners and neurology specialists. Signs and symptoms may suggest benign disorders such as peripheral vestibular dysfunction but then may progress to life-threatening deficits. Because of the small size and complexity of the brainstem and the relatively inaccessible vascular supply in the posterior circulation, treatment of stroke in the vertebrobasilar system has lagged behind treatment of carotid disease and cardioembolic stroke. Newer imaging technologies and endovascular approaches to treatment are leading to rapid advancement in this field.

Case Study 12-1

A 50-year-old male presented with sudden-onset dizziness, dysarthria, dysphagia, and ataxia. A week later while on therapeutic heparin he developed a right hemiplegia, worsening dysarthria, and left-gaze paresis. He was alert and oriented. MRI with diffusion-weighted imaging showed infarcts in the pons and cerebellum. MRA showed no flow in the basilar artery (Figure 12-12). Emergent cerebral

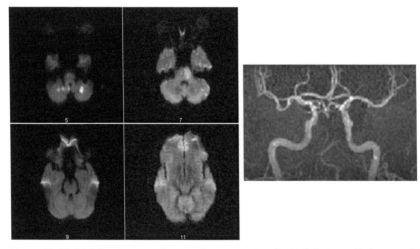

Figure 12-12 Multifocal acute infarcts. Diffusion-weighted MRI (*left 4 panels*) shows multiple bright lesions in the cerebellum and pons consistent with acute ischemia. Magnetic resonance angiography (*right panel*) shows virtually no flow in the proximal and mid basilar artery. Figures 12-13 and 12-14 show the same patient.

angiogram revealed a mid-BA occlusion. The patient underwent intra-arterial administration of t-PA directly into the BA clot with successful recanalization (Figure 12-13). Immediately after the procedure, his neurologic examination remained unchanged. After 6 months of rehabilitation, the patient was left with a spastic right hemiparesis (Figure 12-14). He could ambulate independently with a quad cane and independently engage in activities of daily living. In this case, intra-arterial thrombolysis did not result in immediate neurologic improvement, but it probably prevented the patient from progressing to a locked-in state.

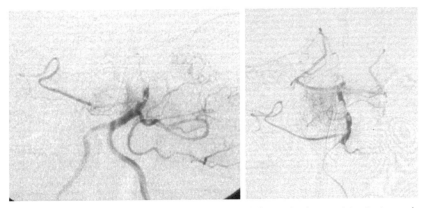

Figure 12-13 Cerebral angiogram (AP view from a left vertebral artery injection) reveals an occluded mid basilar artery (*left*). A microcatheter was threaded into the left vertebral artery up to the point of basilar artery occlusion, and 14 mg of t-PA was slowly infused. Serial repeat angiogram revealed that the basilar artery was partially recanalized from the point of previous occlusion with flow now reaching both posterior cerebral arteries (*right*). See Figures 12-12 and 12-14.

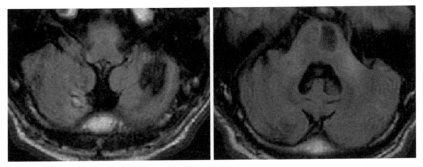

Figure 12-14 MRI at 6 months shows encephalomalacia (*dark signal*) in the left pons and left cerebellum. Note that these regions correspond to infracted areas predicted by the initial diffusion-weighted MRI (Figure 12-12).

REFERENCES

1. **Reivich M, Holling HE, Roberts B, Toole JF.** Reversal of blood flow through the vertebral artery and its effect on cerebral circulation. N Engl J Med. 1961;265:878-85.
2. **Pollock M, Blennerhassett JB, Clarke AM.** Giant cell arteritis and the subclavian steal syndrome. Neurology. 1973;23:653-7.
3. **Caplan LR, Baquis GD, Pessin MS, et al.** Dissection of the intracranial vertebral artery. Neurology. 1988;38:868-77.
4. **Fisher CM.** The arterial lesions underlying lacunes. Acta Neuropathol (Berl). 1968;12: 1-15.
5. **Albuquerque FC, Fiorella D, Han P, et al.** A reappraisal of angioplasty and stenting for the treatment of vertebral origin stenosis. Neurosurgery. 2003;53:607-16.
6. **Eckert B, Kucinski T, Pfeiffer G, et al.** Endovascular therapy of acute vertebrobasilar occlusion: early treatment onset as the most important factor. Cerebrovasc Dis. 2002;14:42-50

Chapter 13

Stroke in Young Patients

LORI C. JORDAN, MD

Key Points

- Risk factors for stroke in young patients include diabetes, hypertension, and cigarette smoking.
- Cardioembolism is the most common cause of stroke in young patients. Patent foramen ovale (PFO) is the most common congenital cardiac abnormality.
- In patients with a combination of patent foramen ovale and atrial septal aneurysm, PFO closure or aggressive medical management is recommended.
- Vasculitis causes 3%-5% of strokes in young patients. Treatment may include glucocorticoids, immunosuppressive therapy, and treatment of an underlying systemic disorder.
- Other causes of stroke in young patients are fibromuscular dysplasia, Moyamoya disease, and arterial dissection.
- Although prognosis after stroke in the young is better than in older patients, the impact of stroke is nevertheless significant because of the increase in years of disability for younger patients.

Stroke in individuals aged 15-44 years is a significant public health problem with an incidence of 9/100,000 (1). Between 5% and 10% of all stroke victims are children and young adults. In the year 2000, cerebrovascular disease was the seventh leading cause of death in Americans 15-24 years of age, and the eighth leading cause of death in those 25-44 years old, accounting for 3315 deaths (2). A significantly greater number suffer disability as a result of stroke. This chapter reviews the causes of stroke in children and young adults, focusing specifically on entities such as patent foramen ovale (PFO), atrial septal aneurysm, vasculitis, arterial dissection, and the impact of migraine and pregnancy on stroke risk.

Risk Factors

Risk factors for stroke at a young age include traditional concerns such as diabetes, hypertension, and cigarette smoking. Cigarette smoking and hypertension are considered the two most modifiable stroke risk factors, and are particularly important in young African Americans (3). Additional risk factors include cardiac/embolic causes, inherited conditions causing early or accelerated atherosclerosis, oral contraceptive use, hypercoagulability, and migraine headaches. Unfortunately, despite careful evaluation, 25%-40% of young adults with stroke will have no specific cause identified; these patients are classified as having cryptogenic stroke (4).

Patent Foramen Ovale and Atrial Septal Aneurysm

Cardioembolism is the most common etiology of stroke in young patients, accounting for one-third of all cerebral infarctions. Many patients have known cardiac disease. However, the recent widespread use of transesophageal echocardiography has revealed a host of more subtle findings.

PFO is the most common congenital cardiac abnormality and can be detected by transthoracic echocardiography in 10%-15% of the normal adult population (Figure 13-1) (5). The association of PFO and cryptogenic stroke has been demonstrated by multiple studies, the majority of which are retrospective (6-10). A meta-analysis of case-control studies found a convincing association of PFO with cryptogenic stroke in patients under the age of 55 years (11).

Because paradoxical emboli are rarely seen crossing the atrial septum during an echocardiogram, a causal relationship between PFO and stroke in an individual patient is difficult to prove. Most authors agree that a PFO

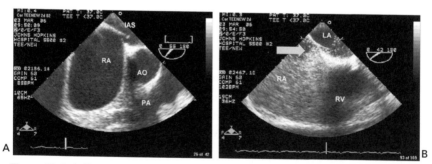

Figure 13-1 A, Transesophageal echocardiogram (TEE) view of the right atrium (RA) and intra-arterial septum (IAS), pre-agitated saline contrast study. Pulmonary artery (PA); aorta (AO). **B,** TEE shows agitated saline contrast study, with right-to-left shunting consistent with PFO (*arrow*). Right atrium (RA); left atrium (LA); right ventricle (RV). (Courtesy of Dr. Mary Corretti, Director of the Johns Hopkins Echocardiography Laboratory.)

by itself is insufficient evidence for diagnosing a paradoxical embolic stroke (i.e., a stroke coming from the venous system in the absence of a deep venous thrombosis [DVT]) or a history placing the patient at increased risk for DVT. Certain settings (e.g., surgery, recent travel with prolonged immobility, cancer) make occult DVT and paradoxical embolism more likely. Evaluation of patients without clinical signs of a DVT by lower extremity noninvasive studies is usually unrevealing. One report revealed occult pelvic vein DVT (using pelvic magetic resonance imaging [MRI] and MRV) in 20% of cryptogenic stroke patients with PFO (12).

Atrial septal aneurysm (ASA) is a congenital, localized bulging of the interatrial septum with excursion into the atrium of at least 10 mm. Putative mechanisms for stroke in patients with ASA include embolization of thrombi formed within the ASA or an association with atrial arrhythmias (7). The ASA multicenter, retrospective, Italian trial evaluated the prevalence of atrial septal aneurysm and the association with PFO in a subgroup of patients with stroke under age 55 and normal carotid arteries (5). ASA and PFO were both more common in patients with stroke than in controls and, in this retrospective review, both ASA and PFO were independent, statistically significant risk factors for stroke.

Impact of Patent Foramen Ovale and Atrial Septal Aneurysm on Stroke Recurrence Risk

The recurrence risk for cerebrovascular events (i.e., stroke or TIA attributed to PFO, ASA, or both while on antiplatelet or anticoagulant therapy) has been addressed in five major studies (6-9a), four of which are summarized in Table 13-1. (The fifth study is discussed below.) With PFO, the average annual recurrence rate was a minimal 1.2%-2.4% for stroke and 2.4%-5.5% for TIA. Patients were followed for an average of 2-3 years.

Table 13-1 Average Annual Recurrent Cerebral Ischemic Events in Patients with Patent Foramen Ovale

Study	No. of Patients	Stroke	Stroke and/or TIA
Mas (6)	132	1.2%	3.4%
Bogousslavsky (9)	140	2.4%	3.8%
De Castro (8)	74	. . .	2.4%*
Nedeltchev (9a)	157	1.8%	5.5%

* In the original article the overall cumulative estimate of risk of cerebrovascular event recurrence is given. Here, the average annual event rate was derived from the overall cumulative estimate of risk of stroke or TIA recurrence at 3 years of follow-up in accordance with the formula $1 - (1 - P)^{1/n}$, where P equals the cumulative event rate at n years of follow-up.

Adapted from Nedeltchev K, Arnold M, Wahl, A, et al. Outcome of patients with cryptogenic stroke and patent foramen ovale. J Neurol Neurosurg Psychiatry. 2002;72:347–50.

A recent, prospective multicenter study was designed to assess the recurrence risk of crytpogenic stroke in 581 patients less than 55 years old who had extensive evaluation, including transesophageal echocardiogram (7). Ninety-two percent of patients in this study were on a standardized dose of aspirin (300 mg), so stroke recurrence was on anti-platelet therapy. Over the 3-year period, the risk of recurrent stroke was 0.8% per year in patients with PFO alone and 5% per year in patients with both PFO and ASA. No patient with ASA alone had a recurrent stroke during the study. Among patients with cryptogenic stroke who had neither PFO nor ASA, the recurrence risk was 4.2% over 3 years, or 1.3% per year. Interestingly, the recurrence risk was lower in patients with a PFO than in those with a normal echocardiogram. This study supports the theory that a strong association of PFO and ASA is a risk factor for recurrent stroke; however, in contrast to other retrospective studies, PFO and ASA were not found to be independent risk factors for stroke recurrence (among young stroke patients).

In addition to ASA, some studies have suggested that increased right-to-left shunting and a large PFO size may increase the risk of recurrent stroke. This has not been confirmed in other studies. Conflicting data may be due to small patient numbers in most of the studies, heterogeneity of cryptogenic stroke, and overall low event rate for stroke during follow-up.

Treatment of Patent Foramen Ovale

The best treatment modality to prevent recurrent stroke in patients with PFO with or without ASA has not been determined. The basic options include medical therapy with antiplatelet drugs or anticoagulants and PFO closure either surgically or via percutaneous transcatheter closure device.

The major advantage of PFO closure is that long-term anticoagulation may be avoided. Surgical closure is accomplished by either primary closure or an autologous pericardial patch. Standard cardiac surgical techniques require cardioplegic arrest and cardiopulmonary bypass. The morbidity of surgery is an obvious disadvantage but is very low in young patients. Several retrospective reviews have looked at outcome after surgical closure of PFO (13,14). No mortality was found, and morbidity included atrial fibrillation (11%), pericardial effusion (6%), and post-operative bleeding or wound infection (13,14). Approximately 2 years later, one-half of patients were on anti-platelet or anti-coagulant drugs, one-third of patients were on aspirin therapy alone, 7% were on warfarin, and 5% were on both warfarin and aspirin. Eight patients (8.7%) had recurrent neurologic events despite echocardiogram-confirmed PFO closure, suggesting another mechanism for their cryptogenic stroke.

Transcatheter techniques to close PFO have been used with increasing frequency over the past few years. An umbrella-like device is deployed under angiographic and transthoracic echocardiogram guidance. The device becomes endothelialized over time. The central issues are efficacy and safety. There have been multiple reviews in the cardiology literature (15,16). Martin et al reported their experience with 110 patients (17). After device deployment, full occlusion was achieved in 45% of patients, and 55% had a trivial shunt. In 8 patients (7%), a second device was required to effectively close the PFO. Complications were infrequent but significant when they occurred. One patient (1%) developed the following complications: transient atrial fibrillation, supraventricular tachycardia that resolved with adenosine, device migration into the pulmonary artery requiring immediate surgical intervention, and cardiac tamponade within 24 hours of device deployment requiring pericardiocentesis. There were no deaths. During 2 years of follow-up, 4 patients required re-intervention for significant residual shunt or device malalignment. Recurrent embolic events occurred in only 2.1% of patients over 5 years of follow-up. The results of the foregoing study are slightly more favorable in terms of effective PFO occlusion rate, recurrent events, and complications than earlier reports, which the authors attribute to improvements in patient selection, technical advances, and physician experience. Antiplatelet therapy or anti-coagulation is recommended for 6-12 months after device placement to allow endothelialization of this foreign body. These devices appear to be both safe and effective, but long-term follow-up data are still lacking.

As mentioned, some patients had recurrent neurologic events while on anti-platelet or anticoagulant medication or after closure of their PFO via open-heart surgery or transcatheter device. This situation further illustrates the point that patients with PFO and/or ASA are classified as having cryptogenic stroke, because their initial cerebrovascular event may have been unrelated to their PFO. Again, PFO is present in 10%-15% of the general population and may be an incidental finding. At present, in patients with PFO only or ASA only, there are no prospective data to support closure of the PFO or long-term anti-coagulation without other compelling risk factors. In patients with both PFO and ASA, there are prospective data that point to a significant risk of stroke recurrence (7). Therefore, in patients with a combination of PFO and ASA, PFO closure or aggressive medical management is recommended by this author. Several clinical trials of PFO closure versus medical therapy are underway, and, given the clinical equipoise of this issue, enrollment of patients in studies is urged.

Case Study 13-1 discusses a patient with PFO.

Vasculitis

Vasculitis is an inflammation of the blood vessels with or without necrosis of the vessel wall. Vasculitides affecting the central nervous system (CNS) are classified as primary or secondary (i.e., related to a systemic disorder known to cause blood vessel inflammation). Distinguishing primary from secondary CNS vasculitis may be difficult because some systemic disorders

(SLE, sarcoidosis, and various infections) may present initially with symptoms of nervous system vasculitis without other systemic manifestations (Table 13-2).

Vasculitis is often reported to cause 3%-5% of strokes in those younger than 50 years (18). There is no "diagnostic test" for vasculitis, and routine screening for vasculitis in young people with stroke is not cost effective. Vasculitis should be considered in two types of stroke patients: patients who have systemic signs or already carry a diagnosis of vasculitis and then present with neurologic involvement, and patients who present with stroke and have associated headache and either multifocal neurologic symptoms or diffuse neurologic dysfunction (e.g., encephalopathy) (18,19). Elderly patients, in particular, may have a subacute presentation of progressive dementia (20). Clinical and radiological features may mimic tumor, infection, dementia, or stroke, however, making diagnosis a challenge (20).

Evaluation for vasculitis may include blood work to exclude systemic disease, MRI, cerebrospinal fluid examination to evaluate for inflammation or infection, and potentially cerebral angiography and brain biopsy (Figure 13-2). Unfortunately, no gold standard for the diagnosis of CNS vasculitis exists. All of the tests mentioned above have the potential for false-negative results, including brain biopsy. If the CNS disease is patchy, biopsy may miss the lesion. The diagnostic yield of brain biopsy in idiopathic neurodegenerative disorders, a situation in which CNS vasculitis is generally part of the differential, has been reported to be as low as 20%-36% (22). In the absence of a tissue diagnosis, the diagnosis of CNS vasculitis is based on careful evaluation of clinical signs and symptoms, correlation with radiological findings, and exclusion of other causes.

Table 13-2 Classification of Vasculitis

Primary
  • Primary angiitis of the CNS

Secondary
  • Infection
    —Virus
    —Fungi
    —Bacteria
    —Protozoa
  • Connective Tissue Disease
    —Systemic lupus erythematosus
    —Rheumatoid vasculitis
    —Sjögren's syndrome
    —Scleroderma
    —Dermatomyositis
  • Systemic Vasculitides
    —Giant cell arteritis
    —Takayasu's arteritis
    —Polyarteritis nodosa
    —Wegener's granulomatosis
    —Churg-Strauss
    —Behçet's
    —Drug use (sympathomimetics)

Therapy for vasculitis affecting the nervous system may require gluco-corticoids, immunosuppressive therapy, and, potentially, treatment of an underlying systemic disorder. Given the rarity of primary CNS vasculitis and difficulty confirming diagnosis, treatment has been very difficult to study and has not been subject to large clinical trials.

Primary Angiitis of the Central Nervous System

Primary angiitis of the central nervous system (PACNS), also known as iso-lated angiitis of the CNS and non-infectious granulomatous angiitis of the CNS, is a primarily small-vessel vasculitis restricted to the brain and lep-tomeninges with few systemic symptoms or laboratory findings (18,20). Although PACNS may occur at any age, incidence peaks in the fourth to sixth decades. Stroke or subarachnoid hemorrhage may be the first symp-tom (23). The distribution of pathology may be focal and segmental. Moore and colleagues (23) have suggested the following diagnostic crite-ria for PACNS:

1. Patient must have clinical features consistent with recurrent, multifocal, or diffuse disease.

2. An underlying systemic inflammatory process or infection must be excluded.

3. Neuroradiographic studies, usually cerebral angiography, must support a diagnosis of vasculopathy.

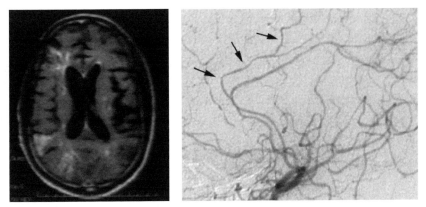

Figure 13-2 Vasculitis. MRI (*left*) shows multifocal areas of ischemia in cortical and sub-cortical regions. High magnification of a cerebral angiogram (*right*) reveals multiple areas of subtle vascular irregularity and narrowing, some of which are indicated by arrows.

4. Brain biopsy must establish the presence of vascular inflammation and exclude infection, neoplasia, or other causes of vasculopathy.

Mortality from PACNS may be due to cerebral ischemia or hemorrhage. Disease may progress rapidly or smolder for years.

Therapy for PACNS generally includes pulse methylprednisolone followed by intravenous or oral cyclophosphamide and oral steroids (18,24). The morbidity of immunosuppressive therapy is significant; in one study, 40% of cases had cytopenia, opportunistic infection, osteoporotic fracture, or cushingoid changes (20). Furthermore, the diagnosis of PACNS is not straightforward. In a recent series, 15 of 30 patients who underwent brain biopsy to "rule out vasculitis" were found to have another diagnosis, including hypertension, amyloid angiopathy, and Alzheimer's disease (20). Only 1 of 30 patients had persistent morbidity (i.e. neurologic deficit after biopsy).

For these reasons, brain biopsy is suggested before committing a patient to immunosuppressive therapy. Although MRI, cerebral angiography, and brain biopsy had similar sensitivities (78%-83%), biopsy had significantly better specificity, 100% in this series, compared with a specificity of 14% for angiography and 19% for MRI (20). False-negative or "non-diagnostic" brain biopsy is possible in up to 20% of patients, given the focal and segmental pathology of PACNS. To minimize this risk, biopsy of both brain parenchyma and the leptomeninges is suggested. Remission and cure have been reported with PACNS (23).

Takayasu's Arteritis

Takayasu's arteritis, originally described in young and middle-aged women of Asian descent, is a large vessel vasculitis affecting the aortic arch and its major branches. Stenosis or occlusion of these great vessels leads to malignant hypertension, subclavian steal, and cerebral hypoperfusion, all of which may cause stroke (18). Patients present with fever, malaise, anemia, and loss of peripheral pulses; the loss of pulses may make hypertension difficult to diagnose via standard blood pressure measurement, hence the common term, "pulseless disease." Although the pathology of Takayasu's seems to be inflammatory, the erythrocyte sedimentation rate (ESR) is not a reliable marker. ESR is elevated in 60%-75% of patients, and values do not seem to correlate with disease activity in all patients. The gold standard for diagnosis is angiography showing narrowing or occlusion of the aorta, its primary branches, or large arteries in the upper and lower extremities, not attributable to other causes. Contrast-enhanced MR angiogram of the aortic arch may also be diagnostic. Treatment may involve immunosuppression (steroids, cytotoxic medication), surgical bypass procedures, and angioplasty of large artery stenoses (25). Long-term follow-up is recommended to monitor for end-organ ischemia and other complications such as stroke, retinopathy, hypertension secondary to renal artery stenosis, and aneurysm formation.

Polyarteritis Nodosa

Polyarteritis nodosa (PAN) is a medium and small vessel necrotizing arterial vasculitis. PAN presents with fever, malaise, and weight loss. The characteristic erythematous, purpuric, and nodular skin lesions may help to differentiate PAN from other vasculitides (19). Up to 70% of PAN has been associated with hepatitis B; however, this number is declining as hepatitis immunization becomes more prevalent (18). Unfortunately, hepatitis C is now replacing hepatitis B as an increasingly common cause of PAN. PAN may involve multiple organs: renal involvement occurs in over 70% of patients, and the CNS is affected in 40% of those with PAN (18,19). The long-term morbidity is due to hypertension affecting the heart and cerebral vessels. Stroke usually occurs later in the course of disease. Frequent presentations of PAN include encephalopathy, multifocal strokes of the brain and spinal cord, and subarachnoid hemorrhage. Immunosuppression is the treatment (19,23,26).

Fibromuscular Dysplasia

Fibromuscular dysplasia (FMD) of the carotid or the intracranial arteries is a disorder of the arterial wall presenting with constricting bands of fibrous material alternating with smooth muscle, resulting in alternating constriction and dilatation of the artery (25). This pattern of involvement leads to the classic "stack of plates" appearance on cerebral angiogram (Figure 13-3). A rare disorder, FMD is found in 0.6% of non-selected angiograms and is most prevalent among middle-aged women (25). One study of 70 patients with cerebrovascular FMD found that 89% of the patients were women (27). Common symptoms at the time of presentation were TIA, pulsitile tinnitus, and, with lesser frequency, stroke (27). Loud carotid bruit is also common, even with a relatively mild degree of stenosis. Patients with FMD have a higher rate of spontaneous carotid artery dissection. In general, the etiology of small strokes and TIA are unclear. FMD is not thought to be an inflammatory disorder.

Treatment of FMD is generally based upon symptomatology. Many cases are now found incidentally on magnetic resonance angiography (MRA). Asymptomatic FMD is often treated with aspirin alone. Carotid endarterectomy is not curative because the vascular disorder is not isolated to the extra-cranial carotid. Intra-arterial angioplasty and stenting has been performed successfully for patients with ischemia and high-grade stenosis. Patients with intracranial FMD are at increased risk for cerebral aneurysms

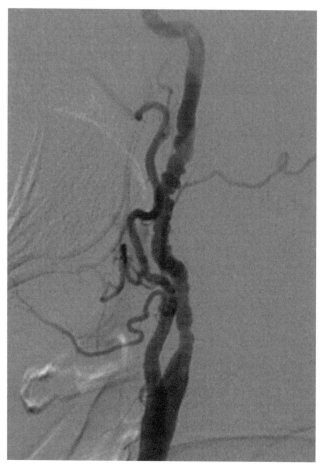

Figure 13-3 Fibromuscular dysplasia. Carotid angiogram starting at the level of the carotid bifurcation reveals a markedly irregular vessel with ripples like a "stack of plates" consistent with fibromuscular dysplasia. (Courtesy of Dr. Philippe Gailloud, Interventional Neuroradiology, Johns Hopkins Hospital.)

and should undergo screening MRA or computed tomography angiography (CTA) (27).

Moyamoya Disease

Moyamoya, the Japanese word for puff of smoke, is a progressive, occlusive vasculopathy primarily involving the intracranial segment of the internal carotid arteries and the proximal portion of the MCA and ACA. Disease is usually bilateral, although it is common for one hemisphere to be more severely affected. Moyamoya can involve the posterior circulation as well, but this is much less common (28). Collateral vessels develop to compensate for lost blood flow; these vessels are diffuse, small and net-like, resembling a puff of smoke on cerebral angiogram (Figures 13-4 and 13-5). Pathologic specimens reveal endothelial hyperplasia and fibrosis, intimal thickening, thinning of the media, and normal adventia with no inflammatory component (29).

Moyamoya is 50 times more likely to occur in women than men and is found more commonly in women who smoke and use oral contraceptives (30,31). The onset of symptoms clusters into two peaks, during the first decade and during the third decade of life. Children present most often with ischemia, either TIA or stroke (32). In young adults, hemorrhages are more common and may be subarachnoid or intraventricular. The presumed etiology for the hemorrhage is aneurysmal thinning of blood vessels and compromise of the very small end vessels from atherosclerotic disease (25). Additional symptoms may include headache, seizure, involuntary movements, and progressive cognitive decline with recurrent strokes. The gold standard for diagnosis is cerebral angiography, but abnormal vessels or flow-voids are often seen on MRI, and MRA may confirm the diagnosis.

Moyamoya disease is idiopathic. The term moyamoya syndrome is used when a secondary cause for the vasculopathy is found. Dozens of associated conditions have been reported. Predisposing factors for Moyamoya include, but are not limited to, protein C or S deficiency, sickle cell anemia, Fanconi's anemia, post-radiation or post-infectious vasculopathy, and Down's syndome (32).

The clinical course of Moyamoya is variable. It may be relentlessly progressive with recurrent TIA, stroke, or hemorrhage in some patients, while more indolent in others. There is no curative therapy, and appropriate treatment is controversial. In younger patients in whom ischemia is more common, anti-platelet therapy may be beneficial. This benefit in adults is less clear because the risk of hemorrhage increases with age. Due to the risk of hemorrhage, anti-coagulation is contraindicated (33). There are also several surgical options. Abnormal cerebral blood perfusion has been demonstrated in patients with Moyamoya with both single photon emission computed tomography (SPECT) and magnetic resonance perfusion imaging (34,35). Poor cerebral perfusion may be the etiology of the bland infarcts associated with the disease. Several surgical procedures have been shown to improve cerebral blood perfusion. Improved neurologic function has been observed in a very small number of patients, but data demonstrating improvement in long-term morbidity and mortality are lacking.

Both artery-to-artery bypass (superficial temporal artery to middle cerebral artery) and encephaloduromyosynangiosis (temporalis muscle flap is placed on top of the dura) have been done with some success, although it may take 6-24 months after the latter procedure for significant angiogenesis

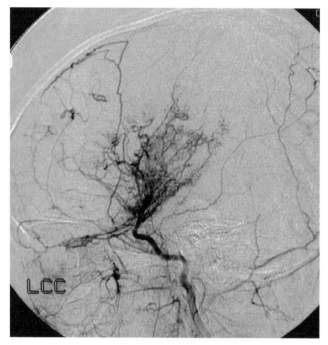

Figure 13-4 Moyamoya. Cerebral angiogram. A carotid injection shows occlusion of the distal intracranial carotid artery with extensive small, fine collateral vessels deep in the brain providing the Moyamoya appearance.

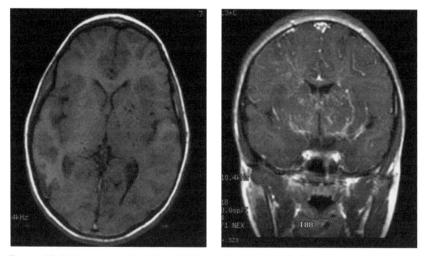

Figure 13-5 Moyamoya. Unenhanced T_1-weighted MRI (*left*) shows flow voids deep in the brain (multiple dark spots) due to abnormal Moyamoya vessels. Coronal section with gadolinium (*right*) from the same patient shows abnormal vessel enhancement.

to occur allowing new vessels to perfuse the hemisphere. The best surgical option depends upon the feasibility of an artery-to-artery anastomosis in an individual patient, and the preference and experience of the surgeon (33).

Case Study 13-2 discusses a patient with Moyamoya.

Arterial Dissection

Arterial dissection is a tear in the vessel intima with tracking of blood into the vessel wall, forming an intramural hematoma (36). Dissection may extend into the subadvential region or remain limited to the media. Dissection into the subadvential space may cause a pseudoaneurysm to form. In a subintimal dissection, the mass effect of the hematoma often narrows the lumen of the vessel, leading to stenosis or occlusion (Figure 13-6) (37,38). When the stenosis involves a long segment of a vessel, the classic "string sign" is seen on cerebral angiogram. In arterial dissection, cerebral angiography may demonstrate areas of stenosis and pseudoaneurysm.

The annual incidence of spontaneous carotid artery dissection is 2.5-3 per 100,000, with spontaneous vertebral artery dissection occurring in 1-1.5 per 100,000. Dissections account for only 2% of all ischemic strokes but may cause 10%-25% of strokes in young and middle-aged patients (37,38). Etiology of dissection is often cryptic. The majority of dissections are thought to be spontaneous, but a history of minor trauma is often found, such as excessive head rotation or hyperextension of the neck (i.e., "the beauty parlor stroke") or chiropractic manipulation of the neck (39,40). There is also an association between recent upper respiratory infection and spontaneous carotid and vertebral artery dissection (41). Genetic factors such as an underlying arteriopathy or structural defect in the arterial wall have been implicated. Elhers-Danlos syndrome type IV, Marfan's syndrome, autosomal dominant polycystic kidney disease, α-1-antitrypsin deficiency, and osteogenesis imperfecta type I are some examples; overall specific connective tissue disorders are found in only 1%-5% of patients with spontaneous arterial dissections (37,38). Additionally, there is a family history of arterial dissection in 5% of patients.

The peak incidence of dissection is between 40 and 45 years, but dissection can occur at any age. Children are more prone to intracranial dissection than adults, although, overall, extracranial dissection is more common than intracranial. The most common site of arterial dissection is the internal carotid at the skull base, opposite C1 and C2 vertebrae. The carotid is tethered to the skull base and likely is stretched with head rotation. Vertebral artery dissections commonly occur at the level of the first and second cervical vertebrae (37) and are associated with spinal manipulative therapy (40) as well as minor trauma.

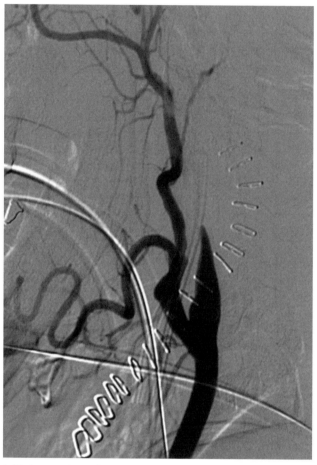

Figure 13-6 Dissection. Carotid angiogram shows a tapered occlusion of internal carotid artery distal to the bifurcation, suggestive of carotid artery dissection. (Courtesy of Dr. Philippe Gailloud, Interventional Neuroradiology, Johns Hopkins Hospital.)

Clinical Manifestations

Recognizing the signs and symptoms of dissection may provide the opportunity to treat patients before cerebral ischemia occurs. The most common clinical manifestation of arterial dissection is pain, which is present in 58%-92% of adults (41a). Localized, unilateral neck pain is reported by one quarter of adults (42). Pain is less common in children, with 1%-11% reporting neck pain and 54% reporting headache (43). Pain may be located in the neck or referred to the head, either around the eye in carotid dissections or the occipital head regions in vertebral dissection. The absence of pain does not rule out dissection. Additional complaints may include pulsatile tinnitus or, in a vertebral artery dissection, the sensation of vertigo, double vision, or unsteadiness. A bruit is auscultated in a small percentage of patients (21).

The classic triad of internal carotid artery dissection is composed of pain on one side of the head, face, or neck and an ipsilateral partial Horner's syndrome (ptosis and miosis), followed hours to days later by cerebral or retinal ischemia. Although this triad is present in less than one-third of patients, two of the three findings strongly suggest the diagnosis (37,38). Cranial nerve palsies are found in 12% of patients with carotid dissection (44). Lower cranial nerves, especially the hypoglossal nerve, are the most commonly affected. Vertebral artery dissections typically present with posterior neck or head pain and symptoms of posterior circulation ischemia. Symptoms of vertebrobasilar ischemia develop in an estimated 60% of patients with vertebral artery dissection (45).

Interestingly, the interval between onset of headache or neck pain and symptoms of cerebral ischemia secondary to dissection may be long. In carotid artery dissection, the median delay is 4 days, and in vertebral artery dissection the median interval is 14 days from onset of posterior neck pain but 15 hours from onset of headache (42).

Imaging

For many years, cerebral angiography was viewed as the imaging study of choice. MRI and MRA have largely supplanted conventional angiography, especially for carotid artery dissection. The resolution of MRA approaches that of conventional angiography and MRI, particularly axial fat-suppressed images of the neck and head, and allows direct visualization of the intramural hematoma (37,38,46). Ultrasound is often not helpful because many dissections occur above the carotid bifurcation; the bifurcation is generally the highest point at which ultrasound can visualize the artery. An abnormal pattern of flow is seen in the majority of cases, but the actual lesion may not be apparent on ultrasound. Diagnostic features such as an intimal flap or intramural hematoma are found in less than one-third of patients (37,38). For all these reasons, a high index of suspicion for dissection is required, and appropriate MR images of the neck should be considered for patients with suggestive features by history, physical exam, or ultrasound.

Treatment

Treatment of arterial dissection has classically been with anti-coagulation, although there have been no randomized controlled trials. This recommendation is based upon imaging studies, which suggest that cerebral infarctions secondary to dissection are embolic in more than 90% of cases (47), as well as transcranial doppler evidence of frequent microemboli (48). Contraindications to anticoagulation include a large cerebral infarction with mass effect or edema, intracranial extension of the dissection, and intracranial aneurysm, all of which increase the risk of hemorrhage (38). Anticoagulation to prevent thromboembolic complications is often recommended for a period of 3-6 months with a target international normalized ratio (INR) of 2.0-3.0.

Prognosis related to cerebral arterial dissection is fairly good. Death secondary to dissection occurs in less than 5% of patients. Approximately 75% of patients with stroke due to dissection make a good functional recovery (36-38). Radiographically, approximately two-thirds of occlusions recanalize, 90% of stenoses resolve, and one-third of aneurysms decrease in size (37,38). Radiographic recovery occurs primarily in the first 2-3 months. Improvement after 6 months is rare. The overall recurrence risk is approximately 5%-10% and may be lower in older patients. Recurrence risk is highest in the first month after dissection (2%), then decreases to about 1% per year for at least a decade. Generally, recurrent dissection occurs in a previously unaffected artery. The use of anticoagulation or anti-platelet therapy does not seem to affect the recurrence risk.

Migraine

Migraine is an established risk factor for stroke in those under age 45, particularly women. Studies suggest that between 1.2% and 14% of ischemic strokes in young adults could be the result of migraine (49). The pathophysiology of migraine-related cerebral infarction is not well defined. Theories include vasospasm-induced ischemia, increased platelet aggregation, and thrombosis due to sludging of blood in narrowed blood vessels (49,50). The International Headache Society criteria for migrainous infarction are quite strict (Table 13-3).

Despite the IHS criteria, strokes do occur in patients who suffer from migraine without aura. The risk is higher in patients with aura (OR = 6.2) than in patients without aura (OR = 3.0) (51). Those at highest risk are women with frequent (more than 12 per year) migraine headaches with aura (52).

Migrainous strokes tend to occur in the posterior circulation, consistent with the usual localization of aura in migraine (49,53). Functional outcomes

---

Table 13-3 International Headache Society Criteria for Migrainous Infarction

A. Patient has previously fulfilled criteria for migraine with aura.

B. The present attack is typical of previous attacks, but neurologic deficits are not completely reversible within 7 days, or neuroimaging demonstrates ischemic infarction in relevant area.

C. Onset of neurologic symptoms occurs during the course of a typical migraine attack.

D. Other causes of infarction ruled out by appropriate investigation.

Adapted from Headache Classification Committee of the International Headache Society. Classification and diagnostic criteria for headache disorders, cranial neuralgias and facial pain. Cephalalgia. 1988; 8(Suppl7):1-96.

after migrainous stroke are quite good (49,53). Stroke size is often small. Preventive therapy for migraine headache is warranted after a migrainous stroke because with fewer migraines there is presumably less chance of recurrent stroke. Preventive anti-migraine medications are myriad; effective therapies may include antihypertensives, anti-epileptics, anti-depressants, and anti-serotonergic drugs (50). Calcium channel blockers such as verapamil have been suggested as logical choices to reduce vasospasm. Abortive therapy for migraines may include nonsteroidal anti-inflammatory drugs (NSAIDs), desirable for their analgesic and anti-platelet properties. Ergotamines should be avoided because they may worsen presumed vasospasm and cerebral ischemia (50).

Recurrence risk after cerebral infarction is thought to be low, perhaps on the order of 1%-2% (53). It cannot be over-emphasized that migrainous stroke is a diagnosis of exclusion. Other etiologies must be carefully investigated and excluded before a stroke may be attributed to migraine. A common misdiagnosis is arterial dissection, which, as described above, may present with a headache and be mistaken for migraine. Migraine is an independent risk factor for cerebral infarction and may be additive with other risk factors, including hypertension, use of oral contraceptives, and smoking (52,54).

Pregnancy

Pregnancy is a hypercoaguable state (55). Logically then, pregnant women should be at increased risk of stroke. Interestingly, a recent population-based study found that the relative risk of ischemic stroke was not increased during pregnancy but was significantly elevated in the puerperium, which was defined as up to 6 weeks post-partum (1). A compilation of 21 studies from 1941 through 1995 found a stroke risk of 4.0 to 38.9 per 100,000 deliveries (56). Other studies subdivided stroke by type and found the risk of ischemic stroke to be 11-13 per 100,000 deliveries (57,58). Again, the greatest risk was during the first post-partum week (58). Intracerebral hemorrhage occurred in 9 per 100,000 deliveries. The risk of subarachnoid hemorrhage was 1 in 2000 to 10,000 deliveries. The greatest risk for subarachnoid hemorrhage is during labor; however, the third trimester and the post-partum period are also high risk. Cerebral venous thrombosis occurs in 11 per 100,000 deliveries (57). Although stroke occurs in only 0.01% of pregnancies, 4%-8.5% of maternal mortality may be attributed to stroke (58a). The two leading causes of maternal mortality, systemic embolism and hypertensive disease, are both risk factors for stroke and may result in an underestimation of stroke as a cause of death (58a,59).

Risk factors for stroke during pregnancy include any of the risk factors associated with stroke in young patients. Additionally, conditions unique to pregnancy may present as a stroke or stroke-like events, including eclampsia, post-partum cerebral angiopathy, amniotic fluid embolism, choriocarci-noma, and peripartum cardiomyopathy (59). As previously mentioned, pregnancy is a hypercoagulable state. The basis for this hypercoagulabil-ity is platelet hyperaggregability, decreased fibrinolysis, increased levels of fibrinogen, and decreased levels of proteins C and S (55,60). Women with undiagnosed hematologic abnormalities may manifest a thrombosis during pregnancy.

Eclampsia is defined as seizures in the setting of hypertension, protein-uria and edema during pregnancy or the immediate post-partum period. Eclampsia can be associated with ischemic or hemorrhagic stroke. The dif-ferential diagnosis of a seizure and focal neurologic deficit during preg-nancy should include ischemic stroke, cerebral venous thrombosis, intracerebral and subarachnoid hemorrhage, meningitis, cerebral neoplasm, and eclampsia, which may produce vasogenic cerebral edema (59,61). The evaluation of stroke during pregnancy should be thorough; stroke should not simply be attributed to eclampsia. To emphasize this point, a recent large US survey found that only 24% of pregnant women with ischemic stroke and 14% with intracerebral hemorrhage actually met criteria for eclampsia (58). In contrast, in a smaller series of women with TIA or nondisabling stroke during pregnancy, 63% of women had a specific hyper-coagulable condition other than pregnancy (62).

With a focal neurologic deficit, a CT scan is the preferred initial diag-nostic test to evaluate for hemorrhage. In eclampsia, CT frequently shows hypodensity, most commonly in the posterior head regions, which may reverse after control of hypertension or termination of pregnancy. It may be difficult to tell initially if hypodensity on CT is due to the reversible edema of eclampsia or due to ischemic stroke. Fortunately, magnetic resonance diffusion-weighted imaging can differentiate vasogenic edema seen in eclampsia from cytotoxic edema representing cerebral infarction (61). With diffusion-weighted imaging, areas of vasogenic edema have increased dif-fusion coefficients and areas of ischemia have decreased diffusion coeffi-cients (Figure 13-7). This distinction is critical for treatment decisions. Edema responds well to blood pressure reduction, and ischemia may be worsened if blood pressure is rapidly reduced. The MRI lesions and neu-rologic deficits of eclampsia are generally reversible with control of blood pressure.

The pathophysiology of eclampsia is unclear. One proposed mecha-nism is cerebral vasospasm, resulting in ischemia and cytotoxic edema. This is based upon MRA and conventional angiogram findings of vasospasm in some patients with eclampsia (63). The most popular theory, however, sug-gests that acute hypertension in eclampsia causes a loss of cerebral autoreg-ulation with passive dilatation of cerebral blood vessels and subsequent extravasation of fluid and proteins into the interstitial space (61). A similar pathophysiology is postulated for reversible posterior leukoencephalopa-thy, which is also associated with acute hypertension and has MRI findings similar to eclampsia (64).

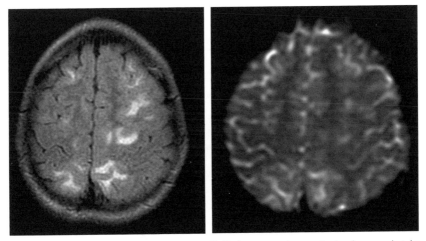

Figure 13-7 Eclampsia. MRI FLAIR image (*left*) shows patchy cerebral edema as bright white. The ADC map (*right*) shows bright rather than dark signal in this region, confirming that this is edema, not infarction.

Cerebral venous thrombosis (CVT) is discussed more comprehensively in Chapter 14. However, because up to one-third of pregnancy-related cerebral infarctions may be caused by intracranial venous thrombosis, mention is warranted here (65). The risk of CVT is approximately 11 per 100,000 deliveries (1,57). The risk is highest in the first post-partum week. Risk factors include: dehydration, tobacco use, an additional hypercoagulable risk factor such as protein C or S deficiency, hypertension, and, for unclear reasons, cesarean section (57,66). A persistent or severe headache in a post-partum woman, particularly with associated papilledema, focal neurologic deficit, or seizures should raise the possibility of cerebral venous thrombosis (59,67). An MRI with magnetic resonance venography and neurology consultation should be requested (67). Differential diagnosis of post-partum headache includes eclampsia, migraine, cerebreal spinal fluid leak after spinal anesthesia (e.g., low-pressure headache), pituitary infarction, and subarachnoid hemorrhage (Table 13-4). Patients who develop pregnancy-related CVT tend to be younger and have a more acute onset of symptoms, faster resolution, and a better prognosis than non-pregnant patients with CVT (57). See Case Study 13-3.

The incidence of non-traumatic intracerebral hemorrhage in pregnancy is approximately 1 in 10,000 (58). Arteriovenous malformation (AVM) and pre-eclampsia/eclampsia are the most common causes when an etiology is found (58). Subarachnoid hemorrhage may be caused by ruptured aneurysm, most commonly, or AVM with extension of the intracerebral hemorrhage into the subarachnoid space. Ideally, ruptured aneurysms should be surgically clipped before delivery because surgical intervention may decrease maternal mortality by as much as 80% (68). Mode of delivery can then proceed according to obstetrical indications. If the aneurysm is not

Table 13-4 Differential Diagnosis of Headache in the Post-Partum Period

Etiology	Distinguishing Features	Diagnostic Tests
Eclampsia	Seizure Increase in baseline BP	MRI
Cerebral venous thrombosis	Seizure Papilledema Focal weakness	MRI/MRV
Pseudotumor cerebri	Papilledema Normal MRI/MRV	Lumbar puncture with opening pressure > 20 Resolution of headache after LP
CSF leak	Positional headache Improved with recumbent position History of spinal anesthesia	Blood patch relieves
Pituitary infarction (Sheehan's syndrome)	Significant blood loss at delivery Lethargy, anorexia, weight loss Unable to produce breast milk	Pituitary hormone levels
Subarachnoid hemorrhage	"Worst headache of life"	Lumbar puncture with RBCs that do not clear Cerebral angiogram

secured, some authors recommend forceps or vacuum-assisted delivery with epidural anesthesia to shorten the second stage of labor (68). Many obstetricians suggest cesarean section to avoid straining during labor. However, recommendations on the optimal means of delivery in a patient with an unruptured aneurysm are anecdotal, and there is no clear evidence that vaginal delivery increases the risk of bleeding (35,59).

AVMs generally come to medical attention with symptoms related to seizure, headache, or hemorrhage but can be an incidental finding. If an AVM presents during pregnancy or during labor and delivery, it tends to present with bleeding rather than seizure (68,69). AVMs present with hemorrhage three times more often in pregnant than non-pregnant women (69,70). These data suggest that pregnancy increases the risk of AVM rupture, although other authors believe the risk of AVM rupture during pregnancy is not increased (71).

AVMs also account for a larger proportion of subarachnoid hemorrhage during pregnancy. In fact, up to 50% of subarachnoid hemorrhages in pregnant women may be due to a bleeding AVM compared with 10% of subarachnoid hemorrhages in non-pregnant women and 6% in the general population (68-70). The reason for this change in AVM presentation with pregnancy is not known. The AVM rebleeding rate may be increased in pregnant women, although studies have been suboptimal. One author documents a 26% risk of rebleeding during the same pregnancy, compared with 3%-6% per year in non-pregnant patients; however, that study defined pregnancy as 2 years before and after the gravid state, so the 26% risk would be over a 4-year interval (72). Neurosurgical criteria guide decision-making about when to operate on ruptured and unruptured AVMs because there is no clear consensus (71). The safest mode of delivery in patients with untreated AVMs has not been well studied; in the published studies, numbers are too small to draw valid conclusions (68,73,74).

Management of stroke, subarachnoid hemorrhage, and cerebral venous thrombosis during pregnancy can be challenging. The first concern should be the hemodynamic stability of both mother and fetus. Therapeutic options for the management of infarction and thrombosis include antiplatelet drug, anticoagulation, and mechanical disruption of the thrombus. Several studies have shown low-dose aspirin (less than 150 mg daily) to be safe after the first trimester of pregnancy (75,76). Aspirin selectively inhibits maternal cyclooxygenase without impairing fetal coagulation (75), although maternal blood loss at the time of delivery may be increased. Heparin does not cross the placenta and is therefore felt to be the safest anticoagulant during pregnancy (77,78). Unfractionated heparin is generally given intravenously to achieve adequate anticoagulation. In addition to the risk of hemorrhage, the long-term use of heparin (longer than 1 month) during pregnancy has been associated with significant loss of bone density in up to one-third of treated women (77). The use of low-molecular-weight heparin (LMWH) during pregnancy has not been well studied, but early experience suggests it is safe and does not cross the placenta (77,78). LMWH may be given subcutaneously, and factor Xa levels may be followed to assess the adequacy of anticoagulation. Due to their short half-lives, both unfractionated and LMWH may be discontinued at the onset of labor.

Warfarin is a well-known teratogen (79,80). The risks of embryopathy are highest during the first trimester, weeks 6 through 12, but it may occur later in pregnancy as well. There is also a significant hemorrhage risk at the time of delivery (81). Therefore attempts should be made to avoid warfarin until after delivery, particularly in the first and third trimesters. If maternal anticoagulation with warfarin is required post-partum, most experts would allow and even encourage breast feeding (77) because there have been several convincing reports that maternal warfarin use does not induce an anticoagulant effect in the breast-fed infant even though it is secreted in breastmilk (82,83).

The risk of stroke recurrence during subsequent pregnancies has not been well studied. One US study and one French study found no increased stroke risk during subsequent pregnancies, but stroke risk was increased during the post-partum period (58). The French Study Group on Stroke in Pregnancy analyzed data from 441 women (337 with arterial ischemic stroke and 68 with cerebral venous thrombosis). During 5 years of follow-up, these women had 187 pregnancies, despite a personal history of stroke.

There were no cases of recurrent cerebral venous thrombosis. Recurrent arterial ischemic stroke occurred in 13 women, or 2.3%, and only 2 of 13 strokes occurred during pregnancy or the post-partum period. Stated differently, the overall stroke recurrence risk was 1% within 1 year and 2.3% within 5 years. Therefore, when counseling women with a history of ischemic stroke regarding future pregnancy, one should advise that the risk of recurrent stroke is low, and that the highest risk period is post-partum. A previous ischemic stroke should not be a contraindication to future pregnancies.

Prognosis

Prognosis after stroke in the young is generally better than in older individuals; however, those with residual deficit have many years of disability ahead of them. The impact of stroke in the young is therefore significant in terms of social, psychological, and economic costs. In an Italian study of 60 consecutive patients with ischemic stroke and TIA between the ages of 17 and 45 years, outcomes at 6 years were quite good (84). Functional disability (Barthel Index) was relatively infrequent: 50% of patients were independent, 39% were partially dependent, and 11% were fully dependent. Almost 70% of these patients were employed, although 27% were working only part-time or in a different job due to stroke-related disability. Swedish neurologists Hindfelt and Nilsson followed 74 young adults with stroke for 13-26 years to assess long-term prognosis (85). At follow-up, 12 patients (16%) were dead, primarily due to significant systemic illness, which in most cases contributed to their original stroke. Among the survivors, 11% had recurrent stroke or TIA, 10% had developed a seizure disorder, and an additional 10% suffered from depression that was not a pre-morbid condition. Functional outcome was again relatively good, with 80% of patients returning to work and 63% remaining employed a decade later; 11% required significant assistance with daily activities. Only one patient was severely disabled to the point of institutionalization. Long-term mortality was about 1% per year in this series.

Recurrence risk varies with the heterogeneous causes of stroke in the young. On average, the risk of recurrent stroke is 1%-2% per year in young patients (84,85). When compared with the elderly, in whom recurrent ischemic stroke has been estimated at 5%-6% per year, the prognosis in younger patients is favorable (85). As mentioned, however, the cumulative risk in young patients is significant.

Conclusion

Stroke is among the top ten causes of death in persons aged 15 to 44, and those with residual deficit have many years of disability ahead of them. While young people may have traditional stroke risk factors such as hypertension, diabetes, hyperlipidemia, and smoking, a careful search for additional stroke risk factors and potential etiologies is indicated. Stroke in the young is a challenging area, because there have not been good treatment trials to guide management in a number of major areas: arterial dissection, vasculitis, Moyamoya, and patent foramen ovale. It is hoped that forthcoming studies will provide much-needed information.

Case Study 13-1

A 33-year-old woman with a past history of Graves' disease who takes oral contraceptives presented with a 12-hour history of acute-onset left arm and leg clumsiness, heaviness, and numbness, followed by a severe bi-frontal headache. She also had mild dizziness, but no true vertigo. The headache improved but did not remit, and the left-sided symptoms persisted. Physical examination was notable for 4+/5 power at the left deltoid and iliopsoas. She had dysmetria on the left and slowed fine finger movements. Her gait was normal. Head CT showed a left cerebellar hypodensity. MRI confirmed the presence of an acute stroke in the left superior cerebellar hemisphere, as well as an old area of infarction in the right thalamus. MRA of the head and neck was unremarkable.

Detailed work-up, including extensive serologic testing for autoimmune and hypercoagulable disorders, revealed only an 8-mm-diameter patent foramen ovale (PFO) with a spontaneous right-to-left shunt and an associated atrial septal aneurysm. Closure of the PFO was recommended, because the patient eschewed long-term anticoagulation therapy. After meeting with interventional cardiologists and cardiothoracic surgeons regarding options for PFO closure, she chose to have her PFO surgically closed. She has done well post-operatively and has discontinued her anticoagulant. She is off oral contraceptives and takes an aspirin daily.

Case Study 13-2

A 17-year-old female presented with right-sided focal seizures and difficulty using her right hand. MRI revealed multiple areas of old infarction bilaterally and a subacute left parietal infarction. MRA was suggestive of Moyamoya syndrome. Cerebral angiography confirmed the diagnosis. Testing revealed no evidence of sickle cell disease or hypercoaguability as a secondary cause of Moyamoya. She continued to have TIAs with hyperventilation or exercise despite aspirin therapy. Magnetic resonance perfusion imaging revealed significantly compromised blood flow in the left MCA territory. She underwent a left encephaloduromyosynangiosis. Her TIAs resolved over the next 6-12 months.

Case Study 13-3

A 22-year-old post-partum female with sickle cell disease presented with 5 days of severe headache and blurred vision. She had delivered a full-term infant by cesarean section 7 days earlier. While undergoing evaluation by her obstetrician, she developed left arm weakness and difficulty speaking. Her initial head CT showed a small right frontal intracerebral hemorrhage affecting the motor strip (Figure 13-8).

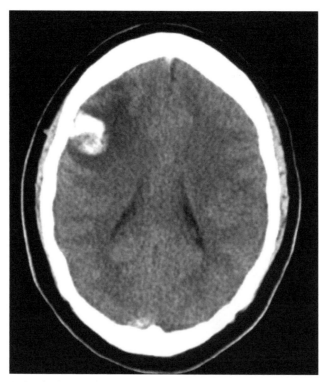

Figure 13-8 Cerebral venous thrombosis. CT shows a right frontal intracerebral hemorrhage in a patient with sagittal sinus thrombosis.

Urgent MRI/MRV revealed thrombosis of the superior sagittal sinus and right transverse sinus (Figure 13-9) as well as hemorrhagic venous infarction of the right frontal lobe. Interestingly, the patient had undergone evaluation for cerebral venous thrombosis 3 months earlier

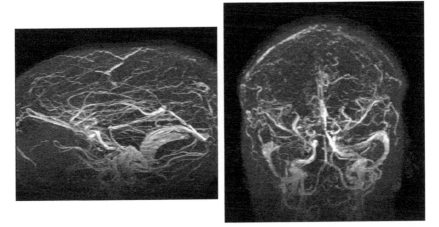

Figure 13-9 Cerebral venous thrombosis. Magnetic resonance venogram (*lateral view on left, coronal view on right*) reveals the presence of deep cerebral veins but conspicuous absence of the superior sagittal sinus, which should be the largest venous structure seen (see Figure 13-10).

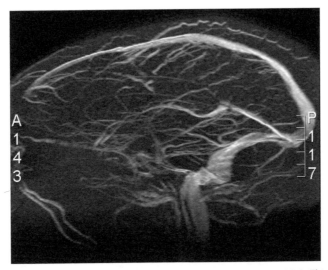

Figure 13-10 Cerebral venous thrombosis. Same patient as in Figure 13-9. This magnetic resonance venogram was taken 3 months before her stroke. Note the presence of a large, sickle-like structure at the top of the image, which is a normal superior sagittal sinus.

when she had complained of headaches. Her (normal) magnetic resonance venogram from that time is shown in Figure 13-10.

The patient was started on heparin drip and loaded with prophylactic phenytoin. She was also given IV fluids and supplemental oxygen. Her strength in the left upper extremity improved from 1/5 at presentation to 4/5 over 7 days. Her phenytoin was discontinued; additional anticonvulsants were not prescribed because she had not had a seizure. An extensive evaluation for hypercoagulabilty was unremarkable, including testing for proteins S and C deficiency, factor V Leiden mutation, antithrombin III, Russell's viper venom, anti-cardiolipin antibodies, and homocysteine. She was transitioned from heparin to warfarin. She did well and was discharged with home physical and occupational therapy. She was seen in clinic 1 month later and was given clearance to return to work. A repeat MRV to evaluate for recanalization of cerebral venous thromboses was planned for the 3-month follow-up. At that time, a decision will be made regarding the duration of warfarin therapy and the possibility of chronic transfusion therapy, which is generally offered to patients with sickle cell disease and stroke.

REFERENCES

1. **Kittner SJ, Stern BJ, Wozniak M, et al**. Cerebral infarction in young adults. The Baltimore-Washington Cooperative Young Stroke Study. Neurology. 2000;54:371-8.
2. **Minino AM, Smith BL**. Deaths: preliminary data for 2000. National Vital Statistics Report. 2001;49:26. www.cdc.gov/nchs/data.
3. **Rohr J, Kittner S, Feeser B, et al**. Traditional risk factors and ischemic stroke in young adults. The Baltimore-Washington Cooperative Young Stroke Study. Arch Neurology. 1996;53:603-7.
4. **Devuyst G, Bogousslavsky J**. Status of patent foramen ovale, atrial septal aneurysm, atrial septal defect and aortic arch atheroma as risk factors for storke. Neuroepidemiology. 1997;16:217-23.
5. **Mattioli AV, Bonetti L, Aquilina M**. Association between atrial septal aneurysm and patent foramen ovale in young patients with recent stroke and normal carotid arteries. Cerebrovasc Dis. 2003;15:4-10.
6. **Mas JL, Zuber M**. Recurrent cerebrovascular events in patients with patent foramen ovale, atrial septal aneurysm, or both and cryptogenic stroke or transient ischemic attack. Am Heart J. 1995;130:1083-8.
7. **Mas JL, Arquizan C, Lamy C, et al**. Recurrent cerebrovascular events associated with patent foramen ovale, atrial septal aneurysm, or both. N Engl J Med. 2001;345:1740-6.
8. **De Castro S, Cartoni, D, Fiorelli M, et al**. Morphological and functional characteristics of patent foramen ovale and their embolic implications. Stroke. 2000;31:2407-13.
9. **Bogousslavsky J, Garazi S, Jeanrenaud X, et al**. Stroke recurrence in patients with patent foramen ovale. The Lausanne Study. Neurology. 1996;46:1301-5.
9a. **Nedeltchev K, Arnold M, Wahl A, et al**. Outcome of patients with cryptogenic stroke and patent foramen ovale. J Neurol Neurosurg Psychiatry. 2002;72:347-50.
10. **Hanna JP, Sun JP, Furlan AJ, et al**. Patent foramen ovale and brain infarct: echocardiographic predictors, recurrence, and prevention. Stroke. 1994;25:782-6.
11. **Overell JR, Bone I, Lees KR**. Interatrial septal abnormalities and stroke: a meta-analysis of case-control studies. Neurology. 2000;55:1172-9.

12. Cramer SC, Rordorf G, Maki JH, et al. Increased pelvic vein thrombi in cryptogenic stroke: results of the Paradoxical Emboli from Large Veins in Ischemic Stroke (PELVIS) study. Stroke. 2004;35:46-50.

13. Dearani JA, Baran Ugurlu BS, Danielson GK, et al. Surgical patent foramen ovale closure for prevention of paradoxical embolism-related cerebrovascular ischemic events. Circulation. 1999;100[Suppl1]:171-5.

14. Homma S, Sacco RL, Di Tullio MR. Effect of medical therapy in stroke patients with patent foramen ovale. Circulation. 2002;105:2625-31.

15. Bridges ND, Hellenbrand W, Latson L, et al. Transcatheter closure of patent foramen ovale after presumed paradoxical embolism. Circulation. 1992;86:1902-8.

16. Windecker S, Wahl A, Chatterjee T, et al. Percutaneous closure of patent foramen ovale in patients with paradoxical embolism: long-term risk of recurrent thromboembolic events. Circulation. 2000;101:893-8.

17. Martin F, Sanchez PL, Doherty E. Percutaneous transcatheter closure of patent foramen ovale in patients with paradoxical embolism. Circulation. 2002;106:1121-6.

18. Siva A. Vasculitis of the nervous system. J Neurol. 2001;248:451-68.

19. Moore PM, Fauci AS. Neurologic manifestations of systemic vasculitis: a retrospective study of the clinicopathologic features and response to therapy in 25 patients. Am J Med. 1981;71:517-24.

20. Chu CT, Gray L, Goldstein LB, et al. Diagnosis of intracranial vasculitis: a multidisciplinary approach. J Neuropathol Exp Neurol. 1998;57:30-8.

21. Stern B, Wityk RJ, Pullicino P, Chan R. Vasculitis, arterial dissection, and other causes of stroke. Continuum. 2003;1-11.

22. Javedan SP, Tamargo RJ. Diagnostic yield of brain biopsy in neurodegenerative disorders. Neurosurg. 1997;41:823-30.

23. Moore PM, Richardson B. Neurology of the vasculitides and connective tissue diseases. J Neurol Neurosurg Psychiatry. 1998;65:10-22 .

24. Calabrese LH. Therapy of systemic vasculitis. Neurologic Clin. 1997;15:973-91.

25. Caplan LR, ed. Caplan's Stroke, 3rd ed. Boston: Butterworth-Heinenmann; 2000:315-7.

26. Ford RG, Siekert RG. Central nervous system manifestation of periarteritis nodosa. Neurology. 1965;15:114-22.

27. Chiche L, Bahnini A, Koskas F, et al. Occlusive fibromuscular disease of arteries supplying the brain: results of surgical treatment. Ann Vasc Surg. 1997;5:496-504.

28. Yamada I, Himeno Y, Suzuki S, et al. Posterior circulation in moyamoya disease: angiographic study. Radiology. 1995;197:239-46.

29. Fukui M, Kono S, Sueishi K, Ikezaki K. Moyamoya disease. Neuropathology. 2000;20:S61-4.

30. Ueki K, Meyer FB, Mellinger JF. MoyaMoya disease: the disorder and surgical treatment. Mayo Clin Proc. 1994;69:749-57.

31. Bruno A, Adams HOP, Bilbe J, et al. Cerebral infarction due to moya-moya disease in young adults. Stroke. 1988;19:826-33.

32. Yilmaz EY, Pritz MB, Bruno A, et al. Moyamoya: Indiana university medical center experience. Arch Neurol. 2001;58:1274-8.

33. Scott RM. Surgery for Moyamoya syndrome? Yes. Arch Neurol. 2001;58:128-30.

34. Kim SK, Wang KC, Oh CW, et al. Evaluation of cerebral hemodynamic with perfusion MR in childhood moyamoya disease. Pediatr Neurosurg. 2003;38:68-75.

35. Wityk RJ, Hillis A, Beauchamp N, et al. Perfusion-weighted magnetic resonance imaging in adult Moyamoya syndrome: characteristic patterns and change after surgical intervention: case report. Neurosurgery. 2002;51:1499-505.

36. Hart RG, Easton JH. Dissections of cervical and cerebral arteries. Neurologic Clin. 1983;1:155-82.

37. Schievink W. Spontaneous dissection of the carotid and vertebral arteries. N Engl J Med. 2001;344:898-906.

38. Schievink W. The treatment of spontaneous carotid and vertebral artery dissections. Curr Opin Cardiol. 2000;15:316-21.

39. Weintraub MI. Beauty parlor stroke syndrome: report of five cases. JAMA. 1993;269:2085-6.

40. Haldeman S, Kohlbeck FJ, McGregor M. Stroke, cerebral artery dissection, and cervical spine manipulation therapy. J Neurol. 2002;249:1098-104.

41. Grau AJ, Brandt T, Buggle F, et al. Association of cervical artery dissection with recent infection. Arch Neurol. 1999;56:851-6.

41a. Zetterling M, Carlstrom C, Konrad P. Internal carotid artery dissection. Acta Neurol Scand. 2000;101:1-7.

42. Silbert PL, Mokri B, Schievink W. Headache and neck pain in spontaneous internal carotid and vertebral artery dissections. Neurology. 1996;46:356-9.

43. Fullerton HJ, Johnston SC, Smith WS. Arterial dissection and stroke in children. Neurology. 2001;57:1155-60.

44. Mokri B, Silbert PL, Schievink WI, et al. Cranial nerve palsy in spontaneous dissection of the extracranial internal carotid artery. Neurology. 1996;46:356-9.

45. Chang AJ, Mylonakis E, Karanasias P, et al. Spontaneous bilateral vertebral artery dissections: case report and literature review. Mayo Clin Proc. 1999;74:893-6.

46. Kirsch E, Kaim A, Engelter S, et al. MR angiography in internal carotid artery dissection: improvement of diagnosis by selective demonstration of the intramural haematoma. Neuroradiology. 1998;40:704-9.

47. Lucas C, Moulin T, Deplanque D, et al. Stroke patterns of internal carotid artery dissection in 40 patients. Stroke. 1998;29:2646-8.

48. Srinivasan J, Newell DW, Sturzenegger M, et al. Transcranial Doppler in the evaluation of internal carotid artery dissection. Neurology. 2000;54:2159-61.

49. Milhaud D, Bogousslavsky J, Melle G, Liot P. Ischemic stroke and active migraine. Neurology. 2001;57:1805-11.

50. Bartleson JD. Transient and persistent neurologic manifestations of migraine. Stroke. 1984;15:383-6.

51. Tzourio C, Tehindrazanarivelo A, Iglesias S, et al. Case-control study of migraine and risk of ischaemic stroke in young women. Br Med J. 1995;310:830-3.

52. Donaghy M, Chang CL, Poulter N. Duration, frequency, recency and type of migraine and the risk of ischaemic stroke in women of childbearing age. J Neurol Neurosurg Psychiatry. 2002;73:747-50.

53. Broderick JP, Swanson JW. Migraine related strokes: clinical profile and prognosis in 20 patients. Arch Neurol. 1987;44:868-71.

54. Schwaag S, Nabavi DG, Frese A, et al. The association between migraine and juvenile stroke: a case-control study. Headache. 2003;43:90-5.

55. Cernenca F, Ricci G, Simeone R, et al. Coagulation and fibrinolysis changes in normal pregnancy: increased levels of procoagulants and reduced levels of inhibitors during pregnancy induce a hypercoagulable state, combined with a reactive fibrinolysis. Euro J Obstet Gynecol. 1997;73:31-6.

56. Lanska DJ, Kryscio RJ. Stroke and intracranial venous thrombosis during pregnancy and the perperium. Neurology. 1998;51:1622-8.

57. Lanska DJ, Kryscio RJ. Risk factors for peripartum and postpartum stroke and intracranial venous thrombosis. Stroke. 2000;31:1274-82.

58. Kittner SJ, Stern BJ, Feeser BR, et al. Pregnancy and the risk of stroke. N Eng J Med. 1996;335:768-74.

58a. Rochat RW, Koonin LM, Atrash HH, et al. Maternal mortality in the United States: report from the maternal mortality collaborative. Obstet Gynecol. 1988;72:91-7.

59. David EP, Wityk RJ. Cerebrovascular disorders. In: Cohen WR, ed. Cherry and Merkatz's Complications of Pregnancy, 5th ed. Philadelphia: Lippincott Williams & Wilkins; 2000:465-85.

60. Lee RV. Thromboembolic disease and pregnancy: are all women created equal? Ann Intern Med. 1996;125:1001.

61. Schaefer PW, Buonanno FS, Gonzalez RG, et al. Diffuion-weighted imaging discriminates between cytotoxic and vaogenic edema in a patient with eclampsia. Stroke. 1997;28:1082-5.

62. Kupferminc MJ, Yair D, Bornstein NM, et al. Transient focal neurological deficits during pregnancy in carriers of inherited thrombophilia. Stroke. 2000;31:892-5.

63. Sengar AR, Gupta RK, Dhanuka AK, et al. MR imaging, MR angiography, and MR spectroscopy of the brain in eclampsia. Am J Neuroradiol. 1977;18:1485-90.

64. Stern B. Stroke in pregnancy and the postpartum period. Continuum. 2003;1-10.

65. Grosset D, Bone I, Warlow C. Stroke in pregnancy and the puerperium: what magnitude of risk? J Neurol Neurosurg Psych. 1995;58:129-31.

66. Lindquvist P, Dahlback B, Marsal K. Thrombotic risk during pregnancy: a population study. Obstet Gynecol. 1999;94:595-9.

67. Bousser MG. Cerebral venous thrombosis: nothing heparin, or local thrombolysis? Stroke. 1999;30:481-3.

68. Dias MS, Sekhar LN. Intracranial hemorrhage from aneurysms and arteriovenous malformations during pregnancy and the puerperium. Neurosurgery. 1990;27:855-66.

69. Robinson JL, Hall CS, Sedzimir CB. Subarachnoid hemorrhage in pregnancy. J Neurosurg. 1972;36:27-33.

70. Sadasivan B, Malik GM, Lee C, Ausman JI. Vascular malformations and pregnancy. Surg Neurol. 1990;33:305-13.

71. Ogilvy CS, Stieg PE, Awad I, et al. Recommendations for the management of intracranial arteriovenous malformations. Statement of Health Care Professionals from a Special Writing Group of the Stroke Council, American Stroke Association. Stroke. 2001;32:1458-71.

72. Robinson JL, Hall CS, Sedzimir CB. Arteriovenous malformations, aneurysms, and pregnancy. J Neurosurg. 1974;41:63-70.

73. Tuttleman RM, Gleicher N. Central nervous system hemorrhage complicating pregnancy. Obstet Gynecol. 1981;58:651-7.

74. Laidler JA, Jackson IJ, Redfern N. The management of caesarean section in a patient with an intracranial arteriovenous malformation. Anaesthesia. 1989;44:490-1.

75. CLASP Collaborative Group. Low dose aspirin in pregnancy and early childhood development: follow up of the collaborative low dose aspirin study in pregnancy. Br J Obstet Gynecol. 1995;102:861-8.

76. Imperiale TF, Stollenwwek-Petrulis A. A meta-analysis of low dose aspirin for the prevention of pregnancy-induced hypertensive disease. JAMA. 1991;266:260-4.

77. Ginsberg JS, Hirsh J. Use of antithrombotic agents during pregnancy. Chest. 1998;114(Suppl):524S-30S.

78. Hirsh J, Warkentin T, Raschke R, et al. Heparin and low-molecular weight heparin: mechanism of action, pharmacokinetics, dosing considerations, monitoring, efficacy, and safety. Chest. 1998;114(Suppl):489S-510S.

79. Hall JAG, Pauli RM, Wilson KM. Maternal and fetal sequelae of anticoagulation during pregnancy. Am J Med. 1980;68:122-40.

80. Born D, Martinez EE, Almeida PAM, et al. Pregnancy in patients with prosthetic heart valves: effects of anticoagulation on mother, fetus, and neonate. Am Heart J. 1992;124:413-7.

81. Gilmore J, Pennell PB, Stern BJ. Medication use during pregnancy for neurologic conditions. Neurol Clin. 1998;16:189-206.

82. Orme ML, Lewis PJ, de Swiet M, et al. May mothers given warfarin breast-feed their infants? Br Med J. 1977;1:1564-5.

83. McKenna R, Kale ER, Vasan U. Is warfarin sodium contraindicated in the lactating mother? J Pediatr. 1983;103:325-7.

84. Musolino R, La Spina P, Granata A, et al. Ischaemic stroke in young people: a prospective and long-term follow-up study. Cerebrovasc Dis. 2003;15:121-8.

85. Hindfelt B, Nilsson O. Long-term prognosis of ischemic stroke in young adults. Acta Neurol Scand. 1992;86:440-5.

Chapter 14

Other Causes of Stroke

MATTHEW A KOENIG, MD
LUCAS RESTREPO, MD
MICHEL TORBEY, MD, MPH
ROMERGRYKO GEOCADIN, MD

Key Points

- Less common stroke etiologies include cerebral venous stroke, acquired and hereditary thrombophilic states, stroke due to proximal aortic atherosclerosis, and hemodynamic strokes.
- Functional outcome after cerebral venous thrombosis (CVT) is generally favorable.
- When a secondary hypercoagulable state is identified, treatment should target the underlying cause.
- Aortic arch atherosclerosis is best evaluated with TEE. Optimal treatment of significant aortic arch atheroma remains unclear.
- Watershed strokes may be readily recognized on CT or MRI. Treatment is directed at the underlying cause.

The less common causes of stroke may lead to atypical or subacute clinical presentations. This chapter describes several less common stroke etiologies, their manner of presentation, and their management. These causes of stroke include cerebral venous stroke, acquired and hereditary thrombophilic states, stroke due to proximal aortic atherosclerosis, and hemodynamic strokes.

Cerebral Venous Thrombosis

Pathophysiology

The venous sinuses draining the brain parenchyma are composed of thin-walled folds of dura mater (Figure 14-1). Thrombosis of this system may involve superficial cortical veins or the deep venous system of the brain.

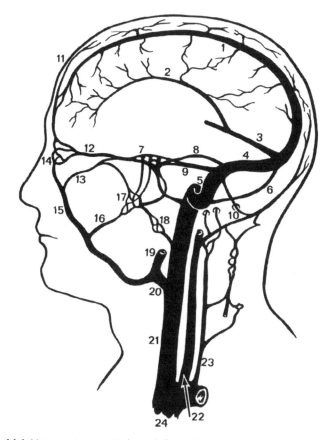

Figure 14-1 Venous sinuses. (Adapted from Osborn AG. Introduction to Cerebral Angiography. New York: Harper & Row; 1980:328.)

Cerebral venous thrombosis (CVT) may be difficult to diagnose because of its protean manifestations and variable clinical course. CVT may cause benign, transient elevation of the intracranial pressure (ICP), leading to headache or devastating hemorrhages causing disability and death.

CVT is commonly associated with conditions that precipitate a pro-thrombotic state, such as craniocervical infection, cranial surgery adjacent to a venous sinus, dehydration, puerperium, pregnancy, oral contraceptive use, and local or remote malignancy (Table 14-1). A substantial proportion of CVT (8%-40%) is attributable to local craniocervical infections, which have greatly declined with the widespread use of antibiotics. Children with untreated otitis media and mastoiditis are at risk for developing transverse sinus thrombosis from direct spread of infectious material and inflammation to the adjacent venous sinus. Diabetics and immunocompromised patients with orbital or frontal sinus infections may also present with thrombosis of the superior sagittal sinus (SSS) or the cavernous sinus. CVT may also be

Table 14-1 Risk Factors for Cerebral Venous Thrombosis

- Thrombophilic disorders (prothrombin G20210A mutation, factor V Leiden, etc.)
- Dehydration
- Occlusion by local mass effect (malignancy, meningioma, etc.)
- Remote malignancy
- Inflammatory bowel disease
- Sickle cell disease
- Polycythemia vera
- Pregnancy and puerperium
- Local sinus, orbit, or ear infection
- Oral contraception
- Skull fracture and trauma
- Protein-losing enteropathy or nephropathy

precipitated by head trauma, most commonly fracture of the vertex leading to SSS thrombosis or basilar skull fracture involving the transverse sinuses.

The diagnosis of CVT is also closely associated with thrombophilic states. Twenty percent of CVT cases are associated with the G20210A prothrombin gene mutation, while an additional 18% of patients have the factor V Leiden gene (1). Another small series (2) identified prothrombotic states in 75% of patients, the most common of which was elevation of factor VIII plasma levels (75%). The etiology of CVT, however, remains unexplained in 20%-35% of cases despite all diagnostic efforts (3). Other factors associated with CVT and systemic venous thromboses include malignancy, inflammatory bowel disease, protein-losing nephropathy or enteropathy, thrombocytosis, polycythemia vera, sickle cell disease, and oral contraceptive use (especially in smokers).

Clinical Features

CVT remains a relatively rare condition, accounting for 1%-9% of deaths due to cerebrovascular disease in autopsy series. Patients with CVT tend to be younger than those with arterial strokes, with a mean age of presentation between 30 and 40 years. CVT may also develop in the setting of dehydration in neonates and the elderly. Women have a small preponderance, especially in younger age groups. Signs and symptoms of increased ICP include headache, vomiting, papilledema, and decreased consciousness.

Headache, usually the earliest and most prominent symptom, occurs in 31%-91% of patients. The headache may be chronic or sudden in onset and has no characteristics specific to the diagnosis of CVT. Seizures occur in 10%-63% of patients and can be focal or generalized, depending on the patient population. Decreased level of consciousness often occurs at some point in the clinical course but is uncommon at presentation. Papilledema is a common, but not universal, finding. CVT should always be considered in the differential diagnosis of benign intracranial hypertension or pseudotumor cerebri. Conventional venography demonstrates CVT in 25%-38% of patients with pseudotumor cerebri, and newer magnetic resonance venography

(MRV) techniques can demonstrate some abnormality in venous drainage in the majority of patients with this condition.

The clinical evolution of the signs and symptoms associated with CVT is generally more gradual compared with stroke caused by arterial occlusion. The delay in presentation is believed to be due to the initial compensation of venous drainage by the extensive collateralization of the cerebral venous system. In one study, the time between symptom onset and presentation to the hospital was up to 14 days (4). The onset of clinical signs and symptoms of CVT is believed to coincide with the exhaustion of compensation by venous collaterals. About 20% of CVT may present with clinically significant ICP elevation. Occasionally, isolated ICP elevation may be the only finding (5). This elevation is primarily due to the obstruction of the venous drainage leading to the increase in local blood volume in sites where drainage is impaired. As the CVT progresses to cause neuronal injury and death, cytotoxic edema may contribute to the increase in ICP. As intraluminal pressure builds, cerebral veins may rupture, leading to intracerebral hemorrhage (ICH), which may further elevate ICP. ICH occurs in 15%-49% of patients with CVT (4). The ICH is typically located in a parasagittal location in patients with sagittal sinus thrombosis and in the temporal lobe in patients with lateral sinus thrombosis. The removal of the venous thrombus and promotion of venous flow may reduce intraluminal pressure and prevent further hemorrhage; hence, paradoxically, use of anticoagulation in the presence of an ICH may actually reduce the risk of recurrent bleeding (see below).

Diagnosis

The first imaging study performed in most patients is a non-contrast head CT, which can appear normal in 25%-40% of all patients in whom stroke is suspected. CT may demonstrate venous infarctions in the territory drained by the occluded venous sinus. These infarctions are usually hemorrhagic and appear as hypodensities mixed with hyperdense blood in the brain parenchyma that do not respect typical arterial distributions. Infarcts involve the temporal lobes in transverse sinus thrombosis, bilateral midline parenchyma in SSS thrombosis, and bilateral thalami and basal ganglia in deep venous occlusions. Enhancement of the tentorium and falx may be seen after administration of contrast. Fresh thrombus may be visible as hyperdensity of the involved sinus on a non-contrast scan. An "empty delta sign" can be seen on axial contrast-enhanced CT of SSS. The "empty delta" refers to contrast enhancement with a triangular configuration surrounding the central hypodense clot (filling defect) in the involved sinus.

MRI is important to better define the lesion in CVT (Figure 14-2). MRI can be used to demonstrate subtle hemorrhage within the infarct, especially on a gradient echo (T_2^*) sequence. MRI is more sensitive than CT for vasogenic edema and sinusitis. Unlike arterial infarcts, venous infarcts often do

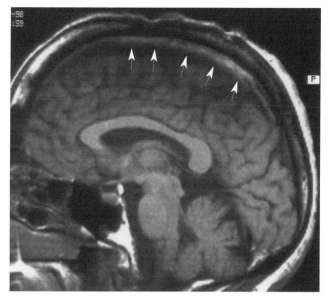

Figure 14-2 MRI better defines the lesion in cerebral venous thrombosis (*arrows*).

not show a pattern of restricted diffusion on diffusion-weighted MRI and apparent diffusion coefficient maps. MRV is more sensitive to CVT than conventional MRI and can display the resultant flow void in three dimensional reconstructions (Figure 14-3). Many normal patients have irregular dural venous sinuses such as unilateral hypoplastic transverse sinuses, so MRV abnormalities are not specific to the diagnosis of CVT. Conventional venography is the gold standard for diagnosis (Figure 14-4) but is invasive and subject to the same diagnostic pitfalls as MRV. In addition, a complete hypercoagulable evaluation is necessary in patients with cerebral venous thrombosis.

Treatment and Prognosis

Anticoagulation with heparin has been used for CVT for many years. It was not until 1991 that a randomized controlled trial compared dose-adjusted unfractionated heparin with placebo (4). This study was stopped after 20 patients because of the dramatic difference with eight full recoveries in the heparin-treated group compared with one full recovery in the placebo group. The use of heparin did not worsen the outcome of patients presenting with ICH in CVT. In the retrospective arm of this study, of those patients treated with heparin after ICH, 15% died, while 52% recovered completely. Of those who did not receive heparin after ICH, 69% died and only 23% recovered completely.

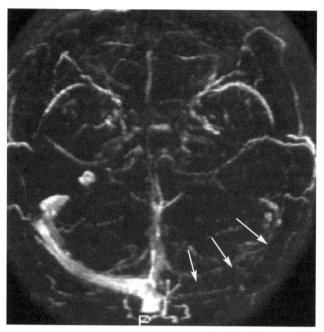

Figure 14-3 Absence of the left transverse sinus (*arrows*) demonstrated by MRV in a patient with dural venous sinus thrombosis.

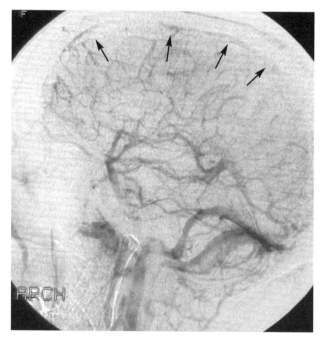

Figure 14-4 Absence of the superior sagittal sinus (*arrows*) demonstrated in the venogram phase of conventional angiography in a patient with dural venous sinus thrombosis.

Low-molecular-weight heparin was investigated in another prospective randomized trial (6). Subcutaneous nadroparin was followed by oral anticoagulation (international normalized ratio [INR], 2.5-3.5) in the treatment group. There was no significant difference in outcome between the treatment group and the placebo group. Despite the question raised by the nadroparin study, it is evident that anticoagulation does not increase the morbidity and mortality in patients with CVT, even in the presence of large ICH. The early use of heparin is therefore still recommended for established cases of CVT (7). After the acute treatment, oral anticoagulation has been recommended for 3-6 months. In cases with known prothrombotic conditions, longer-term anticoagulation may be necessary.

Thrombolytic therapy with urokinase or rtPA administered intravenously or directly into the thrombus by selective catheterization has been advocated for CVT (8). Systemic or direct thrombolytic therapy is effective in restoring venous flow in many cases. A recent retrospective study comparing direct administration of urokinase and systemic heparin in cases of SSS thrombosis reported better neurological outcome with direct urokinase treatment (9). Hemorrhagic complications were not significantly more common in the urokinase group. Mechanical thrombectomy has also shown encouraging results. In the absence of well-controlled comparison studies with heparin or placebo, the use of thrombolytics or mechanical clot disruption remains investigational. The applicability of these strategies is limited by the need for highly specialized personnel and equipment to undertake local thrombolysis and mechanical thrombus dissolution.

Headache may become progressive over the course of the illness, especially with the impairment in venous drainage and ICP elevation. During the acute period, headache can be alleviated with the control of ICP and the judicious use of narcotics or non-narcotic analgesics. In the chronic phase, the impairment in venous drainage may also affect CSF drainage. This can be manifested as a form of communicating hydrocephalus or as pseudotumor cerebri. The management of headache needs to focus on the etiologic cause of the headache as well as the patient's clinical presentation. The use of narcotics, non-narcotic analgesics, and acetazolamide provides relief in most patients. Close monitoring of visual fields to prevent optic nerve injury in cases that mimic pseudotumor cerebri is important. ICP monitoring may be needed, along with serial imaging in cases of hydrocephalus. CSF shunting to relieve ICP elevation, treat medically refractory headache, and prevent optic nerve injury may also be required.

The presence of cortical hematoma increases the likelihood of seizures. The prophylactic use of anticonvulsants is justified in the acute phase of treatment. Data on chronic epilepsy in patients with CVT are lacking, and the decision to use long-term anticonvulsants needs to be individualized.

The functional outcome after CVT is generally favorable, with 57%-86% of patients recovering completely and mortality rates of 5%-18% (6,10). Demonstrated normalization of initially pathological venous drainage by transcranial Doppler portends favorable outcome. Factors associated with poor prognosis after CVT include extremes of age, rapid onset of coma, large ICH, and focal neurological deficit. The underlying etiology of thrombosis such as malignancy, sepsis, and prothrombotic disorders also has prognostic relevance.

Hematological Disorders and Thrombophilia

Pathophysiology

The association between arterial stroke and primary hypercoagulable states is not clear. Many strokes have no evident etiology despite intensive diagnostic scrutiny, which has raised suspicions of an underlying primary hypercoagulable state. Thrombophilic states should be considered in stroke patients with a history of recurrent deep venous thrombosis (DVT) and those lacking traditional vascular risk factors. In contrast to arterial ischemic stroke, hypercoagulable states are frequently found in association with CVT (see above). It is estimated that 1% of patients with brain ischemia have a coagulopathy predisposing to thrombosis, although this figure may be four to seven times higher in younger individuals with ischemic stroke (11).

Hemostasis is the physiological mechanism that maintains blood in a fluid state within the circulation. A complex balance between the procoagulant and anticoagulant activities of plasma is actively maintained by cellular and humoral mechanisms. Thrombosis can result from the failure of the regulatory mechanisms of hemostasis, leading to inappropriate coagulation. Hypercoagulable states may be grouped into two broad categories: primary or secondary (acquired). Primary hypercoagulable states are those with abnormalities of the hemostatic process itself. Most of these cases are due to deficiencies of proteins of the coagulation cascade or fibrinolytic system and are usually hereditary. The majority of hereditary disorders are associated with venous rather than arterial thrombosis. The secondary category includes all hypercoagulable states triggered by systemic illness in which no specific abnormality of hemostasis is found. In such instances, thrombosis is probably the result of multiple factors.

Clinical Features

Factor V Leiden

The most common coagulation defect leading to venous thrombosis is the hereditary resistance of activated protein C caused by a single point mutation in the factor V gene (12). This mutation causes exaggerated function of activated factor V, which cannot be properly cleaved by activated protein C (12). Factor V is procoagulant when it is activated by prothrombin and factor X and anticoagulant after cleavage by activated protein C.

Factor V Leiden mutation is found in 1%-15% of normal people, in 20% of patients with a first episode of DVT, and in up to 60% of individuals with recurrent DVTs. Its frequency in the United States is about 5%, and is higher in people of European descent. Only 1%-3% of all individuals with factor V Leiden mutation develop DVT. The presence of this mutation confers a modest risk for venous thrombosis in the heterozygous state (5-fold to 10-fold) and a significant risk in the homozygous state (50-fold to 100-fold). Once venous thrombosis has developed, the cumulative incidence of recurrent events is almost 40%, even in heterozygous carriers of the mutant factor V gene (13).

Factor V Leiden heterozygosity has not been unequivocally shown to confer an increased risk of arterial thrombosis. In a large cohort of 1408 healthy men from the Physician's Health Study, the heterozygous presence of the mutation was not associated with an increased risk for either stroke or myocardial infarction (14). Another study showed that the prevalence of heterozygous factor V Leiden mutation in 161 elderly patients with stroke was not different from age-matched controls without stroke (15). Nevertheless, a retrospective case-control analysis showed a significant association between ischemic stroke and factor V Leiden heterozygosity in children (16).

Factor V Leiden screening should not be undertaken in adults with isolated arterial strokes because the mutation is common in the population at large and unlikely to be causative of the stroke. A positive result could be misinterpreted as indicative of a need for anticoagulation. In stroke patients with recurrent DVTs or in children with arterial stroke, screening for factor V Leiden is probably justified.

Prothrombin G20210A Mutation
The next most common cause of inherited thrombophilia is the G20210A prothrombin mutation, which is found in 6%-8% of patients with venous thrombosis (17). G20210A prothrombin mutation confers a 3-fold to 5-fold increase in the risk for venous thrombosis, and it is present in about 2% of normal Caucasians (12). The prothrombin G20210A mutation may synergistically interact with other risk factors to produce arterial thrombosis. Although most studies have failed to show an association with stroke, one case-control study of 72 young individuals with cryptogenic stroke suggested that the heterozygous presence of the prothrombin G20210A gene confers a 4-fold increase in stroke risk, while the risk is even higher in the homozygous state (18).

Other Hereditary Protein Deficiencies
Hereditary deficiency of protein C, protein S, and antithrombin III are usually associated with venous thrombosis, although anecdotal cases of arterial thrombosis and stroke have been reported. Proteins C and S are vitamin K-dependent anticoagulants. Protein C inhibits the activated form of factors

V and VIII, therefore slowing clot formation. Protein C is activated by thrombin and requires protein S as a cofactor. Heterozygous deficiency of proteins C or S increases the risk of venous thrombosis by about 10-fold, although the actual risk is difficult to estimate because these mutations are rare in the general population (about one in 300 individuals) and occur in only 1%-3% of patients with venous thromboses (12).

Two case-control studies have suggested an association between protein C and protein S deficiency and stroke in childhood (19,20). Large studies have failed to establish an association between protein S, protein C, and antithrombin III deficiency and arterial stroke in adults.

Antiphospholipid Syndrome

The antiphospholipid syndrome (APS) is characterized by the classic triad of thrombosis (venous or arterial), recurrent pregnancy loss, and thrombocytopenia, in association with the presence of antiphospholipid antibodies (APLs). Arterial thrombosis in APS has a particular predilection for the cerebral vasculature, as suggested by the presence of MRI changes suggestive of silent brain ischemia. Ischemic stroke is often the initial manifestation of the syndrome. APS can be classified as either secondary to another autoimmune disease (usually systemic lupus erythematosus) or primary. About 10% of patients with SLE have the full-blown syndrome, whereas 50% of patients with SLE test positive for APLs.

The characteristic laboratory finding in APS is the presence of serum autoantibodies targeting anionic phospholipids. The most familiar target of these antibodies is cardiolipin, which is predominantly found in the mitochondrial membrane. The lupus anticoagulant (LA) is another APL antibody. The presence of LA is demonstrated when a prolonged partial thromboplastin time (PTT) does not correct with the addition of normal plasma in a mixing study or dilute Russell viper venom time study. Despite the lengthening of coagulation tests in-vitro, LA is associated with thrombotic events rather than hemorrhage. The anticardiolipin antibody (ACLA) enzyme-linked immunosorbent assay is the most common method of screening for APL antibodies, but does not identify all relevant antibodies. In one study of middle-aged patients with cryptogenic stroke, antibodies were found against other phospholipids, including phosphatidylinositol (28%), phosphatidylserine (18%), and phosphatidylglycerol (15%) (21). On the other hand, a positive APL antibody test does not necessarily imply that the patient has APS because these antibodies may be present in HIV, bacterial endocarditis, and even in 10% of normal individuals.

An accurate diagnosis is of major importance before embarking on a long-term treatment plan. The diagnostic criteria of APS include at least one episode of thrombosis or spontaneous abortion and moderate-to-high levels of anticardiolipin antibodies (of the IgG or IgM class) or positive LA screen (22). The presence of APLs and LA should be confirmed 6 weeks after the first positive assay.

The pathophysiology of APS has not been fully elucidated. The APLs may be directly responsible for some of the clinical manifestations, as suggested by animal experiments in which the injection of antibodies induces abortion and promotes thrombosis (23). APS should be suspected in patients with SLE who develop ischemic stroke or deep venous thrombosis. It should also be considered in the differential diagnosis of cerebral venous thrombosis and cryptogenic stroke in young individuals without traditional risk factors. LA should be suspected in stroke patients with a prolonged PTT on initial screening lab work.

Hyperhomocysteinemia

The inborn error of metabolism, homocysteinuria, has long been known to cause early atherosclerosis in children and young adults. More recently, minor elevations in serum homocysteine and polymorphism of the gene encoding methylene tetrahydrofolate reductase have been associated with higher risk for ischemic stroke and cardiac disease. Homocysteine is an amino acid derivative of methionine that is metabolized by two alternative metabolic pathways. One pathway involves B_{12}-dependent methylation via N-5-methyltetrahydrofolate or betaine. The other involves B_6-dependent transsulfuration by cystathione β-synthase. Relative deficiencies in folate, B_6, and B_{12} or abnormalities in the involved enzymes may result in mild-to-moderate elevation in serum homocysteine. Other factors associated with elevated homocysteine include tobacco, coffee, renal insufficiency, male gender, older age, postmenopausal status, sedentary lifestyle, hypothyroidism, and treatment with methotrexate, phenytoin, theophylline, and L-dopa (24). The most common cause of hyperhomocysteinemia in adults is hypovitaminosis, either consequent to pernicious anemia or nutritional deficiencies. The prevalence of elevated homocysteine levels in patients with vascular disease ranges from 12% to 47% (24). Homocysteine is believed to cause vascular damage by impairment of collagen metabolism, which results in intimal thickening.

Numerous case-control and anecdotal reports have demonstrated a relationship between elevated serum homocysteine and ischemic stroke. A recent meta-analysis (25) showed that a 25% (3 μmol/L) lower homocysteine level was associated with a 19% lower risk of stroke. One study showed that elevated homocysteine levels were correlated with a risk of recurrent stroke within 15 months of the initial event (26). Whether hyperhomocysteinemia causes stroke or is simply a marker for vascular disease is unclear and controversial. This question is confounded by the finding that homocysteine levels are transiently increased for 2 weeks after an ischemic stroke (24).

Although many clinicians favor screening younger stroke patients as part of a thrombophilic work-up, the prevalence of hyperhomocysteinemia is more common in older patients with traditional risk factors for vascular disease. One study found no discriminating clinical factors that could be used to target homocysteine screening (24). Because the prevalence of hyperhomocysteinemia is high and the medications used to treat it have few adverse effects, many neurologists screen all patients with stroke or TIA for elevated homocysteine.

A recent multicenter trial found that supplementation with folic acid, vitamin B_{12}, and vitamin B_6 was effective in reducing serum homocysteine in stroke patients but did not reduce the risk of subsequent stroke during a 2-year follow-up period. (27) Criticism of the study is that not all patients had large vessel atherosclerosis as the cause of stroke and the time period of follow-up may have been too short to detect a benefit. Another large, multicenter, double-blind, placebo-controlled trial designed to study whether vitamin supplementation prevents stroke, VITATOPS (28), is underway. One earlier study (29), demonstrated slowed progression of extracranial carotid artery stenosis in hyperhomocysteinemic patients receiving vitamin supplementation. The treatment protocol used in the VITATOPS trial includes folate 2 mg, B_6 25 mg, and B_{12} 500 µg per day (28).

Other Hematologic Conditions

Polycythemia vera, multiple myeloma, and Waldenström macroglobulinemia can raise the risk of brain ischemia directly through rheologic mechanisms or indirectly by altering regulatory components of hemostasis. Blood hyperviscosity may be induced either by an increased number of circulating cells (erythrocytes or malignant leukocytes) or through massive elevation of plasma protein. Ischemic stroke may occur in 10%-20% of patients with polycythemia vera. The best laboratory marker for monitoring stroke risk in patients with polycythemia vera is the hematocrit. Thrombocytosis of various etiologies may be associated with thromboembolic phenomena. Nevertheless, modest elevations of the platelet count are nonspecific indicators of systemic inflammatory and thrombotic processes.

Arterial thrombosis also plays a major role in organ damage from sickle cell anemia. Abnormal erythrocyte adhesion, platelet activation, and abnormal endothelial function may lead to arterial thrombosis in sickle cell anemia, which, in combination with hypoxia due to ongoing erythrocyte sickling, are responsible for brain ischemia. Vascular intimal hyperplasia with intracranial stenosis can also lead to infarcts in the watershed territory between the anterior and middle cerebral arteries (30). Ischemic stroke occurs in 15% of patients homozygous for HbSS, with an average presentation at age 10 (11). The frequency of ischemic stroke in individuals with the sickle cell trait appears to be the same as the general population.

Infectious Diseases

Studies have demonstrated that 25%-35% of stroke patients have had a recent infection, particularly involving the respiratory tract (31). The pathophysiology of infection-related stroke can be divided into three broad mechanisms: central nervous system vasculitis, induction of a systemic prothrombotic state, and cardiac embolization from endocarditis.

Infectious vasculitis is a rare disorder caused most commonly by syphilis but also seen in tuberculosis, mucormycosis, and aspergillosis. Cerebral ischemia is a well-known complication of meningitis, including bacterial, fungal, mycobacterial, and parasitic. This complication should be suspected in any patient with meningitis and focal neurological signs. Infective endocarditis may cause ischemic stroke by cardioembolization or hemorrhagic stroke by rupture of a mycotic aneurysm. Although a retrospective study (32) linked Chlamydia pneumoniae infection to stroke, a prospective study could not substantiate that serological evidence for prior infection is a risk factor for ischemic stroke among patients with pre-existing vascular disease (33).

The association between HIV and stroke is unclear. The annual incidence of ischemic stroke in HIV patients was 216 per 100,000 in a large cohort, which is less than the stroke incidence of the general population (34). Stroke does, however, increase in frequency as the CD4 count declines, particularly in the context of opportunistic CNS infections. One confounding factor is that HIV-infected patients often have concomitant stroke risk factors, particularly illicit drug use (35). CSF examination and thrombophilia screens are not routinely recommended in HIV-infected patients with stroke, but the decision to perform a lumbar puncture or evaluate for coagulopathy should be based on clinical suspicion. CSF interpretation in the setting of stroke may be difficult because of the non-specific elevation of protein and lymphocytic pleocytosis seen after stroke.

Diagnosis

Diagnostic strategies for evaluating potential thrombophilic states differ from institution to institution (Table 14-2). In general, evaluations should be limited to young patients and those without traditional vascular risk factors. Evaluation of arterial strokes in adult patients should be limited to screening for hyperhomocysteinemia and APS if any thrombophilic evaluation is

Table 14-2 Evaluation of Thrombophilic Disorders

Arterial Strokes with Suspicion for Thrombophilic State

• Antiphospholipid antibody panel	• Dilute Russell viper venom time
• Mixing study	• Homocysteine

Venous Strokes, or Arterial Stroke and Systemic Venous Thromboses, or Any Stroke in Children

• Antiphospholipid antibody panel	• Prothrombin G20210A mutation
• Mixing study	• Antithrombin III
• Dilute Russell viper venom time	• Protein S
• Homocysteine	• Protein C
• Factor V Leiden	• Hemoglobin electrophoresis (children)

undertaken. Many physicians screen for hyperhomocysteinemia in all patients with stroke or TIA, but the cost-effectiveness of this practice is untested. Screening for APS or LA should be limited to patients who lack traditional risk factors, have known or suspected rheumatological disorders, have elevated PTT on routine lab work, or have had recurrent abortion or DVT. Other hereditary prothrombotic conditions have not been linked to arterial strokes in adults. Venous strokes or strokes associated with systemic venous thrombosis have been causally linked to other hereditary states, and evaluation may include APS, factor V Leiden, homocysteine, protein C, protein S, antithrombin III, factor VIII, mixing study, and prothrombin G20210A mutation. A similar evaluation may be warranted for arterial and venous strokes in children.

Treatment

When a secondary hypercoagulable state is identified, treatment should target the underlying cause. The best strategy to prevent vascular occlusions in patients with polycythemia vera is to keep the hematocrit around 45% through serial phlebotomies. The optimal treatment of prothrombotic states has not been subjected to rigorous scientific scrutiny. The duration of therapy is particularly unclear. When a specific primary hypercoagulable state is identified or a secondary cause cannot be treated, long-term therapy with warfarin is generally the treatment of choice, with a target INR of 2 to 3. Some argue that a higher target INR > 3 is indicated in the APS, on the basis of a retrospective study (36). Before a decision about the intensity of anticoagulation is made, the physician must consider that most trials indicate that an INR > 3 significantly increases the risk of systemic bleeding.

Aortic Arch Atherosclerosis

Pathophysiology

Aortic arch atherosclerosis results from deposition of lipids in the subintimal layer of the involved vessel. Over a lifetime, lipids accumulate within the vessel wall, giving rise to an enlarging fatty streak. Lipid accumulation leads to infiltration of circulating macrophages and hypertrophy and hyperplasia of the underlying smooth muscle of the vascular media. With time, a fibrin cap covers the atheroma, which eventually calcifies. The ratio of fibrous tissue and smooth muscle to lipid material and inflammatory cells relates to stability of the plaque. Those plaques with dense, calcified fibrin plaques, minor lipid and macrophage content, and greater smooth muscle density tend to have lower risks of rupture. Plaques with greater inflammatory cell and lipid contents are prone to rupture.

Unstable plaques tend to have greater echolucency by TEE because of the higher water content of the lipid-laden material. Rupture of the overlying endothelium exposes thrombogenic material to the circulation and activates the coagulation cascade with subsequent platelet and fibrin adhesion. The resulting thrombus may then embolize distally. Embolic material from the ascending aorta and aortic arch may enter the anterior or posterior cerebral vasculature and result in TIA or large vessel stroke. Prospective studies have demonstrated that aortic plaque initially forms in the descending aorta, then extends sequentially to involve the aortic arch and ascending aorta (37).

Risk factors for plaque formation are believed to be similar to atherosclerosis elsewhere: hypertension, diabetes mellitus, tobacco use, and hypercholesterolemia. Studies have failed to demonstrate a statistically significant difference in the presence of vascular risk factors in patients who have progression of plaque size and those whose plaque remains stable or regresses (37). This paradox may reflect the low power of the small studies that have been performed and the limited time of follow-up as well as the inherent dynamism of plaque morphology. The natural history of aortic plaque includes periods of spontaneous progression, regression, and relative stability that reflect plaque hemorrhage, thrombosis, rupture, lipid accumulation, and inflammation. In a 1-year follow-up study of asymptomatic, untreated aortic plaque (38), progression occurred in 23%, regression in 10%, and stability in 67%. In stroke patients, progression of aortic plaque occurred in 37% and regression in 22% (37), possibly reflecting greater plaque instability with stroke. Accordingly, sessile or mobile components of the plaque may be evanescent in patients who are evaluated serially by TEE. One study (37) showed a correlation between homocysteine levels ≥ 14 μmol/L and progression of aortic plaque in stroke patients.

Clinical Features

Until recently, proximal aortic atheroma was not recognized as a risk factor for ischemic stroke. We now know that the prevalence of severe atheroma in stroke is similar to that of coronary artery disease and atrial fibrillation. The 1-year risk of stroke in patients with large aortic arch plaques is 12%, which is 50% greater than the highest risk group of patients with non-valvular atrial fibrillation (39,40). Whether aortic arch atherosclerosis causes stroke by direct embolization or merely reflects general vasculopathy is not fully established. Complex atheroma morphology is commonly found in stroke patients. In one study (41), 13% of stroke patients had plaque thickness ≥4 mm in the ascending aorta or proximal arch, 22% had plaque ulcerations, 40% had plaque calcification, and 9% had hypoechoic plaque indicative of high lipid content. Aortic arch atheroma ≥4 mm has now been demonstrated as an independent risk factor for new and recurrent stroke in several case-control studies. The frequency of large aortic atheromas is greater in patients with stroke (26%) than controls matched for vascular risk factors (13%) (42).

Other studies have suggested that plaque ulceration, lack of calcification, greater lipid density, and freely mobile or sessile components correlate with increased risk of embolic stroke, but these data have been less uniformly validated in the literature. In one case-control study (42), ulcerated or mobile atheromas occurred more frequently in stroke patients (12%) compared with non-stroke patients matched for vascular risk factors (5%). These differences were entirely attributable to patients aged 60 or older, in whom ulcerated and mobile plaques occurred much more commonly in patients with stroke (22%) compared with controls (8%). Another study (41) found that the presence of plaque ulceration was associated with stroke, but the correlation was entirely attributable to the greater incidence of complex plaque morphology in patients with plaque thickness ≥ 4 mm. The only independent risk factor for stroke not related to plaque thickness appears to be the absence of plaque calcifications, which confers a 10-fold risk relative to patients with calcified plaques (41).

In summary, the only independent risk factors for stroke related to aortic atheroma appear to be thickness ≥ 4 mm and absence of calcification. Although various other morphological findings appear to confer greater risk of stroke, this correlation is confounded by the greater frequency of morphological complexity in thicker plaques. Although mobile plaque has a dramatic appearance on TEE that would logically seem to increase the risk of embolic stroke, this speculation has not been borne out by the literature. The natural history of aortic plaque includes spontaneous appearance and disappearance of mobile components. The presence or absence of mobile plaque at a single time point on TEE may, therefore, have limited clinical relevance.

Diagnosis

Cortical strokes are usually attributed to large artery atherosclerosis and cardioembolism, while subcortical strokes have been historically attributed to small vessel disease. Accordingly, TEE is rarely performed in the evaluation of subcortical strokes. In a retrospective study (43) of TEE findings in patients with strokes of both subtypes, there was no difference in the prevalence of atherosclerotic plaque at any level of the aorta, nor was there a difference in the thickness of the plaque or the presence of complex morphology. Although these data are limited, they suggest that aortic arch atheroma is an equal risk factor for cortical and subcortical stroke.

Aortic arch atherosclerosis is best evaluated with TEE. For further details, see Chapter 4. TEE should be performed in patients with high likelihood of atherosclerosis or other indications for invasive echocardiography. Location of the stroke in the cortex versus the subcortical tissue should have limited impact on the decision to perform TEE in patients with risk factors for large vessel atherosclerosis.

Treatment

Optimal treatment of significant aortic arch atheroma remains unclear. Patients with cryptogenic stroke and the presence of ascending aortic or arch atheroma thicker than 4 mm, especially with complex morphology, are often treated with antiplatelet agents and warfarin, either separately or in combination. The data to support this practice is limited and contradictory. Three small retrospective studies of aspirin and warfarin demonstrated a potential benefit of warfarin (44-46). In a larger retrospective study (47) of patients with stroke or TIA who were found to have severe proximal aortic atherosclerosis, patients were treated with statins, warfarin, or antiplatelet agents separately and in combination. In a matched-paired analysis, recurrent embolic events occurred in 29% of patients not taking statins and 12% of patients taking statins ($P = 0.0004$) over an average of 34 months of follow-up. Conversely, there was no difference in event rates between those taking antiplatelet agents or warfarin and those not taking these medications over the same period of follow-up. These findings may reflect the relative importance of plaque stabilization in preventing embolization from the aorta. The optimal medical treatment of these patients, however, awaits larger, prospective studies, and treatment strategies must be individualized to reflect the risk-benefit ratio and medical co-morbidities of a given patient.

Watershed Infarctions

Pathophysiology

Watershed strokes are caused by regional hypoperfusion in the territory between two vascular beds. The most common watershed infarcts lie in the middle cerebreal artery (MCA)–anterior cerebral artery (ACA) border-zone; the MCA–posterior cerebral artery (PCA) border-zone; and the internal border-zone between the deep and superficial perforators of the MCA. Less common sites include the border-zone between the superior and anterior inferior cerebellar arteries and the spinal border-zone in the mid-thoracic region.

Watershed infarcts can occur in the setting of compromised blood flow to tissue from either systemic or local hemodynamic processes. Equivalent to watershed infarcts in the mesenteric circulation, those border-zone territories most distal to the large feeding arteries are at the highest risk for damage. Cerebral autoregulation allows the brain to provide optimal perfusion between mean arterial pressures of 50 to 150 mm Hg. Outside this range, the autoregulatory mechanism begins to falter and perfusion becomes linearly related to flow. As the MAP declines below 50 mm Hg in the affected arterial beds, hypoperfusion in the vascular border-zones ensues. Above 150 mm Hg, injury to the cerebral vasculature with hemorrhages and cerebral edema may be noted.

Watershed infarcts are commonly seen in two clinical scenarios: 1) systemic hypotension secondary to cardiac arrest, arrhythmia, sepsis, blood loss, profound orthostatic hypotension, or aggressive use of antihypertensive medications; and 2) occlusive, near-occlusive, or tandem lesions in the internal carotid artery (Table 14-3). Watershed infarcts can particularly occur in patients with a combination of systemic hypotension, which may be subtle, and severe occlusive carotid disease.

For the chronically hypertensive patient, functional autoregulatory ranges are shifted higher such that higher than ordinary MAPs are required to maintain perfusion. In the setting of tight carotid stenosis or chronic hypertension, abrupt reduction in blood pressure from the compensatory range may result in watershed ischemia. Older patients with traditional vascular risk factors are at the highest risk for watershed strokes because of impaired autoregulatory mechanisms in the aging brain, reset autoregulatory limits, and atherosclerotic disease of small perforating vessels that limits vasodilation. In these patients, small decrements in systemic blood pressure may be sufficient to collapse perforating vessels and result in ischemia.

Clinical Features

Based on small case series, the frequency of watershed infarction ranges from 8% to 53% of ischemic stroke depending on the clinical setting and criteria for diagnosis. Documented hypotension is reported in only about half of cases, the remainder of which is inferred from syncope or presyncope preceding the event, the pattern of infarction on imaging, or the presence of occlusive carotid disease. Classically, clinical deficits follow a stuttering, progressive course with accumulation of neurological deficits over hours to days. This is especially true of occlusive carotid disease. Infarcts related to myocardial infarction or arrhythmia, however, may be precipitous and monophasic. The clinical manifestation of stroke depends on location. The classic bilateral MCA-ACA border-zone stroke results in quadriparesis of the proximal extremities, the so-called "man-in-barrel" syndrome, which may be clinically mistaken for a myopathic process, especially when progressive.

One case series (48) reported the frequency of watershed strokes as 9.6% of consecutive admissions for ischemic stroke. Cardiac disorders and

Table 14-3 Causes of Watershed Infarction

• Cardiac arrhythmia	• Carotid sinus hypersensitivity
• Severe hemorrhage	• Exaggerated vagal response
• Myocardial infarction	• Internal carotid occlusion or near-occlusion
• Orthostatic hypotension	• Septic shock
• Intraoperative hypotension	• Excessive antihypertensive medication use

orthostatic hypotension were seen or clinically suspected in all patients. Progressive deficits were seen in 72% of patients, many of whom had stereotyped responses to recurrent episodes of hypotension. Cardiac arrhythmias required repeated telemetric monitoring to diagnose in a few cases. Carotid stenosis of >50% was found in 69% of patients. Of the visible watershed strokes on CT, 48% involved the internal border-zone, 30% involved the MCA-PCA border-zone, and 19% involved the MCA-ACA border-zone. The majority of patients were older than 60.

The literature on internal border-zone infarcts is even more limited. One case series (49) reported a frequency of 6% of consecutive admissions for ischemic stroke. The majority of patients had unilateral involvement and were found to have tight internal carotid stenosis. Prodromal syncope or near-syncope was present in 75%. Most patients with complete internal border-zone strokes had hemiparesis, hemisensory loss, and cognitive and behavioral dysfunction. Most patients with partial infarcts had brachiofacial sensorimotor deficits resembling the dysarthria-clumsy hand lacunar syndrome. The course was more commonly stuttering and progressive in complete lesions, but was monophasic in partial lesions. Cardiac disease, carotid disease, and diabetes mellitus were significantly more prevalent in these patients than in typical stroke patients.

Diagnosis

Watershed strokes may be readily recognized on CT or MRI. On MRI, hyperintensities are visible in the deep subcortical white matter (centrum semiovale and corona radiata) in a linear fashion between the MCA-ACA (Figure 14-5) and MCA-PCA territories. Unlike large artery occlusive strokes, the cortex and deep gray matter are generally spared. Lesions may be unilateral or bilateral, contiguous or patchy. MRA or CTA of the extracranial vasculature may reveal tight stenosis of the internal carotid artery, and intracranial MRA may reveal tandem lesions in the circle of Willis.

When the diagnosis of watershed stroke is suspected, a diagnostic evaluation should be undertaken to reveal treatable causes. The work-up should be directed toward cardiac and carotid disease. An echocardiogram should be performed to rule out regional wall motion abnormalities and depressed cardiac output. Telemetry should be performed in the hospital followed by cardiac event monitoring in the outpatient setting to carefully exclude episodic cardiac arrhythmia. The internal carotid circulation should be evaluated by Doppler, MRA, or conventional angiogram as indicated. Vascular risk factors, including lipids and fasting glucose, should be investigated. Orthostatic blood pressure should be monitored and, if indicated, tilt table testing and evaluation for carotid sinus hypersensitivity performed. When excessive vagal responses are suspected (e.g., in the setting of diabetic autonomic dysfunction or multiple system atrophy), a careful history should be taken to evaluate for eating, coughing, or micturition directly

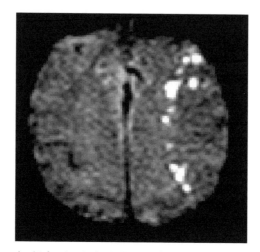

Figure 14-5 Watershed infarction in the MCA-ACA border-zone demonstrated by diffusion-weighted MRI in a patient with severe internal carotid stenosis.

preceding the onset of symptoms. Blood pressure should be monitored at the peak response period for antihypertensive medications to exclude exaggerated responses. Intraoperative records should be reviewed for periods of relative hypotension where appropriate.

Treatment and Prognosis

Treatment must be directed toward the underlying cause. Patients with cardiac arrhythmias or excessive vagal responses should be referred to a cardiologist or electrophysiology specialist. Causes of orthostatic hypotension should be identified and corrected. Patients should be cautioned against sudden postural changes. Morning orthostasis can be lessened by sleeping in a semi-upright position. Strategies for managing more profound orthostatic hypotension include constrictive hosiery, abdominal binders, volume expanders such as fludricortisone and salt supplementation, and vasoconstrictors such as midodrine. The benefits of these strategies must be weighed against patient discomfort and poor compliance with binders and hosiery as well as supine hypertension with the pharmacological agents. Blood pressure medications should be discontinued or decreased in the setting of tight carotid stenosis.

The carotid artery should be evaluated by MRA or Doppler; if a complete occlusion of the internal carotid artery is found, one should consider a conventional angiogram. Patients with complete carotid occlusion and poor collateral supply are at high risk for further ischemic events, particularly with hypotension. Extracranial to intracranial bypass surgery may be an option in selected patients. Patients with near-occlusive carotid stenosis should be considered for carotid endarterectomy. Many clinicians will maintain patients with carotid near-occlusion on dose-adjusted unfractionated heparin until surgery is performed, although strong evidence for doing so is lacking. Non-surgical candidates (due to concomitant medical disorders) and patients with tandem lesions in the intracranial circulation may benefit from consultation with an interventional neuroradiogist or endovascular neurosurgeon for consideration of angioplasty and stent placement.

In one case series (48) of watershed strokes in all territories, 24% of patients experienced recurrent or new neurological deficits after the initial event was identified. Three of the seven patients who underwent carotid endarterectomy suffered from hyperperfusion syndrome. The 1-year mortality rate was 9%, reflecting the older age, underlying cardiac and vascular disease, and stroke-related disability in these patients. Only half of the patients with complete internal border-zone strokes achieved independence, most of whom continued to have severe disability (49). The majority of patients with partial internal border-zone strokes regained independence.

REFERENCES

1. **Martinelli I, Sacchi E, Landi G, et al.** High risk of cerebral-vein thrombosis in carriers of a prothrombin-gene mutation and in users of oral contraceptives. N Engl J Med. 1998;338:1793-7.
2. **Cakmak S, Derex L, Berruyer M, et al.** Cerebral venous thrombosis. Clinical outcome and systematic screening of prothrombotic factors. Neurology. 2003;60:1175-8.
3. **Ameri A, Bousser MG.** Cerebral venous thrombosis. Neurol Clin. 1992;10:87-111.
4. **Einhaupl KM, Villringer A, Meister W, et al.** Heparin treatment in sinus venous thrombosis. Lancet. 1991;338:597-600.
5. **Leker RR, Steiner I.** Isolated intracranial hypertension as the only sign of cerebral venous thrombosis. Neurology. 2000;54:2030.
6. **de Bruijn SF, Stam J.** Randomized, placebo-controlled trial of anticoagulant treatment with low-molecular-weight heparin for cerebral sinus thrombosis. Stroke. 1999;30:484-8.
7. **Bousser MG.** Cerebral venous thrombosis: diagnosis and management. J Neurol. 2000;247:252-8.
8. **Spearman MP, Jungreis CA, Wehner JJ, et al.** Endovascular thrombolysis in deep cerebral venous thrombosis. Am J Neuroradiol. 1997;18:502-6.
9. **Wasay M, Bakshi R, Kojan S, et al.** Nonrandomized comparison of local urokinase thrombolysis versus systemic heparin anticoagulation for superior sagittal sinus thrombosis. Stroke. 2001;32:2310-7.
10. **Villringer A, Mehraein S, Einhaupl KM.** Pathophysiological aspects of cerebral sinus venous thrombosis (SVT). J Neuroradiol. 1994;21:72-80.
11. **Hart RG, Kanter MC.** Hematologic disorders and ischemic stroke: a selective review. Stroke. 1990; 21:1111-21.
12. **Dahlback B.** Blood coagulation. Lancet. 2000;355:1627-32.
13. **Simioni P, Prandoni P, Lensing AWA, et al.** The risk of recurrent venous thromboembolism in patients with an Arg506-Gln mutation in the gene for factor V (factor V Leiden). N Engl J Med. 1997;336:399-403.
14. **Ridker PM, Hennekens CH, Lindpaintner K, et al.** Mutation in the gene coding for coagulation factor V and the risk of myocardial infarction, stroke, and venous thrombosis in apparently healthy men. N Engl J Med. 1995;332:912-7.
15. **Press RP, Liu XY, Beamer N, Coull BM.** Ischemic stroke in the elderly: role of the common factor V mutation causing resistance to activated protein C. Stroke. 1996;27:44-8.

16. **Kenet G, Sadetzki S, Murad H, et al.** Factor V Leiden and antiphospholipid antibodies are significant risk factors for ischemic stroke in children. Stroke. 2000;31:1283-8.
17. **Nguyen A.** Prothrombin G20210A polymorphism and thrombophilia. Mayo Clin Proc. 2000;75:595-604.
18. **De Stefano V, Chiusolo P, Paciaroni K, et al.** Prothrombin G20210A mutant phenotype is a risk for cerebrovascular ischemic disease in young patients. Blood. 1998;91:3562-5.
19. **De Veber G, Monagle P, Chan A, et al.** Prothrombotic disorders in infants and children with cerebral thromboembolism. Arch Neurol. 1998;55:1539-43.
20. **Nowak-Gottl U, Stratter R, Heinecke A, et al.** Lipoprotein(a) and genetic polymorphisms of clotting factor V, prothrombin and methylene tetrahydrofolate reductase are at risk factors for spontaneous ischemic stroke in childhood. Blood. 1999;94:3678-82.
21. **Toschi V, Motta A, Castelli C, et al.** High prevalence of antiphosphatidylinositol antibodies in young patients with cerebral ischemia of undetermined cause. Stroke. 1998;29:1759-64.
22. **Levine JS, Branch W, Rauch J.** The antiphospholipid syndrome. N Engl J Med. 2002; 346:752-63.
23. **Pierangeli S, Barker JH, Stikovac D, et al.** Effect of human IgG antiphospholipid antibodies on an in vivo thrombosis model in mice. Throm Haemost. 1994;71:670-4.
24. **Bushnell CD, Goldstein LB.** Homocysteine testing in patients with acute ischemic stroke. Neurology. 2002;59:1541-6.
25. **The Homocysteine Studies Collaboration.** Homocysteine and the risk of ischemic heart disease and stroke. JAMA. 2002;288:2015-22.
26. **Boysen G, Brander T, Christensen H, et al.** Homocysteine and risk of recurrent stroke. Stroke. 2003;34:1258-61.
27. **Toole JF, Malinow MR, Chambless LE, et al.** Lowering homocysteine in patients with ischemic stroke to prevent recurrent stroke, myocardial infarction, and death: the Vitamin Intervention for Stroke Prevention (VISP) randomized controlled trial. JAMA. 2004;291:565-75.
28. **The VITATOPS Trial Study Group.** The VITATOPS (vitamins to prevent stroke) trial: rationale and design of an international, large, simple, randomized trial of homocysteine-lowering multivitamin therapy in patients with recent transient ischemic attack or stroke. Cerebrovasc Dis. 2002;13:120-6.
29. **Hackam DG, Peterson JC, Spence JD.** What level of homocyst(e)ine should be treated? Effects of vitamin therapy on progression of carotid atherosclerosis in patients with homocyst(e)ine levels above and below 14 µmol/L. Am J Hypertens. 2000;13:105-10.
30. **Rothman SM, Fulling KH, Nelson JS.** Sickle cell anemia and central nervous system infarction: a neuropathological study. Ann Neurol. 1986;20:684-90.
31. **Grau AJ, Buggle F, Heindl S, et al.** Recent infection as a risk factor for cerebrovascular ischemia. Stroke. 1995;26:373-9.
32. **Elkind MS, Lin IF, Grayston JT, Sacco RL.** Chlamydia pneumoniae and the risk of first ischemic stroke. The Northern Manhattan Stroke Study. Stroke. 2000;31:1521-5.
33. **Tanne D, Haim M, Boyko V, et al.** Prospective study of Chlamydia pneumoniae IgG and IgA seropositivity and risk of incident ischemic stroke. Cerebrovasc Dis. 2003;16:166-70.
34. **Evers S, Nabavi D, Rahmann A, et al.** Ischemic cerebrovascular events in HIV infection. Cerebrovasc Dis. 2003;15:199-205.
35. **Malouf R, Jacquette G, Dobkin J, Brust JC.** Neurologic disease in human immunodeficiency virus-infected drug abusers. Arch Neurol. 1990;47:1002-7.
36. **Khamashta MA, Cuadrado MJ, Mujic M, et al.** The management of thrombosis in the antiphospholipid-antibody syndrome. N Engl J Med. 1995;332:993-7.
37. **Sen S, Oppenheimer SM, Lima J, Cohen B.** Risk factors for progression of aortic atheroma in stroke and transient ischemic attack patients. Stroke. 2002;33:930-5.
38. **Montgomery DH, Ververis JJ, McGorisk G, et al.** Natural history of severe atheromatous disease of the thoracic aorta: a transesophageal echocardiographic study. J Am Coll Cardiol. 1996;27:95-101.

39. Tunick PA, Rosenzweig BP, Katz ES, et al. High risk for vascular events in patients with protruding aortic atheromas: a prospective study. J Am Coll Cardiol. 1994;23:1085-90.
40. The French Study of Aortic Plaques in Stroke Group. Atherosclerotic disease of the aortic arch is a risk factor for recurrent ischemic stroke. N Engl J Med. 1996;334:1216-21.
41. Cohen A, Tzourio C, Bertrand B, et al. Aortic plaque morphology and vascular events. Circulation. 1997;96:3838-41.
42. Di Tullio MR, Sacco RL, Gersony D, et al. Aortic atheromas and acute ischemic stroke: a transesophageal echocardiographic study in an ethnically mixed population. Neurology. 1996;46:1560-6.
43. Falcone RA, Shapiro EP, Jangula JC, Johnson CJ. Transesophageal echocardiographic findings in subcortical and cortical stroke. Am J Cardiol. 2000;85:121-4.
44. Dressler FA, Craig WR, Castello R, Labovitz AJ. Mobile aortic atheroma and systemic emboli: efficacy of anticoagulation and influence of plaque morphology on recurrent stroke. J Am Coll Cardiol. 1998;31:134-8.
45. The Stroke Prevention in Atrial Fibrillation Investigators Committee on Echocardiography. TEE correlates of thromboembolism in high-risk patients with nonvalvular atrial fibrillation. Ann Intern Med. 1998;128:639-47.
46. Ferrari E, Vidal R, Chevallier T, Baudouy M. Atherosclerosis of the thoracic aorta and aortic debris as a marker for poor prognosis: benefit of oral anticoagulants. J Am Coll Cardiol. 1999;33:1317-22.
47. Tunick PA, Nayar AC, Goodkin GM, et al. Effect of treatment on the incidence of stroke and other emboli in 519 patients with severe thoracic aortic plaque. Am J Cardiol. 2002;90:1320-5.
48. Bladin CF, Chambers BR. Frequency and pathogenesis of hemodynamic stroke. Stroke. 1994;25:2179-82.
49. Bladin CF, Chambers BR. Clinical features, pathogenesis, and computed tomographic characteristics of internal watershed infarction. Stroke. 1993;24:1925-32.

Chapter 15

Intracerebral Hemorrhage

CONNIE L. CHEN, MD
ANISH BHARDWAJ, MD

Key Points

- Neurological signs typically correlate with the anatomic location of the bleed.
- Initial assessment for rapid diagnosis and management is essential for optimal patient outcome.
- Hemorrhages continue to increase in size after initial presentation. After initial stabilization, effort is concentrated on preventing clot expansion and reducing secondary brain damage from clot mass effect.
- After initial patient stabilization, patients with acute intracerebral hemorrhage (ICH) should be admitted and observed in a monitored setting.
- Patients at risk for developing elevated intracranial pressure (ICP) from large clot size, edema formation, and expanding hematoma from uncontrolled blood pressure or coagulopathy should be admitted to an intensive care unit.
- Other causes of decline in neurological status are increased size of hemorrhage, edema formation, new stroke, or obstructive hydrocephalus.
- After the patient is stabilized, an etiological diagnosis should be established.
- Surgical evacuation remains controversial but in selected patients may be life-saving.
- ICH carries a higher risk for morbidity and mortality than ischemic strokes.

Intracerebral hemorrhage (ICH), defined as bleeding within the brain parenchyma, is a term used interchangeably with "hemorrhagic stroke" and encompasses non-traumatic causes of hemorrhage in the cranium. ICH accounts for 10%-15% of all strokes, although its incidence is higher (20%-30%) in certain ethnic groups (blacks, Asians) (1,2). It afflicts approximately 40,000 individuals per year in the United States (1,2). ICH has a higher morbidity and mortality than other forms of stroke, with death occurring in 35%-52% patients within 1 month of presentation, half being within the first 2 days, and only 20% surviving with functional independence at 6 months (1,2).

Etiology and Pathophysiology

Hypertensive arteriopathy, resulting from long-standing hypertension, is the most common cause of primary ICH (3). Fifty to seventy-five percent of patients with ICH have a history of hypertension. Uncontrolled hypertension carries a two- to six-fold increased risk of developing ICH; patients who are non-compliant with antihypertensives carry an even higher risk of ICH than those patients who were never started on medication. High risk of ICH is thought to be secondary to weakening of the vessel wall of smaller cerebral vessels by long-standing damage to the media layer. Histopathological studies on brain sections from patients who had hypertensive hemorrhages demonstrate thin-walled vessels with smooth muscle degeneration and a classic "moth eaten" appearance (3).

Other associated risk factors for ICH include alcohol use, first-degree relatives with ICH, Asian and Hispanic heritage, use of anticoagulants or coagulation disorders, aspirin use with concomitant history of epistaxis, drug abuse, and presence of the ApoE2 or ApoE4 allele. Low serum cholesterol levels, though debatable, have also been noted as a risk factor for ICH. Factors notable for *not* increasing risk of ICH are smoking and diabetes. Vascular malformations and vasculopathies such as aneurysms, arteriovenous malformations (AVMs), cavernous angiomas, cerebral amyloid angiopathy, infection, intraparenchymal tumors, and head trauma are important secondary causes of ICH. Venous thrombosis with outflow obstruction and subsequent venous infarction may also cause development of ICH. Similarly, ischemic infarctions resulting from arterial thromboembolism may undergo subsequent hemorrhagic conversion and present as ICH.

Aneurysm rupture typically presents as subarachnoid hemorrhage (SAH). However, depending upon the location of the aneurysm, ICH as well as subdural hemorrhage may develop. Upon aneurysmal rupture, a jet of blood may extravasate into the adjacent brain parenchyma and adjacent tissues. Drug use, cocaine, and amphetamines, in particular, are thought to increase the risk of ICH through early rupture of pre-existing aneurysms. Although typically larger aneurysms (>10 mm) have a propensity for spontaneous rupture, smaller aneurysms (<5 mm) are prone to rupture in drug users of a younger population. Average age upon rupture is 50 years old. Smoking, pregnancy, and oral contraceptives increase the risk of aneurysm rupture.

ICH is frequently the presenting symptom of AVMs. Risk of bleeding is estimated at 1%-4% per year, and, in contrast to aneurysmal rupture, AVMs tend to occur in a younger population (average age, 20 years). High pressure systems confer higher risk of rupture. Previously, smaller AVMs were thought to have the highest risk of bleeding, but recent studies suggest that large AVMs in deep locations also carry a higher than previously perceived risk of bleeding (4). Literature on AVMs remains controversial on risk factors for bleeding but has included presence of deep draining veins, venous occlusion, and presence of aneurysms. Like AVMs, cavernous angiomas, malformations that are less well studied, frequently present as ICH. In one large autopsy series, cavernous angiomas were present in approximately 0.1% of the patients studied. However, risk of bleeding is believed to be less than that of AVMs.

Cerebral amyloid angiopathy (CAA), a frequent cause of ICH in the elderly, is found in 50% of patients older than eighty years of age (5). In these affected individuals, amyloid deposition in medium to smaller cerebral vessels leads to weakening of the vessel wall and subsequent spontaneous rupture. Small studies investigating the recurrent bleeding risk of ICH after the initial hemorrhage report a rate of 21% over a period of 2 years. The presence of ApoE2 and ApoE4 alleles is associated with a higher risk of bleeding (6).

Cerebral sinus thrombosis (CST) increases risk of ICH through development of venous outflow obstruction followed by venous stasis with subsequent venous infarct and hemorrhage. Approximately 50% of patients with CST develop ICH (7). Risk factors for CST are numerous, ranging from vasculopathies and sickle cell disease to severe dehydration, trauma, endocrinopathies, infection, and medications.

Nonvascular causes of ICH are less common than hypertension-induced ICH. Infection may precipitate ICH through formation of mycotic aneurysms and subsequent rupture or through development of CST. Intraparenchymal tumors, both metastatic and primary, may also hemorrhage, although ICH incidence is less than 15% (8). Of the metastatic tumors, renal cell carcinoma, melanoma, bronchogenic carcinoma, choriocarcinoma, and thyroid cancer are especially likely to be associated with hemorrhage. Traumatic brain injury may lead to ICH from direct injury and contusion or from development of CST.

Clinical Presentation

ICH presents with diverse neurological and constitutional symptoms. Typically, symptoms and signs are sudden in onset, and a high index of suspicion is warranted in patients with rapid onset of neurological deficit and rapid decline in the level of consciousness (LOC). Common initial signs, other than neurological deficits, may include headache, vomiting, or decreased LOC. Headache occurs in approximately 40% of patients with ICH and vomiting in 49% with supratentorial hemorrhage (9,10). Decreased LOC is perhaps the most important sign because it can be secondary to increased intracranial pressure (ICP) from the hematoma. Lastly, elevated blood pressure may be a presenting sign in up to 90% of patients with ICH (11).

Patients present with neurological signs that typically correlate with the anatomical location of the bleed. A large lobar hemorrhage in the left parietal lobe may present with left parietal lobe signs of right-sided weakness and hemisensory loss, right visual field defects, right-sided neglect, or language deficits (Figure 15-1). Smaller and deeper hemorrhages in the basal

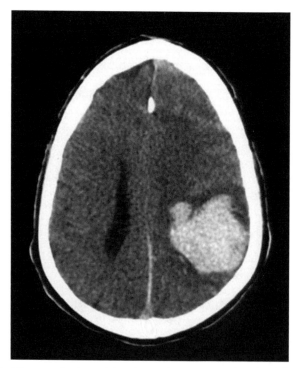

Figure 15-1 CT scan of a large lobar hemorrhage centered in the left parietal lobe. Clinical symptoms include right-sided weakness and hemisensory loss, right visual field defects, right-sided neglect, and language deficits.

ganglia may present with hemiplegia and hemisensory loss. ICH involving the pons may cause cranial nerve deficits, leading to diplopia, dyspahgia, dysarthria, and motor deficits. Massive pontine ICH results in coma, bilateral extensor posturing, and, inevitably, death (Figure 15-2). ICH involving the cerebellum and its connections may present as dysmetria, nystagmus, and ataxia but may rapidly progress to rapid diminution in the LOC due to brain stem compression or development of obstructive hydrocephalus (Figure 15-3).

Clinical exam in a majority of ICH patients will deteriorate from their initial presentation as hemorrhage size grows or edema ensues. Stroke registries have reported that, of the ICH patients who presented, 51%-63% continued to progress in their symptoms while only 34%-38% remained stable (12). Interval CT scans demonstrates that hematoma expansion occurs in approximately 40% of patients within 24 hours of their initial presentation (Figure 15-4) (13). Other reasons for deterioration include development of obstructive hydrocephalus and occurrence of seizures (6%-7%), more commonly in patients with lobar hemorrhages than with deeper basal ganglia location.

Differential Diagnosis

A differential diagnosis can be inferred based on the location of the ICH on neuroimaging studies. To aid in this classification, hemorrhage location is divided into lobar and non-lobar categories. Non-lobar ICHs typically occur in the basal ganglia and thalamus, brainstem, and cerebellum (Figure 15-5).

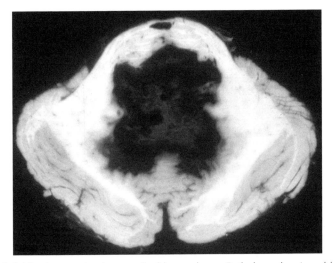

Figure 15-2 Massive pontine intracerebral hemorrhage. Pathology showing obliteration of the central pons by hematoma with extension into the fourth ventricle.

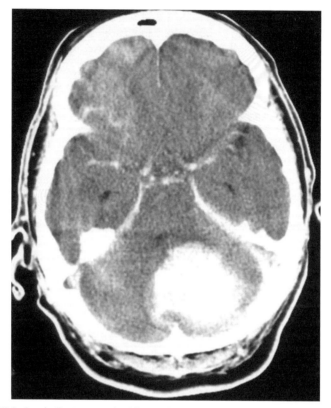

Figure 15-3 Cerebellar intracerebral hemorrhage. Large ICH into left cerebellum compresses and displaces the fourth ventricle. Further enlargement of the mass effect by rebleeding or edema can lead to direct compression of the pons as well as secondary obstructive hydrocephalus.

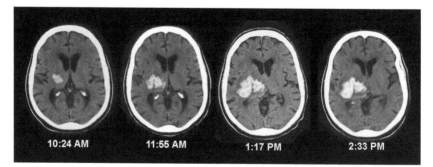

Figure 15-4 Intracerebral hemorrhage expansion. Serial CT images of a patient who presented with left arm clumsiness shows progressive ICH enlargement over 3 hours. The patient deteriorated to hemiplegia and a decreased level of consciousness during this period of time.

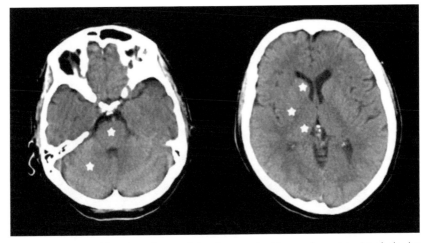

Figure 15-5 Typical locations for non-lobar intracerebral hemorrhage (*stars*) include the pons, cerebellum, caudate, putamen, and thalamus. ICHs in these locations are commonly due to hypertension.

Primary ICH caused by uncontrolled hypertension is typically non-lobar. Classic sites include the caudate, putamen, thalamus, pons, and cerebellum (Figure 15-6). ICH not involving these structures or with disproportionate amount of edema is most likely secondary to non-hypertensive etiologies. Cavernous angiomas, AVMs, venous infarct, and tumor may occasionally present in this manner. Lobar hemorrhages, on the other hand, are usually caused by CAA, ruptured AVMs or aneurysms, cavernous angiomas, venous infarcts with hemorrhage, arterial infarct with hemorrhagic transformation, tumor-associated hemorrhage, or head trauma. History of illness may help narrow the differential. ICH secondary to CAA may be confirmed by hemosiderin sequences on MRI and may reveal multiple sites of old hemorrhages that may have been clinically "silent." Venous infarct and tumor hemorrhage usually present with a disproportionately large amount of vasogenic edema. Infarctions with hemorrhagic conversion typically respect arterial territories. Only rarely does hypertension cause lobar hemorrhages.

Management

Management on Initial Presentation

Patients with ICH usually present first to the emergency department. Initial assessment for rapid diagnosis and management is essential for optimal patient outcome. Early treatment centers on control of airway, breathing, and circulation ("ABC's") for patient stabilization. Decision for endotracheal intubation is based on rapid evaluation of patient's LOC and integrity of airway reflexes. Delay in securing and protecting the airway may lead to

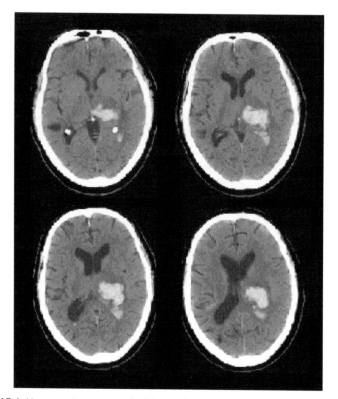

Figure 15-6 Hypertensive intracerebral hemorrhage. Patient is a 62-year-old male who presented with a sudden onset of right hemiparesis, aphasia, and left gaze deviation. Initial blood pressure upon presentation was 210/118. Head CT reveals a 20 cm³ left thalamic ICH with intraventricular extension and perihematoma edema.

hypoxemia, aspiration pneumonia, and hypercapnia, resulting in poorer clinical outcome. Because most of the management of ICH is supportive and neurosurgical, patients with ICH should be admitted to an intensive care unit with expertise in management of neurological emergencies. Otherwise, the patient should be transferred to an institution with critical care expertise and a neurosurgeon on call.

Secondary survey includes neurological assessment focused on ongoing herniation with or without signs of elevated ICP. Because rapid reversal of brain herniation can lead to good clinical outcome, prompt recognition and treatment of this potentially lethal consequence of ICH is paramount. Cardinal signs of increased ICP are decreased or diminishing LOC, Cushing's triad of hypertension, bradycardia, and respiratory variation, with or without the presence of cranial nerve dysfunction composed of anisocoria, absent corneal reflexes, eye movement abnormalities, diminished gag, and cough reflexes. Isolated blood pressure elevation with ICH may be a sign of the initial hemorrhage or an indirect indication of elevated ICP. In a patient whose initial presentation is a decreased LOC, or in a patient whose LOC is deteriorating rapidly, increased ICP should be anticipated and treated promptly.

If increased ICP is a concern, the patient should be intubated for airway protection and ICP control measures (including elevated head position [30–60 degrees] with head midline and internal jugular veins made clear of any external pressure, hyperventilation, and osmotherapy) should be instituted immediately. Of note, there is no evidence to support the use of prophylactic measures for ICP control such as hyperventilation or osmotherapy in the absence of signs indicating elevated ICP. Once the patient is stabilized, clinical diagnosis is confirmed rapidly with a non-enhanced CT of the brain (CT is extremely reliable in detecting acute ICH), to indicate initial size and location of ICH, presence and extent of hydrocephalus, extension into the ventricles, intracranial compartmental, or midline shifts and brain herniation. Laboratories should be drawn at this juncture to check the patient's hematocrit, platelets, liver function, and coagulation function.

After initial stabilization, effort is then concentrated on preventing clot expansion and reducing secondary brain damage from clot mass effect causing decreased cerebral perfusion pressure (CPP) and cerebral blood flow, exacerbating ischemic brain injury. Contrary to previous belief, hemorrhages continue to increase in size after initial presentation (13). Any coagulation abnormality should be immediately and rapidly reversed with vitamin K, and fresh frozen plasma for prolongation in prothrombin time, protamine in heparin overdoses, or platelet transfusions for thrombocytopenia (Table 15-1). Likewise, because most ICHs are secondary to uncontrolled hypertension, blood pressure management becomes foremost in patient management. Change in clinical exam should heighten the suspicion that the hemorrhage is expanding, or, if the patient is presenting subacutely, that edema may be worsening.

The American Heart Association has recommended that mean arterial blood pressure (MAP) be maintained at <130 mm Hg in patients with a history of hypertension (11). In patients with increased ICP, a goal CPP of >70 mm Hg should be maintained (CPP = MAP – ICP). Blood pressure should be monitored at least every 5 minutes during treatment with medication and should be controlled as rapidly as possible.

An ideal anti-hypertensive agent in the acute setting should be easily titratable, given parenterally with minimal side effects, and have a short half-life (14). Anti-hypertensives are usually selected by their ability to not cause cerebral vessel dilation, which would theoretically worsen ICP. Labetolol and enalaprilat are thus intravenous agents of choice in this situation and may be used as intermittent intravenous boluses. In patients not responsive to these medications, hydralazine is usually the next drug of choice, although it is not titratable as a continuous infusion (Table 15-2). Nitrates (nitroprusside and nitroglycerine) are potent vasodilators and

Table 15-1 Rapid Coagulopathy Reversal

Coagulation Abnormality	Correction Time	Adverse Treatment	Reactions
INR > 20 or serious bleeding	Immediate	• Vitamin K 10 mg by slow IV infusion • Fresh-frozen plasma or prothrombin complex concentrate • Monitor INR q 2 hr • Repeat vitamin K q 12 hr as needed	Hemodynamic instability, fever, flushing, diaphoresis, dyspnea, hypertension
Prolonged aPTT, bleeding, heparin administered minutes ago	Immediate	• Protamine 1-1.5 mg/100 U heparin	Hypotension, bradycardia, pulmonary hypertension, dyspnea, flushing, urticaria, angioedema, anaphylaxis
Prolonged aPTT, bleeding, heparin administered 30–60 minutes ago	Immediate	• Protamine 0.5-0.75 mg/100 U heparin	
Prolonged aPTT, bleeding, heparin administered ≥2 hours ago		• Protamine 0.25-0.375 mg/100 U heparin	
tPA administration	Immediate	• Cryoprecipitate 6-8 U	Transfusion reaction
Thrombocytopenia (<50,000), bleeding	Immediate	• 1 U platelets for every 5000/mm^3 platelets below 50,000/mm^3	Transfusion reaction

Adapted from Hirsh J, Fuster V, Ansell J, Halperin JL. AHA/ACC Foundation Guide to Warfarin Therapy. AHA/ACC. 2003;41:1633-52; and Administration of protamine sulfate. In: Chan ED, Terada LS, Kortbeek J, Winston BW, eds. Bedside Critical Care Manual. Philadelphia: Hanley & Belfus; 2002:24.

hence less ideal in the setting of ICH secondary to the possibility of increasing ICP through cerebral vasodilation and increased blood volume in the cranium. However, in patients refractory to labetolol, enalaprilat, and hydralazine, it is more important to lower blood pressure than to avoid these agents out of concern for ICP. In patients not responsive to any anti-hypertensive medication, anesthetic agents such as propofol should be considered.

Management in the Intensive Care Unit

Following initial patient stabilization, patients with acute ICH should be admitted and observed in a monitored setting. At our institution, all patients with acute ICH admitted within 12 hours of onset of symptoms are admitted to an ICU. Even patients with small bleeds and minor deficits may progress substantially in the first 6 to 12 hours after onset. In patients with

Table 15-2 Blood Pressure Management in Intracranial Hemorrhage

Agents for Control of Hypertension

- Labetalol 5-100 mg/hr by intermittent bolus of 10-40 mg IV (maximum dose, 300 mg) or continuous infusion at 2-8 mg/min or 20-60 mg/hr
- Enalaprilat 0.625-1.2 mg IV q 6 hr; maximum dose, 5 mg/dose
- Hydralazine 2.5-10 mg q 20 min; maximum dose, 40 mg/dose
- Nitroprusside 0.5-10 µg/kg/min; maximum dose, 3.5 mg/kg

Agents for Management of Hypotension

- Volume replacement with isotonic saline or colloids, as appropriate
- Vasopressors are recommended if hypotension persists after intravascular volume repletion; these agents can be titrated to the desired MAP > 90 or CPP > 70 mm Hg, if ICP value is available
- Phenylephrine 2-10 µg/kg/min; maximum dose, 200 µg/min
- Dopamine 2-20 µg/kg/min; maximum dose, 50 µg/kg/min
- Norpinephrine 0.05-0.2 µg/kg/min

From Broderick JP, Adams HP Jr, Barsan W, et al. Guidelines for the management of spontaneous intracerebral hemorrhage: a statement for healthcare professionals from a special writing group of the Stroke Council, American Heart Association. Stroke. 1999;30:905-15; with permission.

Table 15-3 Medical Management of Intracranial Hemorrhage

- Intubate prophylactically if GCS ≤ 8 or with compromised airway protective mechanisms
- Control BP to a target MAP of < 130 mm Hg with labetalol, enalaprilat, or hydralazine
- Maintain MAP > 90 and CPP > 70 mm Hg (if ICP value is available)
- Check coagulation profile: correct coagulopathy
- Cardiopulmonary monitoring in ICU
- Neurologic monitoring q 30 min to 1 hr
- 0.9% NaCl as IVF (1.0-1.5 mL/kg/hr)
- Serum Na+ goal: normonatremia to 140-145 mEq/L (serum osmolality, 310-320 mOsm/L)
- ICP-lowering therapies
  —*General:* avoid agitation, maintain normothermia and midline head position at 30-60°
  —*Specific:* controlled hyperventilation, external CSF drainage for hydrocephalus, osmotherapy, metabolic suppression (barbiturates, propofol), steroids (for tumor-associated ICH, consider hypothermia and surgical decompression)
- GI and DVT prophylaxis
- Seizure prophylaxis for supratentorial ICH
- NPO: close monitoring for aspiration
- Initiate work-up for possible etiology

ICH, the goal of management is to prevent brain herniation and further secondary neurological injury (Table 15-3). ICU care therefore centers on blood pressure control to prevent expansion of the hematoma and on early recognition and treatment of increased ICP. Thus, foremost in ICU care is monitoring of any change in neurological status.

Neurological Monitoring

Upon patient admission, ICU staff should establish "baseline" exam and be alerted that a worsening exam may represent worsening ICH, edema, or hydrocephalus. Bedside neurological exams are the cornerstone and strongest indicators of patient's neurological status (15). Neurological monitoring is established through hourly neurological checks for at least the first 48 hours. These neurological checks are based on a modified neurological exam that includes assessments of LOC, orientation, ability to follow commands, cranial nerve exam, motor strength, and sensation. In comatose patients, a diligent neurological assessment is especially crucial because a decline in exam is often difficult to ascertain. In these patients greater emphasis should be placed on determining:

1. The degree of stimulation (voice, light shaking, sternal rub, or deep nail bed pressure) required to elicit a response of eye opening, movement, command following, or verbal response
2. Notation of response, such as vocalization, purposeful movement to command, localizing, withdraw, flexion, extension, or absent
3. Pupil size, shape, brisk or sluggish, or non-reactive to light
4. Presence of corneal reflexes, occulocephalic reflexes, cough, gag, or spontaneous breathing over the ventilator, if intubated

A decline in exam in the comatose patient is therefore indicated by:

1. Increased stimulus needed to elicit a response (sternal rub/nail bed pressure is greater stimulus than "light shaking," which is more than "response to voice")
2. Patient response declines from vocalization and purposeful movement to localization, from localization to flexion, flexion to extension, or from extension to no response
3. Any change in pupil size, shape, or reaction
4. Reduced response or absence of the rest of the cranial nerve exam

Additional monitoring can be done through placement of an ICP monitor in patients whose Glasgow Coma Scale (GCS) score is <8. ICP monitors, in general, are placed by neurosurgery and are composed of fiberoptic devices placed in the subdural, subarachnoid, parenchymal, or intraventricular space. Fluid coupled devices, such as intraventricular monitors, are typically and commonly used therapeutically to drain CSF for ICP control but carry the highest risk for infection. Normal ICP ranges from 5 to 10 mm Hg. ICP is considered high if ICP is sustained above 20 mm Hg for >10 minutes.

Intracranial Pressure Control

Once a neurological decline is detected, elevated ICP and imminent herniation must be first ruled out as the cause. If signs of Cushing's triad and/or new anisocoria are present with a decreased LOC, the patient should be treated for elevated ICP immediately. A non-contrast head CT may be obtained only after the patient is stabilized.

Patient position is essential in the treatment of elevated ICP, and is often overlooked. The patient should be maintained with the head of the bed at least at 45 degrees, with the patient's head midline without compression of the internal jugulars, even by tape or a securing device for the endoctracheal tube. The endotracheal tube may instead be secured by taping around the patient's mouth and cheeks. This upright and head midline positioning of the patient ensures unimpeded venous outflow from the cranium.

Specific therapies in the treatment of elevated ICP are targeted towards reducing the volume of one or more of the three compartments in the cranial vault: brain, blood, and CSF (16,17). Hyperventilation is the most rapid and efficacious method in reducing ICP emergently. It causes vasoconstriction and is achieved by initially "bagging" a patient for approximately 2 minutes, then setting the ventilator to a rate of 16-22/minute, depending upon the tidal volume. Target $PaCO_2$ is 25-30 with a pH > 7.5. There should be caution in "overbagging" the patient because it may lead to severe vasoconstriction and cerebral ischemia.

Brain parenchymal volume is reduced through osmotherapy. Steroids have no role in reducing edema-associated ICH unless tumor is a component of the mass effect. Osmotherapy with mannitol (0.25-1 g/kg) is currently the agent of choice. Alternatively, intravenous bolus infusion (30 mL over 15-20 minutes) of 23.4% hypertonic saline via central venous access has been shown to be efficacious in reducing ICP (16,17). Rapid infusions of hypertonic saline may lead to transient hypotension and hemolysis. Osmotherapy should be targeted to achieve and maintain serum osmolality of 310-320 mOsm/L, or serum Na^+ of 145-155 mEq/L with use of hypertonic saline. Continuous intravenous infusions of 2%-3% hypertonic saline (50:50 chloride:acetate, to avoid hyperchloremic acidosis) given at 1-1.5 mL/kg/hr have been shown to be safe and efficacious in lowering ICP and ameliorating cerebral edema.

Anesthetic agents may also rapidly reduce ICP. If the patient does not respond to the above measures, thiopental at a dose of 250 mg, or propofol at a dose of 100-150 mg, may be given as intravenous bolus. These agents rapidly reduce ICP through reduction of CBF and coupled to reduce cerebral metabolism. Propofol, however, is very short acting, and continuous infusion of 50-150 µg/kg/min may be required until other means may be found to reduce ICP. Blood pressure support to meet CPP goals will be needed with the use of these agents because hypotension is a known side effect.

Evaluation and Treatment of Other Causes of Worsening Neurological Status

Once increased ICP is ruled out as the cause for the decline in neurological status, a head CT may be obtained to evaluate the patient and formulate a differential diagnosis. Possible structural reasons for the decline in exam may include increased size of hemorrhage, edema formation, new stroke, or obstructive hydrocephalus in the patient with blood in the ventricles. Non-structural reasons for decline in exam may include metabolic encephalopathy or seizures.

Hemorrhage size is unstable in 20%-50% of patients presenting with acute hemorrhage (13). Several studies investigating hemorrhage size following acute presentation have found that the majority of ICH expansion occurs within the first few hours of presentation. A lesser percentage of patients with ICH will have hemorrhage expansion up to 20 hours after presentation. Hypertension and coagulopathy are thought to play a role in clot expansion. If coagulopathy is identified as the cause, its rapid correction is recommended.

Edema formation usually peaks 2-4 days after the initial insult. Patients with large amounts of vasogenic edema upon presentation that is disproportionate to the size of ICH should be suspected of having an underlying tumor. Unless an underlying tumor is present, there is no role for treatment of edema with steroids. On the contrary, steroids have been noted to raise morbidity through increased infection risk.

Seizures may be a source for neurological deterioration in any comatose patient. An electroencephalogram (EEG) should be performed because seizures may occur despite "therapeutic" levels of anticonvulsant medications. Seizure activity occurs in 2%-10% of patients with ICH. In patients with lobar hemorrhages, the risk for seizure is higher than in patients with non-lobar hemorrhages. Prophylactic use of anti-epileptic medication, therefore, should be considered in all patients with lobar hemorrhages. The American Stroke Association guidelines suggest that anti-epileptic use be continued up to 1 month after ICH.

Metabolic encephalopathy should not be overlooked as a source for neurological deterioration. Standard work-up includes screening for infection, thyroid function panel, ammonia level, anticonvulsant levels, and urine and serum toxicology screen. An EEG may be helpful not only to evaluate for seizures but to identify global slowing, which is suggestive of metabolic encephalopathy.

Blood Pressure Control

As previously discussed, blood pressure control is essential to maintain adequate CPP and prevent further expansion of the ICH. Thus too aggressive control of blood pressure may reduce CPP in a baseline hypertensive patient whose cerebral autoregulation curve is shifted to accommodate higher pressures. This may lead to infarctions in watershed regions if overly aggressive treatment is instituted. In addition, although still highly debated, an ischemic penumbra is thought to surround the hemorrhage, which may be more susceptible to ischemia with lower CPP (18). The lower limit of blood pressure control has thus been to maintain a CPP of 70 mm Hg. In patients without an ICP monitor, blood pressure or MAP goal may be extrapolated from an estimate of ICP on neuroimaging studies, the normal range being 5-10 mm Hg.

As mentioned earlier, the goal for the upper range of blood pressure has been recommended by the American Stroke Association to be an MAP of 130 mm Hg in patients who are hypertensive at baseline. There are no guidelines, however, for patients who are not hypertensive at baseline. Hypertension in ICH, therefore, is often treated as a hypertensive emergency. Goal decrements of blood pressure are 20% per day.

In the first 24 hours of the ICU stay, blood pressure should be controlled with intravenous medications only (see section on Management at Initial Presentation). During this time, the patient is often unstable, and it is not desirable to initiate longer-acting oral medications. Once the patient is stabilized and no longer at risk for increased ICP, oral agents should be started. The patient is then transitioned from intravenous to oral medications over the following days in the ICU.

Investigation of Etiology

Once the patient is stabilized, an etiological diagnosis should be ascertained. For many patients, the location of the ICH combined with the presentation of hypertension is diagnostic. Other patients presenting in a non-typical manner for hypertensive hemorrhages, such as hemorrhages outside of the caudate, putamen, thalamus, pons, or cerebellum and presentation with disproportionate amount of edema or absence of hypertension, require further work-up. Cavernous angiomas, AVMs, venous infarct, and tumor are possible causes with these presentations. Magnetic resonance imaging (MRI) with and without gadolinium should be obtained to detect accompanying underlying brain tumor. MR angiography and venography may also be useful in patients suspected of having a vascular or venous etiology. A hemosiderin sequence with the MRI may reveal sites of old bleeding that may be consistent with CAA or cavernous angiomas. In patients who remain undiagnosed after MRI/angiography/venography, conventional four-vessel cerebral angiography should be considered. According to a prospective study of angiograms in ICH, diagnostic angiograms had the highest yield in patients younger than 45 years of age without a history of hypertension (19).

Fluid Management

The fluid status goal for patients with ICH is euvolemia. This is especially important in individuals treated for increased ICP because the use of osmotic agents or the concomitant use of diuretic to excrete free water may render the patient dehydrated. It is important to replace volume even in those patients with elevated ICP. The therapeutic effect of osmotic agents on ICP (by the egress of water from the brain to the vascular compartment) is not based on fluid status but on the osmotic gradient between the intravascular compartment and the brain.

Deep Venous Thrombosis Prophylaxis

Deep venous thrombosis (DVT) prophylaxis is important in patients with ICH in particular due to their prolonged immobility. Prophylactic heparin and enoxaparin have not been shown to increase hemorrhage size in patients with ICH. DVT prophylaxis should be initiated 24 hours after admission once it has been ascertained that the patient does not have an underlying coagulopathy.

Surgical versus Medical Treatment

There are no data to support surgical over medical approach for the treatment of supratentorial ICH. Numerous small studies have investigated the feasibility and efficacy of clot resection by both craniotomy and endoscopic approaches. None, however, have conclusively shown any improvement in patient function or outcome (20). Meta-analysis of randomized controlled trials of surgical evacuation of supratentorial ICH demonstrates higher mortality and dependency rates compared with medical treatment only. An ongoing prospective randomized study, Surgical Trial in Intracerebral Hemorrhage (STICH), is evaluating patient outcome with surgical evacuation versus conservative medical treatment. Projected enrollment for this study is 1000 patients, which should be of sufficient power to address the study's hypothesis. A randomized study of endoscopic evacuation of ICH was also performed, the Stereotactic Treatment of Intracerebral Hematoma by Means of a Plasminogen Activator (SICHPA) trial. This study was closed before the full projected enrollment of subjects. Although the study found significant clot reduction by steoreotactic aspiration versus medical management, no significance was found in patient outcome by modified Rankin score.

Large infratentorial hemorrhages may have improved outcome with surgical treatment. Cerebellar hematomas are particularly amenable to surgical evacuation and demonstrate good outcomes, especially with ICH > 3 cm in size. CSF drainage (if hydrocephalus is present) with intraventricular catheter and surgical evacuation or its combination is the recommended treatment of choice.

Prognosis

ICH carries a higher risk for morbidity and mortality than ischemic strokes and subarachnoid hemorrhages. The highest morbidity and mortality period is within the first 30 days of hemorrhage (21). Multiple factors have been identified to prognosticate which patients have the highest risk of death or vegetative state and which will have a good functional outcome. These factors are incorporated into an ICH score (see below), which may be used to guide decision making for treatment upon presentation. However, caution must be taken to avoid the use of the worse prognosticators as a self-fulfilling prophecy of mortality (22).

One of the main prognostic factors identified in ICH patients is the GCS score upon presentation. Hemphill et al have reported that patients with a GCS score of ≤ 4 on presentation have worse prognosis, whereas patients with a GCS ≥ 13 have the best prognosis (23). Other studies group patients differently and have noted that patients with a GCS ≤ 8 have a worse prognosis.

Following initial GCS score, size of ICH is a significant predictor of outcome (20). Hemorrhage size is divided into ≤ 30 cm^3, 30-60 cm^3, and ≥ 60 cm^3; ≤ 30 cm^3 is associated with the best prognosis, whereas ≥ 60 cm^3 is associated with poor prognosis. Size of hemorrhage is calculated by the $(A+B+C)/2$ method. This method is based upon calculation of hemorrhage size on head CT as if it were in the shape of an ellipse. A refers to the length of the hemorrhage in the largest cross section; B refers to the width in the largest cross section when measured perpendicular to A; and C refers to the depth of the bleed in centimeters. This value is taken by calculating the centimeters from the first CT axial image of the hemorrhage to the last.

Presence and volume of IVH have also been noted to affect morbidity and mortality, although it is a less significant prognosticator than the volume of hemorrhage (24). A large amount of IVH also carries a poorer prognosis than a smaller volume. Perhaps related to this finding is that the development of hydrocephalus is also a prognosticator of worse outcome (23).

Other identified prognostic factors are related to the patient's vital signs and glucose level. Both a first-day MAP >145 mm Hg and a body temperature >37.5°C for >24-hour duration have been associated with greater morbidity and mortality. Likewise, patients with a higher glucose upon presentation have also been found to have a higher morbidity (25). It remains unclear, however, whether there is a cause or effect relationship to these findings.

Combining all of these prognostic factors gives the ICH score (23), which has been developed to assist practitioners in the treatment of patients with ICH through risk stratification. Similar to the calculation of GCS score, the ICH score is based on a score added from various categories: GCS score, ICH volume, infratentorial location of ICH, presence of IVH, and age. The total score ranges from 0 to 6. GCS scoring is as follows: GCS score 3-4 (2 points), 5-12 (1 point), and 13-15 (0 points). ICH volume is scored by ≥30 cm³ (1 point), whereas <30 cm³ (0 points). Infratentorial origin: yes (1 point), no (0 points). IVH presence receives 1 point; no IVH receives 0 points. Age ≥80 years receives 1 point; <80 years receives 0 points. An ICH score of ≥3 has 79% sensitivity and 90% specificity for predicting 30-day mortality, with a positive and negative predictive value of 71% and 93%, respectively. A score of <3, on the other hand, has 93% sensitivity and 61% specificity for good outcome (patients able to care for themselves with only slight disability or better).

Conclusion

Intracerebral hemorrhage can be a devastating condition that carries a high morbidity and mortality. A high index of clinical suspicion and a rapid diagnosis are paramount in prevention of hematoma expansion and secondary brain injury. Critical care management in a controlled, monitored setting includes blood pressure control, intracranial pressure (ICP)-lowering therapies, and management of accompanying hydrocephalus. Surgical evacuation remains controversial, but in select patients, depending on patient age and hematoma size and location, it may be a life-saving measure.

REFERENCES

1. Qureshi AI, Tuhrim S, Broderick JP, et al. Spontaneous intracerebral hemorrhage. N Engl J Med. 2001;344:1450-60.
2. Qureshi AI, Suri MA, Safdar K, et al. Intracerebral hemorrhage in blacks: risk factors, subtypes, and outcome. Stroke. 1997;28:961-4.
3. Brott T, Thalinger K, Hertzberg V. Hypertension as a risk factor for spontaneous intracerebral hemorrhage. Stroke. 1986;17:1078-83.
4. Stefani MA, Wallace MC, et al. Large and deep brain arteriovenous malformations are associated with risk of future hemorrhage. Stroke. 2002;33:1220-24.
5. Vonsattel JP, Myers RH, Hendly-Whyte ET, et al. Cerebral amyloid angiopathy without and with cerebral hemorrhages: a comparative histological study. Ann Neurol. 1991;30:637-49.
6. Woo D, Sauerbeck LR, Broderick JP, et al. Genetic and environmental risk factors for intracerebral hemorrhage. Stroke. 2002;33:1190-6.
7. Ameri A, Bousser MG. Cerebral venous thrombosis. Neurol Clin. 1992;10:87-111.
8. Wakai S, Takakura K, et al. Spontaneous intracranial hemorrhage caused by brain tumor: its incidence and clinical significance. Neurosurgery. 1982;10:437-44.
9. Gorelik PB, Caplan LR, Langenberg P. Headache in acute cerebrovascular disease. Neurology. 1986;36:1445-50.
10. Caplan L. General symptoms and signs. In: Kase CS, Caplan LR, eds. Intracerebral Hemorrhage. Boston: Butterworth-Heinemann; 1994:31-43.

11. Broderick JP, Adams HP Jr., Barsan W, et al. Guidelines for the management of spontaneous intracerebral hemorrhage: a statement for healthcare professionals from a special writing group of the Stroke Council, American Heart Association. Stroke. 1999;30:905-15.

12. Mayer SA, Sacco RL, Shi T, Mohr JP. Neurologic deterioration in noncomatose patients with supratentorial intracerebral hemorrhage. Neurology. 1994;44:1379-84.

13. Brott T, Broderick J, Kothari R, et al. Early hemorrhage growth in patients with intracerebral hemorrhage. Stroke. 1997;28:1-5.

14. Torbey MT, Bhardwaj A. How to manage blood pressure in critically ill neurologic patients. J Critic Illness. 2001;16:179-92.

15. Minahan RE, Bhardwaj A, Williams MA. Critical care monitoring for cerebrovascular disease. New Horiz. 1997;5:406-21.

16. Harukuni I, Kirsch JR, Bhardwaj A. Cerebral resuscitation: role of osmotherapy. J Anesth. 2002;16:229-37.

17. Bhardwaj A, Ulatowski JA. Cerebral edema: hypertonic saline solutions. Curr Treat Options Neurol. 1999;1:179-87.

18. Powers WJ, Zazulia AR, Videen TO, et al. Autoregulation of cerebral blood flow surrounding acute (6 to 22 hours) intracerebral hemorrhage. Neurology. 2001;57:18-24.

19. Zhu XL, Chan MSY, Poon WS. Spontaneous intracranial hemorrhage: which patients need diagnostic cerebral angiography? A prospective study of 206 cases and review of the literature. Stroke. 1997;28:1406-9.

20. Hankey GJ, Hon C. Surgery for primary intracerebral hemorrhage: is it safe and effective? A systematic review of case series and randomized trials. Stroke. 1997;28:2126-32.

21. Broderick JP, Brott TG, Duldner JE, et al. Volume of intracerebral hemorrhage: a powerful and easy-to-use predictor of 30-day mortality. Stroke. 1993;24:987-93.

22. Becker KJ, Baxter AB, Cohen WA, et al. Withdrawal of support in intracerebral hemorrhage may lead to self-fulfilling prophecies. Neurology. 2001;56:766-72.

23. Hemphill JC 3rd, Bonovich DC, Besmertis L, et al. The ICH score: a simple, reliable grading scale for intracerebral hemorrhage. Stroke. 2001;32:891-7.

24. Naff NJ, Tuhrim S. Intraventricular hemorrhage in adults: complications and treatment. New Horiz. 1997;5:359-63.

25. Schwarz S, Hafner K, Med C, et al. Incidence and prognostic significance of fever following intracerebral hemorrhage. Neurology. 2000;54:354-51.

Chapter 16

Cerebral Vascular Malformations

GEORGE THOMAS, MD, MPH
KIERAN MURPHY, MD
DANIELE RIGAMONTI, MD

Key Points

- Arteriovenous malformations (AVMs) most commonly present with hemorrhage. Epilepsy, progressive neurological deficit, and headache are less common presentations.
- Treatment options for AVMs include microvascular resection (for those that are accessible) and radiosurgical treatment (for small, inaccessible lesions).
- An emerging treatment is using embolization via endovascular techniques to reduce the size of large AVMs so that they can be more easily treated by surgery or radiosurgery in staged procedures.
- Seizures are the most common presenting symptom of cavernomas.
- Treatment is not necessarily warranted for cavernomas if they are discovered incidentally. Lesions causing seizures, however, may benefit from resection.
- Most venous malformations are incidental findings discovered in the course of work-up for headache.
- Resection of a venous malformation is not only unnecessary but dangerous.
- Capillary telangiectasias are visualized by magnetic resonance imaging (MRI). No treatment is recommended for these lesions.

Cerebral vascular malformations (CVMs) are a group of neurovascular disorders characterized by abnormalities in cerebral blood vessels, including arteriovenous malformations (AVMs), cavernomas, venous malformations, and capillary telangiectasias. In a prospective study,

McCormick examined the incidence of CVMs and established that they occur as a group in 4% of the general population (1). Of all the cases, AVMs accounted for 0.6%, cavernomas accounted for 0.4%, capillary telangiectasias accounted for 0.7%, and venous malformations accounted for 2.6% (1). This finding was indirectly corroborated several years later when two large prospective MRI series confirmed that the incidence of cavernomas was between 0.4% and 0.5% of the patients studied (2,3). Knowledge of the classification and natural history of these different conditions helps in the understanding of their symptomatology and in selecting the appropriate therapeutic strategy.

Arteriovenous Malformations

Pathophysiology

The presence of a shunt, or an early abnormal communication between the arterial and venous beds, is the characterizing feature of an AVM. The intervening capillaries normally serve to decrease the blood pressure and velocity by amplifying the vascular bed. The absence of these intervening capillaries in this malformation causes an abnormal flow, which leads to the development of the pathological changes observed in arteries and veins. The arteries and veins are tangled and extremely dilated, and the intervening brain parenchyma is gliotic. Associated aneurysms are frequently found.

Diagnosis

Arteriovenous malformations most commonly present with hemorrhage. Focal neurologic signs and symptoms are related to the mass effect of the hematoma in the case of rupture of the AVM into the parenchyma of the brain. Other patients may have rupture of a superficial portion of the AVM and present primarily with subarachnoid hemorrhage. Epilepsy, progressive neurological deficit, and headache are less common presentations.

Computed tomography (CT) scan and MRI have become the primary tools for the diagnosis of this condition (Figure 16-1). The visualization of one or more early veins on cerebral angiography remains the gold standard for AVM diagnosis (Figures 16-2 to 16-4).

Treatment

The natural history of AVMs was best described in a landmark paper by Ondra reporting the results of the study of a large group of Finnish patients. The study clearly established the notion that AVMs not only tend to bleed with a predictable frequency (4% per year) but that the bleeding is either lethal or catastrophic in half of the cases (4).

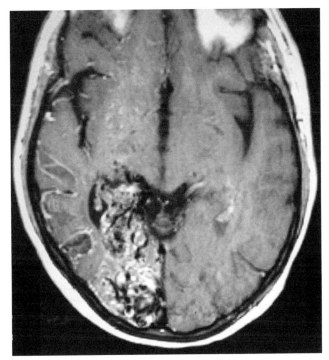

Figure 16-1 MRI shows a prominent arteriovenous malformation (AVM) in the right occipital lobe extending anteriorly along the outline of the optic radiation.

This critical piece of information must weigh very heavily on the selection of the course of action for each patient diagnosed with an AVM. Choosing what to do in every case is not always straightforward. The therapeutic decisions are best derived from a discussion between the interested individuals: the patient and primary doctor on one side; the neurologist, neurosurgeon, radiosurgeon, and interventional radiologist on the other side. Although conservative therapy is not intuitively a reasonable choice given the dismal natural history, it may in some instances be the safest choice. This may apply in the case of elderly patients, patients affected by terminal disease, and patients with AVMs so large and complicated that the risk associated with therapeutic intervention is prohibitively high. In the majority of cases, however, reasonable treatment options are available, and a frank discussion of the risks and benefits associated with each one helps the patient and the team of physicians make the selection. These options include microvascular resection of AVMs that are small and accessible and radiosurgical treatment of small, inaccessible lesions. As AVM size increases, the risks associated with either surgical resection or radiosurgical therapy also begin to rapidly increase, and consideration of endovascular obliteration with glue by the interventional neuroradiologist, which is aimed at

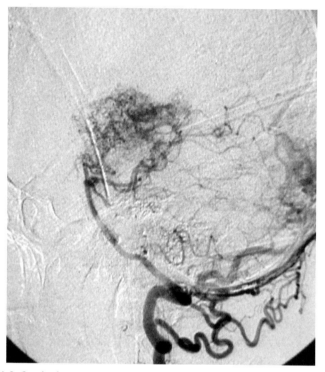

Figure 16-2 Cerebral angiogram of a selective vertebral artery injection shows a large AVM fed by the right posterior cerebral artery. There is evidence of venous congestion.

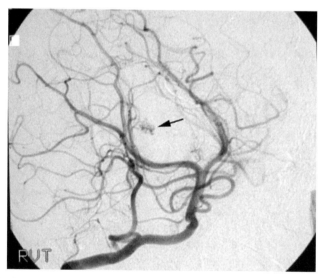

Figure 16-3 Angiogram shows a small vascular anomaly (about 5 mm) in the right mid-brain (*arrow*), suggestive of a small AVM. The lesion is vascularized by a small arterial branch from the right PCA.

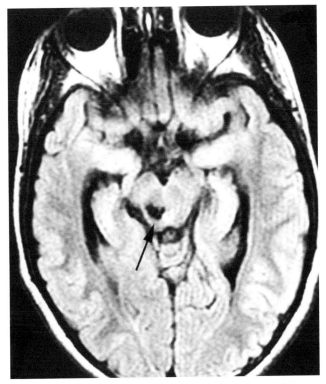

Figure 16-4 MRI shows a small intraparenchymal lesion characterized by signal void in the right midbrain (*arrow*).

eliminating all or part of the AVM, gains momentum (5,6). When the lesion is extremely large and complex, a combination of embolization, surgery, and radiosurgery may provide the therapeutic solution (7). See Case Study 16-1.

Cavernomas (Cavernous Angiomas and Malformations)

Pathophysiology

The pathology of cavernomas is characterized by the presence of extremely dilated and abnormal capillaries, the walls of which are composed of collagen lined by endothelium and devoid of tight junctions. Brain parenchyma is not usually found in the center of the lesion, where the dilated vascular channels are contiguous with one another. Although arteries and veins are present at the periphery of the lesion, they do not possess the features of abnormal tortuosity and extreme dilatation previously described for the AVMs. Thrombosis, hemorrhage, calcification, and even ossification may be present. The characterizing feature of a cavernoma, however, is the presence of large numbers of hemosiderin-laden macrophages.

Cavernomas may occur in families. The true incidence of the hereditary form is not fully established, but it may be as high as 50% of the affected individuals, at least in some populations. Patients with familial disease are more likely to have multiple lesions than patients with sporadic disease (8,9). Several genes responsible for the development of this condition have been described in the past decade, and recent genetic work has begun to elucidate the mechanism by which the genotype leads to the phenotype. Sporadic cavernomas are frequently associated with venous malformations (10,11).

Clinical Features

Seizures have been described as the most common presenting symptom in the past. The probable explanation for this phenomenon is that cavernomas have a much lower tendency to produce a catastrophic bleeding than AVMs. Many minor hemorrhages, however, may occur over the years. These hemorrhages, when occurring in the supratentorial compartment, will lead to accumulation of highly epileptogenic iron-containing metabolites within the brain parenchyma unless the cause is removed.

When the hemorrhage occurs in the brainstem or basal ganglia, it may cause a waxing and waning but generally progressively worsening neurological course, which in the pre-CT era was sometimes attributed to multiple sclerosis.

Diagnosis

CT scan can detect many, but not all, cavernomas. MRI is the diagnostic tool of choice: it is both highly sensitive and specific (see Case Study 16-2). The mature lesion has a characteristic mixed-signal intensity core surrounded by a ring or 'halo' of decreased signal intensity due to the hemosiderin-laden macrophages surrounding the lesion from multiple bleeds (Figures 16-5 and 16-6). When the lesion is immature, it appears as a small area of decreased signal intensity or a "black dot" (only one or two previous microbleeds) (Figure 16-7) (12). The hereditary form of the condition is characterized by a multiplicity of both types of lesions. Because the cavernomas lack a shunt and the flow within it is extremely slow, it is usually angiographically occult. It is therefore not surprising that cerebral angiography does not play an important role in the management of this condition. It is, however, occasionally performed to elucidate the architecture of an associated venous malformation, especially if surgery is contemplated.

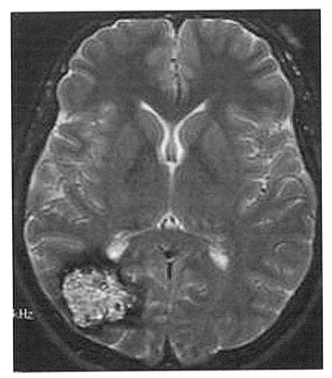

Figure 16-5 MRI shows a large cavernoma lesion in the right parietal-occipital region.

Treatment

The discovery of a cavernoma does not necessarily warrant intervention. Small lesions, discovered incidentally, can be safely watched. However, if the lesion is the cause of seizures, it should be dealt with, because resection of the lesion, especially if single and deemed to be the source, could be curative. If the lesion has bled and caused a neurological symptom besides severe headache, intervention should be considered.

Evidence of repeated bleeding is obviously a stronger indication for intervention. The choice of therapeutic modality is usually surgical, and several reported series documented excellent results even in locations that were considered off-limits just a few years ago, such as the brainstem and basal ganglia (13,14). There is, however, evidence that radiosurgery, which requires careful selection of appropriate technique and dose, may play a role in the management of some of these bleeding-prone cavernomas (15,16). Again, it must be stressed that decisions regarding complicated clinical scenarios should be taken in the context of multidisciplinary team conferences.

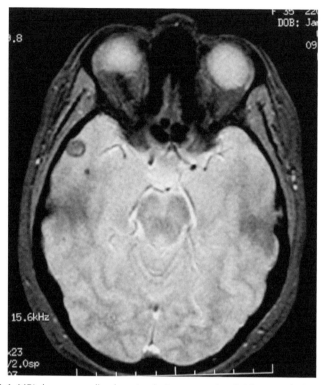

Figure 16-6 MRI shows a small enhancing lesion measuring 8-10 mm with decreased signal on the gradient echo images in the right temporal cortical white matter.

Venous Malformations (Venous Angiomas and Developmental Venous Anomalies)

Pathophysiology

The morphology of venous malformations is characterized by the presence of a tuft of anomalous medullary (i.e., deep white matter) veins converging into an enlarged central trunk that could drain either in the deep or superficial venous system. The complexity of these anomalies varies greatly in size and architecture. The microscopic analysis does not reveal any wall abnormality or the presence of abnormal arteries feeding into the venous malformation. An important finding, however, is the fairly common association of this lesion with sporadic cavernoma. Based on careful follow-up images, it is hypothesized that the presence of the venous malformation may induce the formation of the cavernoma. The mechanism, however, remains speculative at this juncture.

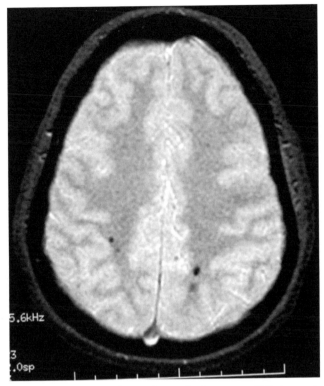

Figure 16-7 Low signal areas on the gradient echo images on MRI demonstrate hemosiderin deposition consistent with cavernous angiomas that have had microhemorrhages in the past.

Clinical Features

The benign appearance of the lesion under the microscope explains the equally benign natural history of this condition. The vast majority of these lesions are discovered in the course of work-up for headache. In the past they have been associated with seizures, progressive neurological deficits, and hemorrhage. Several natural history studies have documented that the risk of bleeding from these anomalies is indeed negligible (17,18). The notion that these lesions, when located in the posterior cranial fossa, had a much less benign course was based on the lack of appreciation of the common association of the venous malformation with the cavernoma. In the absence of a coexisting cause of bleeding, such as a cavernoma, the very rare hemorrhage originating from a venous malformation usually reabsorbs without causing apparent damage (19).

Diagnosis

Venous malformations have a characteristic appearance on CT, MRI, and angiography. On MRI the lesion appears as a linear or curvilinear signal void, and the surrounding parenchyma is usually normal (20) (Figure 16-8). The presence of increased signal intensity in the surrounding parenchyma on T_2-weighted images should raise suspicions about the presence of pathology, such as a tumor. As mentioned above, there is a frequent association between these lesions and cavernomas, and the MRI is exquisitely sensitive in uncovering the presence of a cavernoma. Although all imaging modalities clearly depict the central trunk as a linear or curvilinear structure, the tuft of medullary veins converging on it is best appreciated by cerebral angiography (Figure 16-9). This classic appearance has been called the *caput medusae*, because it reminds one of the snake-covered head of the mythical Greek creature.

Treatment

The resection of a venous malformation is not only unnecessary but dangerous (21). The elimination of a morphologically anomalous, but physiologically competent, venous drainage system inevitably leads to congestion, swelling, and infarct of the brain parenchyma drained by the malformation. In fact, stroke and death have been reported after ill-advised surgical

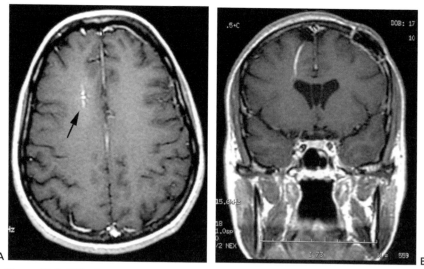

Figure 16-8 MRI of a venous angioma in the right frontal lobe, appearing as a "starfish" on the axial image (**A**, *arrow*) and as a curvilinear enhancing vascular structure on the coronal image (**B**). The venous angioma was discovered incidentally in a 51-year-old woman who presented with adult-onset seizures from another etiology.

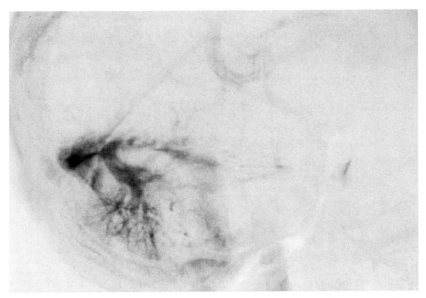

Figure 16-9 Angiogram of posterior fossa venous angiomas. In this late venous phase, starburst-like venous structures drain into large venous sinuses in the posterior fossa.

interventions. If an associated lesion such as a cavernoma is found on images, and if it is thought to be the source of the bleeding, it should be resected with extreme care to avoid interfering with the venous malformation.

Capillary Telangiectasias

Pathophysiology

The morphology of this lesion is that of enlarged capillaries interspersed in normal brain parenchyma. The vessels are devoid of smooth muscles and elastic fibers. They seem to have a predilection for the pontine location. Multiplicity and familial occurrence have been reported. Capillary telangiectasias and cavernous malformations may represent two pathological extremes within the same vascular malformation category (22).

Diagnosis and Treatment

Capillary telangiectasias are generally clinically silent and found incidentally. There is only one reported fatality in the literature. In general, they may be confused with other pathology, and only the benign clinical course helps confirm the diagnosis.

Until recently it was not possible to visualize these lesions in vivo. CT and angiography are unable to detect them, and the MRI appearance was unknown. It is now believed that these lesions have a somewhat characteristic MRI signature (Case Study 16-3) (23). No treatment is recommended in the management of capillary telangiectasias.

Case Study 16-1

A 9-year-old boy presents in the emergency room with complaints of tingling and cold numbness, described as a "fuzzy" feeling, on his left side. At home, he had attempted to walk to the bathroom and fell in the hallway. The patient was noted to be lethargic, wobbly, and had a left facial droop with left-sided weakness.

Angiogram detected a small vascular anomaly in the right midbrain suggestive of a small AVM (Figure 16-3), and MRI identified a small parenchymal lesion in the right midbrain (Figure 16-4). Radiosurgery is an excellent treatment option. Because of the location in a very eloquent part of the brain, the precision of the delivery of the energy is critical to avoid damaging the thalamus or the midbrain.

Case Study 16-2

The patient is a 35-year-old woman with multiple hereditary cavernomas. Her mother has multiple skin lesions, her grandmother had seizures for many years, and her son presented with intracerebral hemorrhage shortly after birth. The patient complains of headache and nausea, episodes of dizziness, and a feeling of being in a "twilight state." MRI shows a small enhancing lesion with mild decreased signal on gradient echo images (Figure 16-6). In addition, there are multiple small foci of decreased signal measuring 2-4 mm in size. The low signal areas on the gradient echo images (Figure 16-7) demonstrate hemosiderin deposition consistent with cavernomas that have had microhemorrhages in the past.

The patient was sent for EEG to rule out the possibility of partial seizures causing her symptoms. If the EEG is negative, the patient should be treated for possible migraine headaches, which are unrelated to the cavernoma. Given multiple lesions seen on MRI, there is little indication for surgical resection or radiosurgery. The patient was advised to avoid anticoagulants and aspirin.

Case Study 16-3

A 27-year-old woman experienced a sudden episode of loss of consciousness that lasted a few minutes, unassociated with tonic-clonic

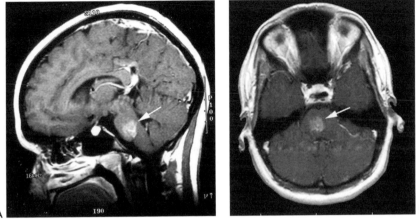

Figure 16-10 MRI shows an approximately 1.5-cm pontine capillary telangiectasia demonstrated as a rather vague area of enhancement (*arrow*) in the right pons (**A,** sagittal image; **B,** axial image).

movement or incontinence. MRI showed an approximately 1.5 cm pontine capillary telangiectasia (Figure 16-10) but no other lesion, and the patient was further evaluated for unexplained syncope. The pontine capillary telangiectasia was felt to be an incidental finding.

REFERENCES

1. McCormick WF. The pathology of vascular ("arteriovenous") malformations. J Neurosurg. 1966;24:807-16.
2. Del CO Jr., Kelly DL Jr, Elster AD, Craven TE. An analysis of the natural history of cavernous angiomas. J Neurosurg. 1991;75:702-8.
3. Robinson JR Jr., Awad IA, Magdinec M, Paranandi L. Factors predisposing to clinical disability in patients with cavernous malformations of the brain. Neurosurgery. 1993;32:730-5.
4. Ondra SL, Troupp H, George ED, Schwab K. The natural history of symptomatic arteriovenous malformations of the brain: a 24-year follow-up assessment. J Neurosurg. 1990;73:387-91.
5. Liu HM, Wang YH, Chen YF, et al. Endovascular treatment of brain-stem arteriovenous malformations: safety and efficacy. Neuroradiology. 2003;45:644-9.
6. Liu HM, Huang YC, Wang YH. Embolization of cerebral arteriovenous malformations with *n*-butyl-2-cyanoacrylate. J Formos Med Assoc. 2000;99:906-13.
7. Soderman M, Andersson T, Karlsson B, et al. Management of patients with brain arteriovenous malformations. Eur J Radiol. 2003;46:195-205.
8. Rigamonti D, Hadley MN, Drayer BP, et al. Cerebral cavernous malformations: incidence and familial occurrence. N Engl J Med. 1988;319:343-7.
9. Zabramski JM, Wascher TM, Spetzler RF, et al. The natural history of familial cavernous malformations: results of an ongoing study. J Neurosurg. 1994;80:422-32.
10. Rigamonti D, Spetzler RF. The association of venous and cavernous malformations: report of four cases and discussion of the pathophysiological, diagnostic, and therapeutic implications. Acta Neurochir (Wien). 1988;92:100-5.

11. Clatterbuck RE, Elmaci I, Rigamonti D. The juxtaposition of a capillary telangiectasia, cavernous malformation, and developmental venous anomaly in the brainstem of a single patient: case report. Neurosurgery. 2001;49:1246-50.
12. Rigamonti D, Drayer BP, Johnson PC, et al. The MRI appearance of cavernous malformations (angiomas). J Neurosurg. 1987;67:518-24.
13. Bertalanffy H, Benes L, Miyazawa T, et al. Cerebral cavernomas in the adult: review of the literature and analysis of 72 surgically treated patients. Neurosurg Rev. 2002;25:1-53.
14. Ziyal IM, Sekhar LN, Salas E, Sen C. Surgical management of cavernous malformations of the brain stem. Br J Neurosurg. 1999;13:366-75.
15. Kim DG, Choe WJ, Paek SH, et al. Radiosurgery of intracranial cavernous malformations. Acta Neurochir (Wien). 2002;144:869-78.
16. Hasegawa T, McInerney J, Kondziolka D, et al. Long-term results after stereotactic radiosurgery for patients with cavernous malformations. Neurosurgery. 2002;50:1190-7.
17. Naff NJ, Wemmer J, Hoenig-Rigamonti K, Rigamonti DR. A longitudinal study of patients with venous malformations: documentation of a negligible hemorrhage risk and benign natural history. Neurology. 1998;50:1709-14.
18. Rigamonti D, Spetzler RF, Medina M, et al. Cerebral venous malformations. J Neurosurg. 1990;73:560-4.
19. Topper R, Jurgens E, Reul J, Thron A. Clinical significance of intracranial developmental venous anomalies. J Neurol Neurosurg Psychiatry. 1999;67:234-8.
20. Rigamonti D, Spetzler RF, Drayer BP, et al. Appearance of venous malformations on magnetic resonance imaging. J Neurosurg. 1988;69:535-9.
21. McLaughlin MR, Kondziolka D, Flickinger JC, et al. The prospective natural history of cerebral venous malformations. Neurosurgery. 1998;43:195-200.
22. Rigamonti D, Johnson PC, Spetzler RF, et al. Cavernous malformations and capillary telangiectasia: a spectrum within a single pathological entity. Neurosurgery. 1991;28:60-4.
23. Lee RR, Becher MW, Benson ML, Rigamonti D. Brain capillary telangiectasia: MR imaging appearance and clinicohistopathologic findings. Radiology. 1997;205:797-805.

Chapter 17

Aneurysms and Subarachnoid Hemorrhage

QUOC-ANH THAI, MD
PHILIPPE GAILLOUD, MD
RAFAEL J. TAMARGO, MD

Key Points

- Aneurysmal subarachnoid hemorrhage (SAH) represents a small proportion of cerebrovascular accidents but accounts for 25% of all cerebrovascular-associated deaths.
- Classic presentation of aneurysmal SAH is sudden onset of severe headache.
- The gold standard in the diagnosis of aneurysms is intra-arterial digital subtraction angiography.
- The major initial complications are hydrocephalus and rebleeding.
- Medical management of hemodynamic status during the first hours after an aneurysmal SAH is essential. Prophylactic management of seizures is necessary to prevent risk of rebleeding.
- Symptoms of vasospasm are ameliorated with hypertensive, hypervolemic, and hemodilution therapy. For refractory cases, angioplasty with intra-arterial balloon dilatation and intra-arterial papaverine should be attempted early.
- Improvements in microneurosurgical techniques have improved outcomes of aneurysm patients.
- Patients requiring aneurysm treatment should be referred to specialized centers at a high-volume institution. The level of experience of the neurosurgeon and the endovascular interventional neuroradiologist has a great impact on patient outcome.

Most subarachnoid hemorrhages (SAHs) are caused by the rupture of intracranial aneurysms, but they can also result from angioma rupture, neoplasms, cortical thrombosis, and subarachnoid extension of parenchymal hemorrhages. Although SAH represents a small proportion of cerebrovascular accidents, it leads to a disproportionately high morbidity and mortality. Twenty-five percent of cerebrovascular mortality is due to SAH (1), which represents only 3% of all strokes (2). The case-fatality rate is reported to be between 25% and 67% (1,3). Of those who survive, 50% have a disability requiring aid in performing activities of daily living (1,4). Furthermore, treatment for these patients uses a disproportionately high number of resources. The average cost of an SAH admission is $23,777, over twice that for other intracranial hemorrhages (ICHs) and over four times that for patients admitted with an infarction (5). The average length of stay for SAH patients is 11.5 days compared with 7.5 days for ICH patients and 5.9 days for patients with infarction (5). Refinements of diagnostic tools, such as computed tomography angiography (CTA) and magnetic resonance angiography (MRA), as well as the advent of therapeutic options in the field of endovascular interventional neuroradiology, have facilitated treatment but have also presented new challenges in management decisions. Therefore, in a patient population with poor outcomes and high costs, coupled with a rapidly changing field, it is crucial for physicians involved in the treatment of these patients to have current knowledge of the disease process, the tools of diagnosis, and the available therapeutic options.

Anatomy

Aneurysm refers to an expansion and dilatation of the vessel wall of an artery involving all three components of the vessel wall, which include tunica intima, tunica media, and tunica adventitia. Aneurysms caused by atherosclerotic disease, infection (mycotic aneurysms), hypertension, or congenital weakness of the vessel wall are referred to as saccular or "true" aneurysms. Aneurysms can also occur secondary to dissection and typically do not involve all three components of the blood vessel wall; these are referred to as "pseudoaneurysms." Saccular aneurysms, in contrast to dissecting or fusiform aneurysms, are also known as "berry" aneurysms and are the "true" intracranial aneurysms that appear as rounded, berry-like out-pouchings. These aneurysmal dilatations from the vessel wall constitute the critical pathological weak point, and they generally arise at the bifurcations of major intracranial arteries. Most of these large bifurcations in the brain occur at the circle of Willis; thus the majority of saccular aneurysms are located there. Approximately 39% occur in the anterior communicating artery, 30% in the internal carotid artery (ICA), 22% in the middle cerebral artery (MCA) bifurcation, and 8% in the posterior circulation (6). Locations outside of the circle of Willis or the MCA bifurcation are uncommon for saccular aneurysms and, when present, are mostly due to trauma or infection (7).

Etiology

The etiology of saccular aneurysms is not fully understood, but it appears to be a combination of congenital and acquired defects. Intracranial arteries consist of three main layers: the outer connective tissue adventitia, the middle tunica media, and the inner internal elastic lamina. The tunica media is notably absent in saccular aneurysms; this observation is the basis for a congenital etiology of saccular aneurysms. These interruptions of the tunica media generally occur at bifurcation points along the vessels and were thought to be the "congenital medial defects" or "medial gaps" responsible for aneurysm formation (8). The site of aneurysmal growth shows abrupt termination of the tunica media at the neck of the aneurysm, and the internal elastic lamina becomes increasingly fragmented as it enters the sac (9,10). However, evidence that these medial gaps are purely congenital and have a causal effect on aneurysm formation is lacking. Thus far, there is only a slight increased association of aneurysm formation in patients with autosomal dominant polycystic kidney disease, Ehlers-Danlos syndrome IV, and pseudoxanthoma elasticum (7).

Other evidence suggests that aneurysm formation may not be due to a congenital absence of the tunica media only. Although medial gaps are found in infants, aneurysms in children are rare. Medial gaps found in infants have been shown to increase in frequency, size, and density with increasing age (10). In adults, medial gaps are equally common in patients with and without aneurysms (10). Older individuals have an increased prevalence of these gaps at bifurcation points, suggesting an acquired mechanical stress factor (11). Extracranial vessels are not subject to the same amount of sheer stress and do not develop saccular aneurysms, as would be expected of a diffuse process in a congenital etiology.

Mechanical stress appears to be the major factor in aneurysm formation. Saccular aneurysms often occur at the branching points of high flow intracranial vessels, where hemodynamic stress is highest. Increased flow stress in experimental models shows enlargement and bulging of the medial gaps (12), and induced hypertension has been associated with aneurysm formation in animal models (13). Contributing factors that alter the hemodynamic stress, such as atherosclerosis, loss of tensile strength, and post-stenotic dilatation, may also contribute to aneurysm formation (10).

The "combination theory" (14) states that prevalence of congenital medial gaps along with degenerative changes are required for aneurysmal formation. The fact that saccular aneurysms lack a medial layer suggests that a congenital absence of the tunica media is a prerequisite for subsequent degenerative changes. However, this appears to have a small contribution to aneurysm formation. Evidence now suggests that degenerative changes are the major contributors to the formation of aneurysms (7,10,15) and that mechanical stress is needed in the presence of medial gaps for aneurysm formation. Other factors contributing to degenerative changes include hypertension, tobacco use, and cocaine use, which have all been shown to increase the risk of aneurysmal rupture (16).

Epidemiology

The prevalence of intracranial aneurysms is 2% in autopsy reviews (17). A systematic review in 1998 by Rinkel and colleagues reported a slightly higher rate of 2.3% (18). The incidence of SAH has remained stable at 6 cases per 100,000 per year (18,19), with recent studies citing ranges from 5.6 to 6.9 cases per 100,000 per year (20,21). The United States Census Bureau reported in 2000 that the population was 281.4 million. This calculates to 5.6 million people with aneurysms and up to 30,000 cases of SAH per year. SAH from a ruptured intracranial aneurysm accounts for 75%-80% of all spontaneous SAH (22).

Non-modifiable risk factors identified in association with aneurysms and aneurysmal rupture are sex, race, seasonal variances, and heritable traits. Aneurysmal SAH occurs in females 1.6 times more than males (20) and in African Americans 2.1 times more than Caucasians (23). And, for reasons that are unknown, SAH has peaks in April and September and troughs in June and July (24). Several familial and heritable traits have also been linked to increased risks of aneurysm and SAH. Familial history of SAH increases the risk of rupture in patients with aneurysms; there is a three- to seven-fold increased risk in patients with a first-degree relative with prior SAH (25). Heritable connective tissue disorders have also been documented to increase risks of aneurysms and SAH, but the associations are weak. The most notable association is with autosomal dominant polycystic kidney disease. Weaker associations have been reported for Ehlers-Danlos syndrome type IV and pseudoxanthoma elasticum (7).

Modifiable risk factors associated with aneurysms and aneurysmal rupture include smoking, hypertension, heavy ethanol use, and cocaine use. Active smoking increases the relative risk of aneurysmal rupture to 1.9 (16). Hypertension has been shown by literature reviews to increase the relative risk to 2.8 (16). Furthermore, a high systolic blood pressure is an independent risk factor for fatal SAH versus non-fatal SAH, with an odds ratio of 1.11 per 1 mm Hg SBP increase (26). Drinking more than 150 g of ethanol per week (15 glasses of wine or standard cans of beer) increases the relative risk to 4.7 (16). Cocaine use has also been implicated in SAH (22), possibly secondary to transient increases in blood pressure. Oral contraceptives, hormone replacement therapy, cholesterol, and strenuous activity have not been strongly associated with SAH.

The size of an aneurysm is a significant independent factor in its propensity to rupture. In general, there is increased risk of rupture in larger aneurysms. It is known, however, that aneurysm size is dynamic and that small aneurysms can increase in size and tendency to rupture. Therefore it is important to know the natural history of unruptured aneurysms.

Unruptured Intracranial Aneurysms

Natural History

The natural history of unruptured intracranial aneurysms (UIAs) is crucial in understanding the risk of rupture associated with an aneurysm. The risk of rupture can then be assessed against the risk of intervention to determine the safest management option. However, the rate of intervention, mainly surgical, has increased rapidly since the advent of the operating microscope in the 1970s; therefore the population with UIA that remains untreated does not accurately reflect the entire population. Modern studies are left with this population, which is biased by surgical selection, making the study of natural history difficult.

The largest study of UIA on a surgically unbiased population is by Juvela and colleagues in Finland and remains the most significant assessment of the true natural history of UIA. This study from Helsinki examined 142 patients with 181 UIA diagnosed from 1956 to 1978 and followed them until death, until the occurrence of SAH, or until 1998 (27). The median follow-up time was 19.7 years (range, 0.8-38.9 years) with a total of 2575 person-years of follow-up. There were 33 SAH from a UIA, giving an annual rupture of 1.3%, which corresponds with the often-cited rupture rates of 1%-2% per year. The cumulative risk of rupture was 10.5% at 10 years, 23% at 20 years, and 30.3% at 30 years after diagnosis. The case-fatality was 52% for this group.

This report of the natural history of UIA found that the patient's age is inversely related to the overall lifetime risk of rupture of an intracranial aneurysm. Younger patients diagnosed with UIA have the greatest life expectancy, which equates to a higher cumulative risk of rupture. Therefore, knowing the patient's age, the estimated life expectancy, and the risk of rupture, one can predict for any given patient the lifetime risk of aneurysmal rupture, independent of other factors, using the multiplicative law of probability in the following formula (28):

$$\text{Lifetime risk of rupture} = 1 - (1 - \text{Annual risk of rupture})^{\text{Expected years of life}}$$

Table 17-1 presents the predicted lifetime risk of rupture and death from birth to 85 years of age, assuming an annual risk of rupture of 1.3% (27) and a case fatality rate of 52% (27). The size of an aneurysm is an independent risk factor in which larger aneurysms have higher risks of bleeding. The rupture rate increased almost linearly according to size category in the paper by Juvela and colleagues (27). In their multivariate analysis

Table 17-1 Lifetime Risk of Aneurysmal Subarachnoid Hemorrhage and Death*

Age at Presentation (years)	Life Expectancy (years)	Cumulative Risk of Rupture (%)	Cumulative Mortality (%)
0	76.9	63	33
5	72.5	61	32
10	67.6	59	31
15	62.6	56	29
20	57.8	53	28
25	53.1	50	26
30	48.3	47	24
35	43.6	43	23
40	38.9	40	21
45	34.4	36	19
50	30.0	32	17
55	25.7	29	15
60	21.6	25	13
65	17.9	21	11
70	14.4	17	9
75	11.3	14	7
80	8.6	11	6
85	6.3	8	4

* Lifetime risk of aneurysmal subarachnoid hemorrhage (SAH) and death based on patient age at time of presentation, annual risk of rupture of 1.3%, and case fatality of 52% (27) using the multiplicative law of probability. Life expectancy estimates are derived from the National Vital Statistics Reports, Vol. 51, No. 3, 19 December 2002, published by the National Center for Health Statistics of the Centers for Disease Control and Prevention.

adjusted for sex, hypertension, and aneurysm group (prior SAH and other groups), the relative risk for rupture was 1.00 for aneurysms with 2-6 mm diameter, 2.57 (95% CI, 0.97-6.81) for 7-9 mm, and 3.38 (95% CI, 1.05-10.93) for 10-26 mm. This equates to a relative risk of 1.11 (95% CI, 1.00-1.23) for each 1 mm, continuously. This is a reasonable finding, given the generally accepted notion that rupture risk increases with increasing size, although the actual relationship between size and rupture risk is not mathematically known. Case Study 17-1 gives a sample use of Table 17-1.

The largest study on the management of UIA is the International Study of Unruptured Intracranial Aneurysm (ISUIA), published in 2003, in which 61 centers from the United States, Canada, and Europe enrolled 4060 patients from 1991 to 1998. Of those enrolled, 1692 were preselected to have conservative management and had a prospective mean follow-up time of 4.1 years, equating to 6544 patient-years of follow-up. From this, the 5-year rupture rate was reported at 0% for aneurysms less than 7 mm, 2.6% for 7-12 mm, 14.5% for 13-24 mm, and 40% for those greater than 25 mm (29).

The prior report by the ISUIA investigators in 1998 reported in their retrospective analysis that the rupture rate for aneurysms less than 10 mm was less than 0.05% per year for those without prior SAH. These results would suggest that the natural history of UIA is more benign than the reports of prior studies (18,27).

The ISUIA papers, which report a much lower risk of rupture amongst small aneurysms, have several inherent weaknesses that render them less reliable. The main fault is the selection bias. In both the retrospective and prospective studies, a selection bias is present at the onset, since enrollment of patients into the conservative management group is only after a preselection of those acceptable for surgery or endovascular interventions. In the retrospective group reported in 1998, a total of 1449 patients were collected during a 22-year period for the 53 centers, representing an enrollment rate of approximately 1 patient per high-volume referral center per year after selection of other patients for treatment. This fraction of the population unlikely represents the true population of UIA, and this is seen by the skewed distribution of aneurysm location and sizes. There were higher numbers of intracavernous aneurysms, which are not associated with the risks of SAH and in general are not treated surgically, and the group is older than expected. This, among other factors, suggests that the preselection has eliminated the aneurysms that are more likely to bleed and those in younger patients who have an overall higher lifetime risk of bleeding. What remains is an unknown sample from the population.

The prospective portion of the ISUIA paper published in 2003 is a large study whose final results remain to be seen. The current results only have a 5-year follow up in a relatively small representation of the patient base. Although this is the largest prospective study of its kind, with 6544 patient years of follow-up, its weakness is, again, a biased population from which the surgical and endovascular candidates are excluded. The exclusion criteria were extensive, and there is no detail on the number or outcome of those who were not included. Furthermore, as in the prior ISUIA report, the number of patients is far fewer than expected from an aggregate of over 60 international referral centers.

Management

The management of unruptured intracranial aneurysms is controversial. The key questions of the natural history of UIA and of their risk of rupture continue to be debated. The available information on their natural history suggests that intervention should be considered in most patients. Patients with aneurysms of any size should be carefully monitored for any change in diameter. Small aneurysms of 6 mm or less have a lower likelihood of rupture, but it is important to note that 70% of all aneurysmal ruptures occur in aneurysms that were initially 6 mm or less (27). Any change in size during follow-up or any presenting aneurysms larger than 6 mm should be strongly considered for intervention, especially in younger patients. Younger patients have an overall higher lifetime risk of rupture, which can be generally estimated as shown in Table 17-1. All the risks of rupture should be considered with the risk of intervention and the type of intervention, which will be discussed in those sections.

Clinical Presentation

The classic clinical presentation of an aneurysmal SAH is the sudden onset of a severe headache. This headache is reported as unusually severe and unrelenting and usually develops in seconds. Approximately 50% of patients with SAH report an instantaneous onset, and the other half describes its onset in seconds or minutes (30). The headache is associated with emesis in 70% of SAH patients compared with 43% in patients with thunderclap headaches (30). Occasionally, patients may not give a classic report of such a headache, but this usually is in the setting of an altered mental status. Changes in mental status and signs of meningismus with complaints of nuchal discomfort often follow the headache in patients with a ruptured aneurysm. These signs and symptoms tend to occur in patients with thicker blood clots, as seen on the head CT. As a result of the thick blood clots, non-communicating hydrocephalus can occur from blockage of the foramina of Magendie and Luschka, giving the characteristic dilatation of all four ventricles (31), and this leads to decreased mental status. The blood can also cause irritations of the meninges and result in photophobia, neck soreness/stiffness, Brudzinski's sign, Kernig's sign, and even a low-grade fever occurring within 6-24 hours after an SAH (22).

Ocular hemorrhage in the subhyaloid (preretinal), intraretinal, and within the vitreous humor occurs in up to 40% of SAH (22). This is believed to be a result of increased intracranial pressure compressing the central retinal vein and the retinochoroidal anastomoses. The result is venous hypertension and disruption of retinal veins. This finding may be associated with a higher mortality rate.

Diagnosis

The first diagnostic test for a suspected SAH is a non-contrast head CT. The sensitivity of detecting SAH within the first 24 hours of hemorrhage is 92%, and it decreases by about 7% each 24 hours post-hemorrhage (7). A false-positive may occur in the rare case of generalized brain edema that causes venous congestion in the subarachnoid space, mimicking an SAH (25). Hemorrhage in the subarachnoid space has a diffuse hyperdense appearance at the basal cistern (Figure 17-1), and concentration of the blood clot or a hematoma in the adjacent parenchyma may reveal the location of the aneurysm. More importantly, mass effect hematomas, intraventricular hemorrhages, and hydrocephalus can be easily seen with a non-contrast head

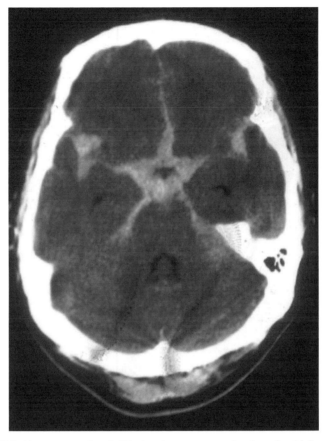

Figure 17-1 Non-contrast head CT showing aneurysmal subarachnoid hemorrhage. Acute blood in the subarachnoid space appears as diffuse hyper-intensities in the chiasmatic, sylvian, and interhemispheric cisterns.

CT, and this is a guide for initial management. Furthermore, the amount of subarachnoid blood seen on head CT may indicate outcome indirectly because vasospasm is more likely to develop with thicker blood clots. The Fisher Scale (Table 17-2) assigns a number and helps predict the risk for vasospasm by grading the amount of blood on initial presentation.

Suspected cases of aneurysmal SAH in which the head CT is not diagnostic require a lumbar puncture. The lumbar puncture remains the most sensitive test for SAH. Once a hemorrhage occurs in the subarachnoid space and blood gets mixed in the cerebral spinal fluid (CSF), it takes 6-12 hours for sufficient lysis of the red blood cells and for bilirubin and oxy-hemoglobin to form (25). This gives the CSF a yellow tinge, or xantho-chromia, after centrifugation. This allows a distinction between a traumatic tap with fresh RBCs in the CSF versus a hemorrhage with lysis of RBCs and resulting xanthochromia. The method of counting red blood cells in serial

Table 17-2 Fisher Scale*

Fisher Grade	Head CT Assessment
1	No subarachnoid blood detected
2	Diffuse or vertical layers < 1 mm thick
3	Localized clot and/or vertical layer ≥ 1 mm thick
4	Intracerebral or intraventricular clot with diffuse or no subarachnoid hemorrhage

*The Fisher Scale grades the amount of hemorrhage on diagnostic head CT (direct measurement, no calibration to actual thickness), which then can be used to assess for risk of vasospasm.

tubes of CSF is highly unreliable and should not be used to rule out an SAH. Furthermore, lumbar puncture ideally should be performed at least 6 hours after suspected hemorrhage and, in addition to routine CSF labs, CSF bilirubin should be checked.

The gold standard in the diagnosis of aneurysms, after CT scan or lumbar puncture confirms SAH, is intra-arterial digital subtraction angiography. This enables visualization of the aneurysm in relation to its parent vessel, definition of the collateral circulation, and assessment for vasospasm. In order to assess all these characteristics thoroughly, it is imperative that the angiogram include contrast injection of both carotid arteries and both vertebral arteries (a four-vessel angiogram) with multiple views (anterio-posterior, lateral, oblique) of each injection. The risk of such a study in experienced centers is very low. One meta-analysis reported a transient or permanent neurological complication risk of 1.8% in patients with SAH and 0.3% in patients without SAH (32). The risk of permanent neurological damage is as low as 0.09%, according to some experienced centers (33).

Procedural risks are eliminated in MRA or CTA, but their detection rate is lower. CTA and MRA are non-invasive (excluding the IV contrast injection) tests that aid in the diagnosis and management of aneurysms. They are especially useful in planning for surgery when definition of the surrounding anatomy is necessary because three-dimensional reconstruction with interactive manipulation of the views is possible. However, they remain inadequate replacements for intra-arterial angiography in the diagnosis of aneurysms at this time. CTA sensitivity and specificity are 91% and 95%, respectively (34). MRA sensitivity and specificity have been reported at 83% and 97%, respectively (35). However, the detection rate decreases dramatically with smaller aneurysms and becomes negligible for sizes less than 3 mm. Direct comparisons of CTA and MRA with intra-arterial angiograms showed that the accuracy of CTA/MRA is around 90% and is improving (36). CTA accuracy is reported at 89%. In the period prior to 1995, CTA accuracy was 84%; in the period subsequent to that, it was 93% (36). MRA accuracy is reported at 90% and has not changed significantly. Further improvements are promising for these non-invasive tests, but intra-arterial angiograms remain the gold standard for detection of intracranial aneurysms. Therefore it is crucial that patients with suspected SAH have the following tests in this order: 1) non-contrast head CT, 2) lumbar puncture if head CT is non-diagnostic, and 3) intra-arterial angiography in cases with confirmed SAH.

Non-Aneurysmal Subarachnoid Hemorrhage

Approximately 15% of patients with documented non-traumatic SAH will have negative findings on intra-arterial angiogram (7). These angiogram-negative SAHs consist mainly of two groups: non-aneurysmal perimesencephalic SAH and non-visualized occult aneurysms. The management of these two groups differs vastly.

Non-aneurysmal perimesencephalic SAH is a diagnosis of exclusion in association with characteristic CT appearance. Non-contrast head CT shows concentration of the SAH in the perimesencephalic, interpeduncular, and prepontine regions (Figure 17-2). There is little or no SAH in the chiasmatic,

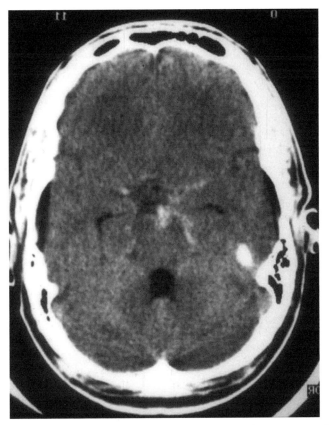

Figure 17-2 Non-contrast head CT showing non-aneurysmal perimesencephalic subarachnoid hemorrhage. Acute blood appears as a focal hyper-intensity in the perimesencephalic, interpeduncular, and prepontine regions. No subarachnoid blood is seen in the chiasmatic, sylvian, or interpeduncular cisterns.

sylvian, or interhemispheric cisterns, and it is not diffuse, as in aneurysmal SAH, because it is thought to originate from spontaneous rupture of small pontine or perimesencephalic veins. A repeat angiogram, usually done 2 weeks after the first, is required before this diagnosis is accepted. As many as 6% of patients with SAH pattern suggestive of perimesencephalic origins had aneurysms on repeat angiogram (37). The prognosis of these patients is excellent, and they do not need further follow-up after the two negative angiograms.

A small percentage of post-hemorrhagic aneurysms are not visualized with the initial angiogram. These angiogram-negative patients have CT patterns that are suggestive of aneurysmal rupture, and the blood deposition is diffuse throughout the chiasmatic, sylvian, and interhemispheric cisterns. However, the aneurysm may not have been visualized secondary to thrombosis, obliteration of the aneurysm from the hemorrhage, inadequate angiogram technique, or vasospasm. A delay of 2 weeks is required for resolution of possible vasospasm prior to a repeat angiogram, which reveals an aneurysm in 21% of cases (38). When the repeat angiogram is positive, the aneurysm is located at the anterior communicating artery in 88% of cases (38). These patients should be treated with routine vasospasm precaution, including blood pressure management IV fluid therapy, and nimodipine.

Grading and Prognosis

The single most important predictor of outcome after an aneurysmal SAH is the presenting level of consciousness. The mental status and consciousness level seen during triage are routinely quantified by health care personnel using the Glasgow Coma Scale (GCS) (Table 17-3). The assessments of eye opening, verbal responses, and motor commands contribute to the initial assessment and reflect the sum of the other prognostic factors associated with SAH, such as extent of hemorrhage, injury to the brain, size of ruptured aneurysm, patient's age, and contributing medical illnesses (28). Proper assessment of this provides an accurate assessment of outcome. Therefore,

Table 17-3 Glasgow Coma Scale

Points	Eye Opening	Verbal Response	Motor Response
6	N/A	N/A	Obeys
5	N/A	Oriented	Localizing
4	Spontaneous	Confused	Normal flexion
3	To speech	Inappropriate	Abnormal flexion (decorticate)
2	To pain	Incomprehensible sounds	Extension (decerebrate)
1	None	None	None

grading the severity of SAH, or the consciousness of the patient, is an important evaluation of prognosis and is necessary in management decisions.

The Hunt and Hess scale (Table 17-4) (39) was introduced to quantify the severity of SAH. This assessment includes signs of SAH such as nuchal rigidity, cranial nerve palsy, and hemiparesis. The scale also relied on patients' subjective report of their headaches. These integrated assessments resulted in a strong predictive factor. However, the subjective components of the scale are vulnerable to variances in interpretation between different examiners and examinees. For example, "mild" versus "moderate" headaches reported by the patient could change the rating of SAH severity. Inter-observer disagreement was less than 44% by several reports (28), which makes the scale less reliable.

The World Federation of Neurological Surgeons (WFNS) scale (Table 17-5) eliminates the subjective aspects of the Hunt and Hess scale and incorporates the GCS score as a main basis for grading SAH. It effectively uses the objective criteria of the GCS to yield a WFNS SAH scale. Although this scale is easier to memorize and use, its categories have not been validated clinically, perhaps one reason why it has not been widely adopted.

In 1997 Oshiro and colleagues introduced the GCS scale for grading SAH (40), which remains the simplest scale to use with the highest predictive value for discharge Glasgow Outcome Score and lowest inter-observer variability. The GCS-SAH scale incorporates the clinically validated Glasgow Coma Score as the objective criteria for grading SAH (Table 17-6). The GCS-SAH scale was the highest predictor of discharge Glasgow Outcome Score.

Table 17-4 Hunt and Hess Subarachnoid Hemorrhage Scale

SAH Grade	Clinical Assessment
I	Asymptomatic or mild headache
II	Moderate-to-severe headache, nuchal rigidity, cranial nerve palsy
III	Lethargy, confusion, mild focal deficit
IV	Stupor, moderate-to-severe hemiparesis, early decerebrate rigidity
V	Deep coma, decerebrate rigidity, moribund

Table 17-5 World Federation of Neurological Surgeons (WFNS) Subarachnoid Hemorrhage Scale

SAH Grade	Glasgow Coma Scale and Clinical Assessment
I	15
II	13–14, without focal deficit
III	13–14, with focal deficit
IV	7–12
V	3–6

Table 17-6 Glasgow Coma Scale Score as Basis for Subarachnoid Hemorrhage
Grade

SAH Grade	GCS Score
I	15
II	14-12
III	11-9
IV	8-6
V	5-3

Furthermore, the GCS SAH had the lowest inter-observer variability (40). In our opinion, the high predictive value, low inter-observer variability, and ease of use make the GCS-SAH scale a preferred scale.

Complications

The major initial complications after an SAH associated with high morbidity and mortality are hydrocephalus and rebleeding. Hydrocephalus is present radiographically in 15%-20% of patients with SAH on admission (41), and an additional 3% develop hydrocephalus within 1 week after SAH (42). This leads to shunt-dependent hydrocephalus in >20% of all SAH (43-46). This is usually associated with intraventricular hemorrhage, which is thought to block drainage at the foramina of Magendie and Luschka, resulting in a non-communicating four-ventricle dilation hydrocephalus (31). However, about half of patients with hydrocephalus do not have radiographically evident intraventricular hemorrhage (41). This non-communicating four-ventricle hydrocephalus is associated with decreased mental status and increased neurological deficit, which may progress to coma. When present on initial evaluation, this equates to a higher SAH grade and less favorable outcome. Mortality within the first month of SAH for patients with hydrocephalus was 32% compared with 9% in patients without hydrocephalus (47). Patients presenting with hydrocephalus or who develop hydrocephalus need intensive monitoring for decreased mental status. When there is decreasing mental status in the setting of hydrocephalus, the standard of care is insertion of an intraventricular catheter for external CSF drainage, which improves the level of consciousness in 78% of patients (42). This can be done under standard sterility at the bedside. The initial pop-off pressure should be set at ≥20 mm Hg to prevent rapid drainage, which can lead to a pressure gradient that could cause a re-rupture of the aneurysm. The rebleeding rate is reported to increase to 43% with intraventricular drainage versus 15% in patients without drainage (42).

Rebleeding is a major risk in all patients with SAH within the first 24 hours and remains high during the first 2 weeks. Rebleeding increases morbidity and mortality significantly. One study reported a mortality rate for rebleeding of 80% compared with 41% in patients without rebleeding (48). The rate of rebleeding is highest during the first 24 hours. The actual rate is unknown, but it has been reported as high as 15% (49) in the initial hours. After the initial 24 hours, the rate of rebleeding drops to 1.5% over the next 24 hours and continues to decline over the next 2 weeks. The total risk of rebleeding for the first 2 weeks has been reported at 19% (49). Considering the high mortality associated with rebleeding and the trends of early rebleeding, prompt medical and surgical management are critical in the setting of an SAH.

Delayed ischemic neurological deficit from chronic post-hemorrhagic vasospasm is the most significant cause of morbidity and mortality in patients who survive the initial rupture. It occurs in one third of patients who survive the initial SAH (22) and is distinct from any transient, acute arterial spasms that may occur during the first 12-24 hours. The onset of vasospasm is around 3 to 4 days after the hemorrhage. Vasospasm generally lasts 2 weeks, but it has been seen for up to 3 weeks (22). During this time of vasospasm, patients may manifest a low-grade fever, mild leukocytosis, decreased level of consciousness, and focal neurological deterioration. The time course, signs, and symptoms suggest that an inflammatory process is involved in the pathogenesis of vasospasm; recent experimental data support these findings (50-55).

Diagnosis of vasospasm includes the clinical assessment that shows deficits occurring within the proper time course and supporting diagnostic tests. Transcranial Doppler (TCD) can assess for vasospasm indirectly by measuring cerebrovascular velocities. TCD results showing an increase in velocity of 50 cm/sec or more in a particular vessel in a 24-hour period suggest vasospasm. However, increased cerebrovascular velocities can also be due to fever, infection, hypovolemia or hypervolemia, improved cardiac output, endocrine abnormalities, sympathetic activation, technical errors or variances, and other factors. The MCA:ICA velocity ratio can also be useful (normal is <3, mild vasospasm is 3-6, severe vasospasm is >6) (22). Angiography remains the most useful diagnostic test for vasospasm; visualization of focal vasoconstriction that correlates with the clinical exam is definitive. Treatment for vasospasm is limited at this time to angioplasty or intra-arterial papaverine injection by interventional radiology specialists. Medical management is limited to "triple-H" therapy, discussed in the medical management section.

Treatment

Medical Management

Medical management of hemodynamic status during the first hours after an aneurysmal SAH is essential while awaiting definitive intervention. The major risk with an unsecured aneurysm is rebleeding, as discussed in the previous section. This rebleeding is known to be associated with a higher blood pressure (56), the only modifiable parameter affecting rebleeding. However, any benefits of aggressive antihypertensive therapy will decrease cerebral perfusion pressure and increase risk of cerebral infarction. A systolic blood pressure of 120-150 mm Hg is used as a guideline, but this should take into account a patient's baseline blood pressure (22). Furthermore, hemodynamic management should be focused on maintaining euvolemia, achieving normal intracranial pressure and perfusion pressure, and normalizing electrolyte abnormalities.

Prophylactic management of seizures is necessary to prevent risk of rupture and worse long-term outcome. The incidence of seizures after SAH is 4%-16% and is an independent predictor of poor outcome (57). Seizure is a manifestation of the extent of neuronal injury, intracranial pressure, focal mass effect, and irritation from blood products, and onset of seizure activity results in high transient increases in blood pressure and intracranial pressures. This can prove disastrous in the setting of an unsecured aneurysm. It is therefore routine to administer phenytoin or other equivalent anticonvulsant medication to all patients diagnosed with SAH.

Chronic post-hemorrhagic vasospasm remains a medical management challenge throughout the hospitalization course because the pathogenesis of vasospasm is not fully understood. One hypothesis proposed that there is a smooth muscle arteriopathy that results in pathological vasoconstriction. To prevent this arterial narrowing, calcium channel blockers have been advocated; nimodipine has been the calcium channel blocker of choice due to its preferential central nervous system action. Although nimodipine does not prevent angiographic vasospasm and there is no statistically significant difference in mortality, there is a slightly improved outcome (58). Better outcome may be the result of dilatation of collateral leptomeningeal arteries (59), anti-platelet aggregating effects (60), and prevention of calcium entry into ischemic cells (61). It is therefore routine to administer nimodipine 60 mg PO q4h on admission for a period of 14-21 days.

Hypertensive, hypervolemic, and hemodilution therapy, also known as "triple-H" therapy, has definite benefits in the acute management of symptomatic chronic post-hemorrhagic vasospasm. The symptoms of vasospasm are ameliorated with triple-H therapy according to a review of the literature in 2003 (62). In comparison to no therapy, triple-H therapy resulted in decreased symptomatic vasospasm with a relative risk of 0.68 (95% CI, 0.53-0.87) (62). This is most likely a result of direct expansion of the circulating volume and thus facilitates flow to hypoxic regions. Triple-H therapy is most efficacious when used early in the course of vasospasm. Early triple-H therapy initiated before neurological deterioration can decrease delayed ischemic neurological deficits by almost 50% (63). In areas where ischemia has developed, triple-H therapy does not appear to be therapeutic. In cases refractory to triple-H therapy, angioplasty for intra-arterial balloon dilatation and intra-arterial papaverine should be attempted early (64). See Case Study 17-2.

Surgical Intervention

The high risks of rebleeding, poor medical management options for treating vasospasm in the setting of an unsecured aneurysm, and time course of vasospasm are all factors in the decision to use prompt, definitive surgical intervention. Neurosurgical treatment of aneurysms began in 1937 when Walter Dandy surgically treated the first aneurysm patient. Modern microsurgical treatment of aneurysm evolved in the 1970s with the advent of the operating microscope. Since then, the techniques of microneurosurgery and skull base surgery have reached maturity, and aneurysm clips are routinely used to occlude the necks of the aneurysm and exclude the weak saccular portion from the cerebral circulation.

Timing of surgery is essential in achieving optimal outcome, and the time course of vasospasm is the major consideration. "Early surgery" has been advocated for several obvious practical reasons. Prompt clipping of an aneurysm eliminates the risk of rebleeding that is associated with significant increased morbidity and mortality. Also, once an aneurysm is secured, treatment of vasospasm is facilitated with the use of triple-H therapy, an option that is dangerous in an unsecured aneurysm. Vasospasm and edema may complicate surgery that is delayed 7-10 days after SAH, when vasospasm is at its peak. Another surgical option is that of "late surgery," in which clipping is done after 12-14 days, when vasospasm has resolved and edema has subsided. We advocate clipping or coiling aneurysms within 24 hours of admission.

The Cooperative Study on the Timing of Aneurysm Surgery showed that the results of early surgery were equivalent to those of late surgery (6,65). This was a prospective observational study involving 3521 patients from 60 centers collected over a period of 2.5 years. Comparable good outcomes were reported for surgery performed on post-SAH day 0-3 (63%) and day 4-6 (60%). Delayed surgery on day 11-14 post-SAH yielded similar results (62%), as well as late surgery on day 15-32 (63%). Surgery during day 7-10 after SAH had the worst outcome, and this coincides with the peak of vasospasm.

Expertise of the aneurysm center is a crucial determinant of good outcome in patients who undergo surgical clipping. Microsurgical techniques of aneurysm clipping are technically demanding and are usually not employed for most neurosurgical cases. The neurosurgical centers that treat the average patient population without a referral bias would typically not encounter a high volume of aneurysm patients, thus limiting the experience of the surgeons. A study on the effects of patient volume on the outcome of craniotomy and aneurysm clipping showed that institutions performing more than 30 craniotomies per year had 43% reduction in mortality rates

(66). Similar results have been noted in other studies, suggesting that patients with SAH would have improved outcome if surgery is performed at a high-volume institution.

Endovascular Intervention

Endovascular intervention for aneurysms is a more recent technique and is a promising minimally invasive option for the treatment of aneurysms. Endovascular interventional neuroradiology began in the 1970s, when Fedor Serbinenko used detachable latex balloons to occlude the supplying artery of the aneurysm or to occlude the aneurysm sac itself (67). Modern endovascular treatment of aneurysms started in 1991 when Guido Guglielmi introduced an electrolytic detachable platinum coil (Guglielmi detachable coils [GDC]) (68,69). These coils are inserted through a femoral artery cannula via a microcatheter that can be threaded to the location of the aneurysm. The coils are then packed into the saccular portion and separated from the microcatheter by electrolysis, thus excluding the aneurysm sac from the cerebral circulation.

The use of endovascular coiling for the treatment of aneurysms is rapidly increasing worldwide. This is a reflection of improved coil design and refinements of techniques as more centers sub-specialize in this area. A few centers are reserving surgery as a back-up option when coiling is deemed unsuitable. In a paper published in 2001, it was estimated that approximately 1500 patients worldwide were being treated by endovascular coiling per month and that over 100,000 patients with aneurysms had been treated with endovascular coiling (70).

Long-term efficacy and outcomes are important aspects of endovascular coiling that are under investigation in this relatively young field. Efficacy in obliterating aneurysms and preventing future hemorrhages is the key aspect of any aneurysm treatment, especially in consideration of devastating results of SAH. Current series of endovascular coiling lack long-term follow-up for obvious reasons. A recent summary of the endovascular and surgical outcome of current reports consisted of a total of 2018 patients, and this showed the rate of incompletely treated aneurysm to be 33.7% for patients in the endovascular group in contrast to 4.6% in the surgical group. Recurrence of aneurysm was reported at a rate of 12.9% for the endovascular group, in contrast to 0.6% in the surgical group (71). Only short-term follow-up is currently available in terms of outcomes, and preliminary data suggest that there is no significant difference in Glasgow Outcome Score (GOS). In a 1-year outcome study, 79% of patients who had endovascular coiling had a good GOS compared with 75% with good GOS in the surgical group (72). However, long-term follow-up is needed to evaluate accurately the efficacy and outcomes of endovascular techniques.

Surgical versus Endovascular Treatment

The decision of treating aneurysms with surgical clipping versus endovascular coiling remains controversial. The main dilemma is a lack of long-term data on the outcome of patients who had endovascular coiling. It is a matter of time before this can be examined because modern endovascular coiling is just over a decade old. Technological refinements made in more recent years will not be appreciated in terms of outcome for several years. Current reports have a wide range of results, a reflection of the still-evolving field. Several studies report equally good outcomes, whereas others report conflicting results.

Outcomes of early surgery and endovascular treatment for patients with SAH are equal according to a study by Koivisto and colleagues (73). This was a prospective randomized study of 109 consecutive patients randomly assigned to either surgical (n = 57) or endovascular (n = 52) intervention. Post-operative follow-up at 1 year showed that good or moderate recovery was similar in both groups. Also, the morbidity and mortality rates were equal. Neuropsychological testing was performed for both groups and showed no difference between the surgical and endovascular groups. The only predictor of worse outcome was the presence of chronic post-hemorrhagic vasospasm, poorer SAH grade, need for permanent shunt, and larger size of aneurysm, and this was independent of the type of intervention. A longer follow-up period is necessary for long-term outcomes. However, because the majority of the morbidity and mortality associated with SAH occurs within the first few months, the long-term results of this study would not be expected to change drastically. Although this was a small study, the consecutive selection of the 109 patients eliminated any biases, and assignment to intervention group was randomized. Other larger studies, such as the International Subarachnoid Aneurysm Trial (ISAT), may not represent the population accurately due to biased selection criteria and a randomization process that allows perceived benefits of endovascular or surgical intervention to enter into the process.

The ISAT compared the safety and efficacy of standard neurosurgical clipping with endovascular coiling. This randomized multi-center trial, published in 2002, assessed 9559 patients with SAH and enrolled 2143 patients for the study (1073 in endovascular treatment arm, 1070 in neurosurgical treatment arm). Follow-up was analyzed at 1 year (801 patients in the endovascular treatment arm, 793 patients in neurosurgical treatment arm). In this highly selected patient sample (17% of the initial patient group) from mostly European centers, the study reported that outcome at 1 year was better in patients who had endovascular coiling. The relative risk of dependence or death was reduced by 22.6%, and the absolute risk reduction was 6.9% (74). These findings have important implications that are, however, valid only for this highly selective patient population.

Improved outcome in the ISAT study for the endovascular group may not be universally applicable to the general population. Most centers in the study were in the UK or European countries, where a high number of practitioners already consider endovascular coiling as the primary treatment option for aneurysms. This situation is likely to result in more experienced interventional radiologists, while neurosurgeons, especially vascular neurosurgeons, are generally not as experienced as their colleagues in other centers that perform a higher volume of aneurysm surgery. The stated criterion for an endovascular operator in ISAT was experience with at least 30 procedures, whereas the criterion for inclusion of a neurosurgeon was that he be "accredited." As was discussed previously, high-volume aneurysm surgery by sub-specialists results in significant improvement in outcome (66). The ISAT neurosurgeons operated on mostly grade I and grade II aneurysms (88% of study group) in which 97.3% was in the anterior circulation. Despite these favorable conditions, the 2-month follow-up reported 36.4% dependent outcome or death; it was 30.6% at 1-year follow-up (74). The intra-operative rupture rate for these neurosurgeons was 19% (75). This is much higher than the reported average of 2.6% mortality and 10.9% morbidity in a recent meta-analysis (76). Additionally, reported intra-operative rupture rates are generally less than half, as in the ISAT study (77,78). This suggests that ISAT neurosurgery does not represent the quality of care that is generally available, thus making an unfair comparison to endovascular techniques.

Another aspect of the ISAT that renders it difficult to generalize to the general population is the highly selected patient group. Of the 9559 patients assessed for inclusion, only 17% are reported at the conclusion. Part of this problem involved the subjective judgment of evaluators, where patients could be excluded if regarded as unsuitable for one or both treatments. This introduces biases for the selected patients by allowing the perceived benefits of endovascular or surgical intervention to enter into the selection process. This is evidenced by a skewed distribution of aneurysms. There were 50% anterior communicating, 33% internal carotid, and 14% MCA aneurysm but only 3% posterior circulation aneurysms (74). As discussed earlier, this is not the normal distribution of aneurysms that would be expected in a sample representative of the population. Therefore conclusions reached by ISAT are important and valid only for the actual study population, not for the general population.

The ISAT study was effective in addressing the outcome of a select group of patients in a short-term follow-up, but a more representative population studied over a longer follow-up period is needed to clarify the actual merits of endovascular and surgical interventions. No such study is available at this time. Therefore, as suggested by past reports showing better outcome in high-volume centers, patients should be referred to centers where there are equally experienced neurosurgeons and endovascular interventional neuroradiologists who perform a high volume of aneurysm treatment. This integrated team approach from experienced physicians would likely eliminate any biases and offer the best outcome for patients.

Conclusion

Aneurysmal subarachnoid hemorrhage remains a devastating problem, with high morbidity and mortality and associated high health care costs. Improvements in CTA and MRA have aided in the detection of aneurysms and have facilitated the planning for intervention. Although their sensitivity and accuracy of detecting aneurysms are each over 90% (rates which have improved during the past decade), the intra-arterial digital subtraction angiogram remains the gold standard for diagnosing aneurysms. Improvements in microneurosurgical techniques since the introduction of the operating microscope have also improved outcome of aneurysm patients. The morbidity and mortality reported by Hunt and Hess (39) before the operating microscope have decreased by more than 50%; recent meta-analysis reported a 2.6% mortality and 10.9% morbidity associated with surgical clipping (76). The advent of endovascular coiling for aneurysms has also supplemented the options for treatment. Refinements in coiling technology and technique have resulted in improved short-term outcomes; however, long-term outcomes are still unavailable.

Patients requiring aneurysm treatment should ideally be referred to specialized centers of excellence that have sub-specialists in both cerebrovascular neurosurgery and endovascular interventional neuroradiology who perform a high volume of cases. The deciding factor is not necessarily the type of intervention but the volume of the center performing the intervention; center expertise can reduce mortality by 43% (66). Advances in the understanding of chronic post-hemorrhagic vasospasm are promising, and prevention of delayed ischemic neurological deficits in the near future will be the key to further reduction of morbidity and mortality associated with aneurysms and SAHs.

Case Study 17-1

A 74-year-old female presented with an incidental right middle cerebral artery aneurysm. The patient had had a transient episode of left facial and left upper extremity numbness of uncertain etiology. Initial studies included MRI, MRA, and CTA. An incidental right middle cerebral artery bifurcation aneurysm was seen. There was no family history of aneurysms or any personal history of SAH. Her medical history was significant for hypertension and smoking. She was referred for neurosurgical consultation, which confirmed the incidental findings of an aneurysm. To fully assess the morphology of the aneurysm for possible surgical intervention, the patient underwent a diagnostic four-vessel cerebral angiogram that showed a 5-mm right MCA aneurysm and, in addition, a 3-mm right ophthalmic artery aneurysm previously unseen by non-invasive studies. Both aneurysms had a benign morphology.

In assessing the risks and benefits of surgical intervention, we can refer to Table 17-1, which shows the lifetime risk of aneurysmal SAH and death based on the patient's age at the time of presentation, annual risk of rupture of 1.3%, and case fatality of 52%. It is therefore estimated that a 75-year-old-patient will have a life expectancy of 11.3 years, a 14% risk of rupture, and a 7% risk of mortality from the rupture. The patient's advanced age and medical problems increase her risk of morbidity and mortality for undergoing general anesthesia, especially for prolonged craniotomy for clipping of aneurysms, which has its own inherent risks. It is estimated that her risk of morbidity and mortality for

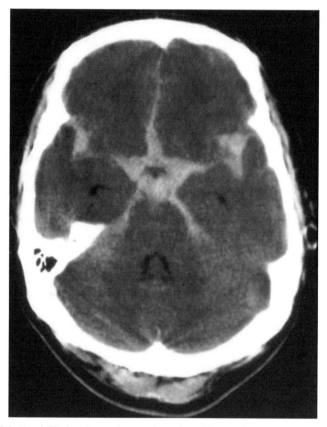

Figure 17-3 Head CT showing a classic subarachnoid hemorrhage, with the acute blood appearing as a hyperdense mass filling the basal cisterns and interhemispheric fissures. See Figure 17-4.

aneurysm surgery at this age is the same as her risk of aneurysmal rupture and death. Thus, because there was no benefit to performing surgery, the aneurysms were observed.

Case Study 17-2

A 30-year-old male developed a sudden excruciating headache after heading a ball while playing soccer. He was taken to the hospital with a GCS score of 15. Neurological exam was intact. Head CT showed a classic SAH, with the acute blood appearing as a hyperdense mass filling the basal cisterns and interhemispheric fissures (Figure 17-3). Hydrocephalus was noted. Angiography showed a left posterior communicating artery, a right posterior communicating artery, and a right anterior choroidal artery aneurysm (Figure 17-4). Close examination of the morphology suggested that the left posterior communicating artery aneurysm had ruptured, so the patient was urgently taken to the operating room for craniotomy and clipping of the left posterior communicating artery aneurysm.

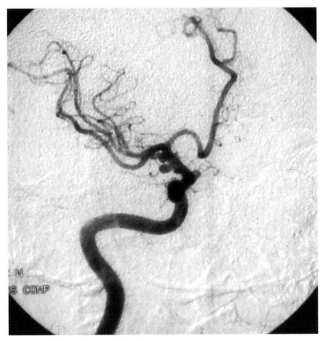

Figure 17-4 Angiogram showing a left posterior communicating artery, a right posterior communicating artery, and a right anterior choroidal artery aneurysm. Same patient as in Figure 17-3.

Post-operatively, the patient had a good recovery from the surgery but had delayed difficulties relating to vasospasm. Daily TCDs were done to monitor for chronic post-hemorrhagic vasospasm. On post-hemorrhage day 4, the patient developed aphasia and right hemiparesis; TCDs showed an increase of >50 cm/sec in a 24-hour period in the left MCA. This suggested chronic post-hemorrhagic vasospasm. He underwent angiography, which confirmed vasospasm that was then treated with angioplasty. Hypervolemic, hypertensive, hemodilution ("triple-H") therapy was initiated. The patient had a full and complete recovery, and the remaining aneurysms were addressed during subsequent elective surgery for clipping.

REFERENCES

1. Wardlaw JM, White PM. The detection and management of unruptured intracranial aneurysms. Brain. 2000;123(Pt 2):205-21.
2. Sudlow CL, Warlow CP. Comparable studies of the incidence of stroke and its pathological types: results from an international collaboration. International Stroke Incidence Collaboration. Stroke. 1997;28:491-9.
3. Hop JW, Rinkel GJ, Algra A, van Gijn J. Case-fatality rates and functional outcome after subarachnoid hemorrhage: a systematic review. Stroke. 1997;28:660-4.
4. Hijdra A, Braakman R, van Gijn J, et al. Aneurysmal subarachnoid hemorrhage. Complications and outcome in a hospital population. Stroke. 1987;18:1061-7.
5. Reed SD, Blough DK, Meyer K, Jarvik JG. Inpatient costs, length of stay, and mortality for cerebrovascular events in community hospitals. Neurology. 2002;57:305-14.
6. Kassell NF, Torner JC, Haley EC Jr., et al. The International Cooperative Study on the Timing of Aneurysm Surgery. Part 1: Overall management results. J Neurosurg. 1990;73:18-36.
7. Osborne AG. Diagnostic Neuroradiology. St. Louis: CV Mosby; 1994.
8. Forbus W. On the origin of miliary aneurysms of the superficial cerebral arteries. Bull Johns Hopkins Hosp. 1930;47:239-84.
9. Sahs A. Observations on the pathology of saccular aneurysms. J Neurosurg. 1966;24:792-806.
10. Stehbens WE. Etiology of intracranial berry aneurysms. J Neurosurg. 1989;70:823-31.
11. Stehbens WE. Aetiology of cerebral aneurysms. Lancet. 1981;2:524-5.
12. Hassler O. Experimental carotid ligation followed by aneurysmsal formation and other morphological changes in the circle of Willis. J Neurosurg. 1963;20:1-7.
13. Hazama F. An animal model of cerebral aneurysms. Neuropathol Appl Neurobiol. 1987;13:77-90.
14. Carmichael R. Gross defects in the muscular and elastic coats of the large cerebral arteries. J Pathol Bacteriol. 1945;57:345-51.
15. Stehbens WE. Pathology and pathogenesis of intracranial berry aneurysms. Neurol Res. 1990;12:29-34.
16. Teunissen LL, Rinkel GJ, Algra A, van Gijn J. Risk factors for subarachnoid hemorrhage: a systematic review. Stroke. 1996;27:544-9.
17. Bannerman RM, Graff CJ. The familial occurrence of intracranial aneurysms. Neurology. 1970;20:283-92.
18. Rinkel GJ, Djibuti M, Algra A, van Gijn J. Prevalence and risk of rupture of intracranial aneurysms: a systematic review. Stroke. 1998;29:251-6.
19. Broderick JP, Brott T, Tomsick T, et al. Intracerebral hemorrhage more than twice as common as subarachnoid hemorrhage. J Neurosurg. 1993;78:188-91.

20. Linn FH, Rinkel GJ, Algra A, van Gijn J. Incidence of subarachnoid hemorrhage: role of region, year, and rate of computed tomography: a meta-analysis. Stroke. 1996;27:625-9.
21. Menghini VV, Brown RD Jr., Sicks JD, et al. Incidence and prevalence of intracranial aneurysms and hemorrhage in Olmsted County, Minnesota, 1965 to 1995. Neurology. 1998;51:405-11.
22. Greenberg M. Handbook of Neurosurgery, vol 2. Lakeland, FL: Greenberg Graphics; 1997.
23. Broderick JP, Brott T, Tomsick T, et al. The risk of subarachnoid and intracerebral hemorrhages in blacks as compared with whites. N Engl J Med. 1992;326:733-6.
24. Lejeune JP, Vinchon M, Amouyel P, et al. Association of occurrence of aneurysmal bleeding with meteorologic variations in the north of France. Stroke. 1994;25:338-41.
25. van Gijn J, Rinkel GJ. Subarachnoid haemorrhage: diagnosis, causes and management. Brain. 2002;124:249-78.
26. Juvela S. Prehemorrhage risk factors for fatal intracranial aneurysm rupture. Stroke. 2003;34:1852-7.
27. Juvela S, Porras M, Poussa K. Natural history of unruptured intracranial aneurysms: probability of and risk factors for aneurysm rupture. J Neurosurg. 2000;93:379-87.
28. Tamargo RJ, Walter KA, Oshiro EM. Aneurysmal subarachnoid hemorrhage: prognostic features and outcomes. New Horiz. 1997;5:364-75.
29. Wiebers DO, Whisnant JP, Huston J 3rd, et al. Unruptured intracranial aneurysms: natural history, clinical outcome, and risks of surgical and endovascular treatment. Lancet. 2003;362:103-10.
30. Linn FH, Rinkel GJ, Algra A, van Gijn J. Headache characteristics in subarachnoid haemorrhage and benign thunderclap headache. J Neurol Neurosurg Psychiatry. 1998;65:791-3.
31. Komotar RJ, Olivi A, Rigamonti D, Tamargo RJ. Microsurgical fenestration of the lamina terminalis reduces the incidence of shunt-dependent hydrocephalus after aneurysmal subarachnoid hemorrhage. Neurosurgery. 2002;51:1403-12.
32. Cloft HJ, Joseph GJ, Dion JE. Risk of cerebral angiography in patients with subarachnoid hemorrhage, cerebral aneurysm, and arteriovenous malformation: a meta-analysis. Stroke. 1999;30:317-20.
33. Grzyska U, Freitag J, Zeumer H. Selective cerebral intraarterial DSA: complication rate and control of risk factors. Neuroradiology. 1990;32:296-99.
34. Pedersen HK, Bakke SJ, Hald JK, et al. CTA in patients with acute subarachnoid haemorrhage: a comparative study with selective, digital angiography and blinded, independent review. Acta Radiol. 2002;42:43-9.
35. Raaymakers TW, Buys PC, Verbeeten B Jr., et al. MR angiography as a screening tool for intracranial aneurysms: feasibility, test characteristics, and interobserver agreement. Am J Roentgenol. 1999;173:1469-75.
36. White PM, Wardlaw JM, Easton V. Can noninvasive imaging accurately depict intracranial aneurysms? A systematic review. Radiology. 2000;217:361-70.
37. Urbach H, Zentner J, Solymosi L. The need for repeat angiography in subarachnoid haemorrhage. Neuroradiology. 1998;40:6-10.
38. Iwanaga H, Wakai S, Ochiai C, et al. Ruptured cerebral aneurysms missed by initial angiographic study. Neurosurgery. 1990;27:45-51.
39. Hunt WE, Hess RM. Surgical risk as related to time of intervention in the repair of intracranial aneurysms. J Neurosurg. 1968;28:14-20.
40. Oshiro EM, Walter KA, Piantadosi S, et al. A new subarachnoid hemorrhage grading system based on the Glasgow Coma Scale: a comparison with the Hunt and Hess and World Federation of Neurological Surgeons Scales in a clinical series. Neurosurgery. 1997;41:140-7.
41. Suarez-Rivera O. Acute hydrocephalus after subarachnoid hemorrhage. Surg Neurol. 1998;49:563-5.
42. Hasan D, Vermeulen M, Wijdicks EF, et al. Management problems in acute hydrocephalus after subarachnoid hemorrhage. Stroke. 1989;20:747-53.

43. **Auer LM, Mokry M.** Disturbed cerebrospinal fluid circulation after subarachnoid hemorrhage and acute aneurysm surgery. Neurosurgery. 1990;26:804-8.

44. **Gjerris F, Borgesen SE, Sorensen PS, et al.** Resistance to cerebrospinal fluid outflow and intracranial pressure in patients with hydrocephalus after subarachnoid haemorrhage. Acta Neurochir (Wien). 1987;88:79-86.

45. **Grant JA, McLone DG.** Third ventriculostomy: a review. Surg Neurol. 1997;47:210-2.

46. **Joakimsen O, Mathiesen EB, Monstad P, Selseth B.** CSF hydrodynamics after subarachnoid hemorrhage. Acta Neurol Scand. 1987;75:319-27.

47. **van Gijn J, Hijdra A, Wijdicks EF, et al.** Acute hydrocephalus after aneurysmal subarachnoid hemorrhage. J Neurosurg. 1985;63:355-62.

48. **Rosenorn J, Eskesen V, Schmidt K, Ronde F.** The risk of rebleeding from ruptured intracranial aneurysms. J Neurosurg. 1987;67:329-32.

49. **Kassell NF, Torner JC.** Aneurysmal rebleeding: a preliminary report from the Cooperative Aneurysm Study. Neurosurgery. 1983;13:479-81.

50. **Clatterbuck RE, Gailloud P, Ogata L, et al.** Prevention of cerebral vasospasm by humanized anti-CD11/CD18 monoclonal antibody administered after experimental subarachnoid hemorrhage in nonhuman primates. J Neurosurg. 2003;99:376-82.

51. **Clatterbuck RE, Oshiro EM, Hoffman PA, et al.** Inhibition of vasospasm with lymphocyte function-associated antigen-1 monoclonal antibody in a femoral artery model in rats. J Neurosurg. 2002;97:676-82.

52. **Oshiro EM, Hoffman PA, Dietsch GN, et al.** Inhibition of experimental vasospasm with anti-intercellular adhesion molecule-1 monoclonal antibody in rats. Stroke. 1997;28: 2031-7.

53. **Sills AK Jr., Clatterbuck RE, Thompson RC, et al.** Endothelial cell expression of intercellular adhesion molecule 1 in experimental posthemorrhagic vasospasm. Neurosurgery. 1997;41:453-60.

54. **Thai QA, Oshiro EM, Tamargo RJ.** Inhibition of experimental vasospasm in rats with the periadventitial administration of ibuprofen using controlled-release polymers. Stroke. 1999;30:140-7.

55. **Tierney TS, Clatterbuck RE, Lawson C, et al.** Prevention and reversal of experimental posthemorrhagic vasospasm by the periadventitial administration of nitric oxide from a controlled-release polymer. Neurosurgery. 2001; 49:945-51.

56. **Voldby B, Enevoldsen EM.** Intracranial pressure changes following aneurysm rupture. Part 3: Recurrent hemorrhage. J Neurosurg. 1982;56:784-9.

57. **Butzkueven H, Evans AH, Pitman A, et al.** Onset seizures independently predict poor outcome after subarachnoid hemorrhage. Neurology. 2000;55:1315-20.

58. **Barker FG 2nd, Ogilvy CS.** Efficacy of prophylactic nimodipine for delayed ischemic deficit after subarachnoid hemorrhage: a metaanalysis. J Neurosurg. 1996;84:405-14.

59. **Auer LM.** Pial arterial vasodilation by intravenous nimodipine in cats. Arzneimittelforschung. 1981;31:1423-5.

60. **Dale J, Landmark KH, Myhre E.** The effects of nifedipine, a calcium antagonist, on platelet function. Am Heart J. 1983;105:103-5.

61. **Schanne FA, Kane AB, Young EE, Farber JL.** Calcium dependence of toxic cell death: a final common pathway. Science. 1979;206:700-2.

62. **Treggiari MM, Walder B, Suter PM, Romand JA.** Systematic review of the prevention of delayed ischemic neurological deficits with hypertension, hypervolemia, and hemodilution therapy following subarachnoid hemorrhage. J Neurosurg. 2002;98:978-84.

63. **Dorsch NW.** The effect and management of delayed vasospasm after aneurysmal subarachnoid hemorrhage. Neurol Med Chir (Tokyo). 1998;38(Suppl):156-60.

64. **Flemming KD, Brown Jr. RD, Wiebers DO.** Subarachnoid hemorrhage. Curr Treat Options Neurol. 1999;1:97-112.

65. **Kassell NF, Torner JC, Jane JA, et al.** The International Cooperative Study on the Timing of Aneurysm Surgery. Part 2: Surgical results. J Neurosurg. 1990;73:37-47.

66. **Solomon RA, Mayer SA, Tarmey JJ.** Relationship between the volume of craniotomies for cerebral aneurysm performed at New York state hospitals and in-hospital mortality. Stroke. 1996;27:13-7.

67. **Serbinenko FA.** Balloon catheterization and occlusion of major cerebral vessels. J Neurosurg. 1974;41:125-45.

68. **Guglielmi G, Vinuela F, Dion J, Duckwiler G.** Electrothrombosis of saccular aneurysms via endovascular approach. Part 2: Preliminary clinical experience. J Neurosurg. 1991;75:8-14.

69. **Guglielmi G, Vinuela F, Sepetka I, Macellari V.** Electrothrombosis of saccular aneurysms via endovascular approach. Part 1: Electrochemical basis, technique, and experimental results. J Neurosurg. 1991;75:1-7.

70. **Hopkins LN, Lanzino G, Guterman LR.** Treating complex nervous system vascular disorders through a "needle stick": origins, evolution, and future of neuroendovascular therapy. Neurosurgery. 2001;48:463-75.

71. **Lawton M, Quinones-Hinojosa A, Sanai N, et al.** Combined microsurgical and endovascular management of complex intracranial aneurysms. Neurosurgery. 2002;52:263-75.

72. **Koivisto T, Vanninen RL, Hurskainen H, et al.** Outcomes of early enovascular versus surgical treatment of ruptured cerebral aneurysms. Stroke. 2000;31:2369-77.

73. **Koivisto T, Vanninen R, Hurskainen H, et al.** Outcomes of early endovascular versus surgical treatment of ruptured cerebral aneurysms. A prospective randomized study. Stroke. 2000;31:2369-77.

74. **Molyneux A, Kerr R, Stratton I, et al.** International Subarachnoid Aneurysm Trial (ISAT) of neurosurgical clipping versus endovascular coiling in 2143 patients with ruptured intracranial aneurysms: a randomised trial. Lancet. 2002;360:1267-74.

75. **Molyneux A, Kerr R.** ISAT correspondence. Lancet. 2003;361:432.

76. **Raaymakers TW, Rinkel GJ, Limburg M, Algra A.** Mortality and morbidity of surgery for unruptured intracranial aneurysms: a meta-analysis. Stroke. 1998;29:1531-8.

77. **Houkin K, Kuroda S, Takahashi A, et al.** Intra-operative premature rupture of the cerebral aneurysms: analysis of the causes and management. Acta Neurochir (Wien). 1999;141:1255-63.

78. **Lin CL, Kwan AL, Howng SL.** Surgical outcome of anterior communicating artery aneurysms. Kaohsiung J Med Sci. 1998;14:561-8.

Chapter 18

Effect of Oral Contraceptives and Hormone Replacement on Stroke Risk in Women

IRENE CORTESE, MD
LOUISE D. McCULLOUGH, MD, PhD

Stroke and Oral Contraceptives in the Pre-Menopausal Woman

Oral contraceptives (OC) are used by more than 10 million women in the United States and by more than 78.5 million women worldwide. Since their introduction in 1960, there have been concerns regarding their safety (1). The first report of thrombosis associated with OC use was a case of pulmonary embolism in 1961. Seven years later, an association between OC use and ischemic stroke was published, and an association between OC and hemorrhagic stroke followed in 1973 (2,3).

Estrogens have a variety of different effects on coagulation, including increasing levels of procoagulant factors VII, X, XII, and XIII and reducing the anticoagulant factors protein S and antithrombin. This leads to a relative hypercoagulable state, whose varied expression in the population may be due to genetic predisposition. OCs do not appear to have atherogenic properties; this is supported by the absence of increased risk of stroke in former OC users (3).

Most OCs contain an estrogen and a progestin. The first oral contraceptive available in the United States contained 250 µg of estrogen. Since then, the estrogen dose has been progressively reduced, first to 50 µg, then to 30–35 µg; some currently available brands contain only 12-20 µg of ethinyl estradiol. Modifications have also been made in the progestin content of OCs. The different progestin molecules contained in OCs are grouped into "generations" based on when they were first produced. Early OCs contained a first-generation progestin, including norethisterone, norethynodrel, lynestrenol, and thynodiol acetate. In the 1970s, the second generation was introduced, including norgestrel, levonorgestrel, and norgestrione. Third-generation progestins, including desogestrel, gesto-dene, and norgestimate, were introduced in the early 1980s in Europe and the 1990s in the United States (3).

While numerous studies have investigated the associations between OC use and stroke, these case-control or cohort epidemiological studies contain unavoidable bias. Early studies examined first-generation OCs containing high doses of estradiol; these showed a significant increase in risk of stroke (1,4). Recently, seven large case-control studies comparing over 3000 women with stroke with nearly 10,000 controls have helped define the risk according to stroke subtype and OC generation (5). Two of these studies were done in the United States. These studies showed that there is a risk for stroke associated with OC use, which is clearly dependent on the estrogen dose. With high-dose preparations, the risk was significant, with an OR between 2 and 4. With the low-dose preparations most commonly used today, the majority of studies showed very low risk of stroke. The two US studies in fact did not show any increased risk of stroke with low-dose OC (2). Of interest, a non-significant increased risk of stroke with low-dose estrogen preparations has been observed in Europe, whereas in developing countries (Africa, Asia, Latin America) there seems to be a significant three-fold increased risk of ischemic stroke associated with use of low-dose estrogen preparations. It is possible that differences in prevalence of associated risk factors, such as smoking and hypertension, are responsible for these differences (5). A recent study from Australia mirrors the US results, with no increase in ischemic stroke with low-dose OC use. Surprisingly, in this study there was no evidence that smoking or hypertension increased the risk of stroke in current OC users. Hypertension, cigarette smoking, diabetes, and a positive family history were all associated with increased stroke risk independently of OC use (6). Most studies do not show increased risk of intracerebral hemorrhage (ICH) among OC users. Only in developing countries has a dose-dependent risk of ICH been described (5).

Cerebral venous sinus thrombosis (CVST) is a rare, potentially under-diagnosed cause of ischemic and hemorrhagic strokes. Although OC use does appear to be significantly associated with CVST, with a RR as high as 15.9 (95% CI, 6.98-36.2), very few studies have been done to investigate this (1). What does appear clear, however, is that the proportion of OC users among patients with CVST is highly variable from country to country. In poorer countries where puerperium and infections remain the major causes of CVST, and where OC use is typically limited, the percentage of OC users among patients with CVST is low. On the other hand, it is very high, reaching over 90%, in rich countries in which aseptic CVST predominates and postpartum CVST has decreased in frequency. Usually, OC use is not the only risk factor identified in the single patient. In fact, the percent of women with CVST who have OC use as their only risk factor is dramatically lower (10%). Association of congenital thrombophilia (i.e., factor

V Leiden and prothrombin 20210A gene mutation) and OC use can greatly increase this risk; the estimated relative risk for CVST in OC users increases six-fold in the presence of the prothrombin gene mutation (5).

Results regarding risk of ischemic stroke with preparations containing different progestins are conflicting. Some studies have reported an increased risk with second-generation progestins, whereas others have found higher risk with third-generation preparations. Yet others have shown no difference in stroke risk between different OC generations (5,7,8).

Associations between OC use and other stroke risk factors have also been explored. The two US studies addressing stroke risk among current users of low-dose OC showed that ischemic and hemorrhagic stroke were more likely in African American women and less likely in Asians. Patients were more likely to be receiving treatment for hypertension, to be current cigarette smokers, obese, and diabetic. Ischemic stroke patients were more likely to have a history of migraine compared with controls (2). The relationships between OCs and hypertension are complex because all OCs induce a small but significant increase in mean blood pressure, which may influence stroke risk. The association of smoking and OC use led to a three-fold increase in risk of ICH and five- to seven-fold increase in risk of ischemic stroke (5).

Migraine was first implicated as an independent risk factor for stroke in 1975. Subsequently numerous studies have confirmed an increased risk of stroke in migraineurs, which appears greater in women and greater in migraine with aura. Regardless of personal history, even a family history of migraine was associated with increased risk of ischemic stroke.

There are an estimated 11 million people in the United States with migraine. Given this high prevalence, up to one third of persons with stroke would be expected to have a history of migraine. Independent of this, however, there are a number of hereditary disorders in which migraine and stroke are both prominent clinical features, including mitochondrial encepahlopathy with lactic acidosis and stroke (MELAS) and cerebral autosomal dominant arteriopathy with subcortical infarcts and leukoencephalopathy (CADASIL). Migrainous infarction, in which the migraine itself evolves into a stroke, has been implicated in up to 20% of strokes in women under the age of 45. The pathogenic mechanism is unclear; however, vasospasm, prolonged cortical spreading depression with oligemia, and in situ thrombosis related to hypercoagulability have all been postulated (9).

The use of OC in migraineurs has been estimated to increase the expected number of strokes per 100,000 women by up to 10 for those with migraine without aura and by up to 20 for those with migraine with aura. This risk is dependent on the estrogen dose, with an OR of 16.9 for high-dose preparations and 6.6 for low-dose formulations. The addition of smoking leads to a dramatic increase in the relative risk to 34.4 (9).

There is general agreement that although there may be a small risk of increased stroke associated with OC use, the contraceptive and non-contraceptive benefits of their use far outweigh their risk. Based on background incidence rates, the absolute risk of stroke in OC users is low. It has been estimated at 6.7 per 100,000 women per year in users of low-dose OCs, and 12.9 in users of high-dose OCs. Women under the age of 35 would have an even lower attributable risk of about 1 in 200,000. Studies indicate that association of OC use with other stroke risk factors, such as increased age, smoking, and hypertension, may lead to greater risk of stroke, and it is reasonable that these remain a relative contraindication to even low-dose OC use (1,2,5).

Current recommendations of the International Headache Society Task Force on Combined Oral Contraceptives and HRT in women with migraine suggest that there is no contraindication for use of OC in women with migraine in absence of aura or other risk factors. There is a potential of increased risk of ischemic stroke in women with migraine who are using OCs and have additional risk factors, which cannot be easily controlled, including migraine with aura. It is not considered generally necessary or cost effective to screen women for thrombophilia before initiating treatment with OCs in absence of a family history of such. In addition, aspirin has not been studied in this setting and therefore its role, if any, in primary prevention of stroke in OC users with or without other stroke risk factors is not known (10).

Observational studies suggest that progesterone-only formulations are not associated with increased risk of ischemic stroke, although quantifiable data are limited; these should be considered in women who are at increased risk for ischemic stroke, including women with migraine with aura (11). At this point, it appears that women who use OCs with low estrogen concentrations are at a minimal increased risk for ischemic stroke (odd ratio, 2) compared with older formulations. Certainly, cautious use in women with other ischemic stroke risk factors such as smoking, hypertension, and diabetes is reasonable, and alternative methods of contraception should be considered, although ischemic stroke in the premenopausal woman remains a rare event.

Stroke and Hormone Replacement Therapy in the Post-Menopausal Woman

Pre-menopausal women have lower rates of stroke and vascular disease than age-matched men and post-menopausal women, a finding attributed to the higher endogenous estrogen levels in young women. By the year 2015, almost 50% of the women in the United States will be over 45 years old and at increasing risk for stroke with its associated disability. Because most strokes occur in post-menopausal women, there is great interest in determining the role of hormone replacement therapy in preventing or reducing cerebrovascular disease.

Over the past 30 years, most cohort, retrospective, and prospective observational studies have demonstrated significant reductions in coronary heart disease (CHD) in postmenopausal women taking estrogen or combined estrogen-progestin therapy (i.e., hormone replacement therapy [HRT]) (12,13). Observational reports for cerebrovascular disease (CVD) were not as clearly positive, but most studies show no increase in risk from HRT (13). Over the past decade, several major randomized clinical trials have been completed that address the role of HRT in both primary and secondary prevention of heart disease and stroke. All trials to date have shown either no effect or, more recently with the Women's Health Initiative (WHI), a negative effect on stroke incidence with hormone treatment.

The Heart and Estrogen-Progestin Replacement Study (HERS) was the first randomized, blinded trial on the effect of HRT (0.625 mg estrogen + 2.5 mg medroxyprogesterone acetate [MPA], daily) on coronary disease progression. After 4 years of HRT therapy, HERS found no reduction in risk for coronary events, stroke, or transient ischemic attack (TIA) but did observe a three-fold increase in venous thromboembolism (14). An important observation was that patients receiving HRT sustained an early increased risk of cardiovascular events that was offset by a lower event rate in subsequent years. It was presumed that this was due to an early pro-thrombotic risk, followed later by protection, and that prolonged follow-up would demonstrate an overall beneficial effect for HRT. However, the release of the 6.8-year follow-up on the HERS cohort (HERS II) in 2002 (15) showed no benefit of prolonged HRT treatment on cardiovascular or cerebrovascular endpoints.

The HERS study was designed to investigate the effects of HRT on coronary disease; stroke and TIA were secondary endpoints. In contrast, the Women's Estrogen for Stroke Trial (WEST) was the first randomized trial designed to examine stroke recurrence as the primary endpoint (16). WEST found no benefit on total stroke incidence and a surprising increase in fatal stroke among women who were assigned to unopposed estradiol therapy. Additionally, nonfatal strokes that occurred in estrogen-treated women were associated with worse neurologic and functional deficits than strokes occurring in the placebo group. This suggests that estrogen increases both the incidence of stroke and damage from stroke once ischemia occurs. The results above led to the recommendation that HRT/ERT should not be prescribed for preventing cerebrovascular disease.

The unexpected findings of the secondary prevention trials are not easily aligned with earlier epidemiological data, suggesting a beneficial effect of estrogen on vascular disease. However, it is important to note that both the HERS trial and the WEST trial enrolled women with known vascular disease who were years past menopause; it was then postulated that estrogen, as in animal models, cannot salvage vessels that have already been damaged by atherosclerosis. The WHI, which is a large randomized trial of primary prevention of stroke and vascular disease (among other endpoints), was designed to address this question.

The NIH-sponsored WHI was the first large randomized trial of primary prevention of stroke and vascular disease among healthy hormone users (WHI Writing Group). In one arm, women with a prior hysterectomy were randomized to receive either conjugated equine estrogen (CEE, 0.625 mg/day/ERT arm) treatment or placebo. A second arm examined women with an intact uterus randomized to either placebo or combined estrogen plus progestin (HRT, MPA) in acknowledgment of the increased risk of endometrial cancer with unopposed estrogen therapy. The combined HRT trial was terminated 3 years early based on recommendations by the WHI Data and Safety Monitoring Board (DSMB). HRT-treated patients had a higher incidence of both invasive breast cancer and stroke and an overall negative effect on health, including increases in cardiovascular events and pulmonary embolism. Although the overall risk of stroke was small (8 more strokes per year for every 10,000 women in the HRT group), the overall outcome was clearly negative and the trial was stopped (17). In further follow-up (5.6 years) of the HRT cohort, there have been 151 strokes in the HRT group (1.8%) vs. 107 strokes (1.3%) in the placebo group; most were ischemic strokes. Women receiving HRT sustained a 31% increased risk of stroke compared with placebo-treated women; this risk was unrelated to interactions with other risk factors, such as hypertension, diabetes, or age (18). Risk was largely evident after year one, reinforcing the concept that short-term HRT for relief of postmenopausal symptoms of vasomotor instability remains low risk in healthy women.

In April 2004, the estrogen-alone arm of the WHI (total subjects, 10,739) was also stopped. After an average follow-up of 6.8 years (planned duration 8.5 years), there was an absolute excess risk of 12 additional strokes per 10,000 person-years in estrogen-treated women (19). Although active treatment produced relief from vasomotor symptoms, oral CEE did not have a clinically meaningful effect on the health-related quality of life. The results of the WHI have led to the current recommendation from the American Heart Association and the FDA that "HRT and ERT should neither be initiated nor continued for prevention or treatment of heart disease or stroke." If replacement therapy is prescribed for post-menopausal symptoms, the lowest effective dose should be used for the shortest possible time to alleviate symptoms.

The results of the WHI were quite unexpected and seem to be in direct contrast to previous large epidemiological studies. Several explanations have been suggested for this dichotomy. In the WHI, although women had no prior history of clinical CVD, because the trial was oriented toward primary prevention, 7.7% of women participants in the WHI had documented vascular disease. Furthermore, many women were enrolled despite relative contraindications to HRT, such as smoking, previous stroke, or venous thromboembolism (17). Women in the WHI trials were, on average, older, more frequently diabetic, obese, and more likely to smoke than women using hormone therapy in the prior observational studies. Most women who took HRT in observational studies began it early in the menopause for control of estrogen-deficiency symptoms (at an average age of 51), whereas in the WHI, HRT was started an average of 12 years after menopause (mean age, 63 years). Less than one third of WHI participants were between the ages of 50 and 59, and women within a year of menopause were excluded (17,20).

Substantial data demonstrate protective effects of estrogen on the vasculature before vascular damage occurs, whereas adverse effects seem to predominate once atherosclerosis is well established (20). In surgically postmenopausal monkeys fed atherogenic diets, coronary atherosclerosis is delayed only if treatment is started immediately after ovariectomy (21,22), suggesting that estrogen's atheroprotective effects are lost with prolonged estrogen deficiency. In areas of atherosclerosis, estrogen seems to promote thrombosis and inflammation, especially if used at supraphysiological doses. These detrimental effects were seen in the Nurses' Health Study; high doses of CEE were less protective against vascular disease and actually increased stroke risk (23). The pro-inflammatory effects of estrogen were well documented in a recent trial examining the effects of treatment on C-reactive protein (CRP), an inflammatory marker associated with increased risk for cardiovascular disease. Healthy women over age 65 were randomized to one of three doses (0.25, 0.5, and 1 mg/day) of 17 beta-estradiol (E2) or placebo. After 12 weeks of treatment, CRP decreased 59% in the 0.25 mg/day E2 group and increased 65% in the 1 mg/day E2 group compared with placebo. The CRP level continued to be elevated (92%) in the 1 mg/day E2 group, even 12 weeks after treatment was discontinued (24).

Oral estrogen is metabolized by the liver and has numerous effects on clotting mechanisms, producing a relative hypercoagulable state. These effects account for the increase in venous thromboembolism seen with treatment in previous trials (HERS). Transdermal E2 does not appear to have these adverse effects (25,26), and CRP levels in patients treated with transdermal formulations were similar to untreated women.

In response to these concerns, the Kronos Early Estrogen Prevention Study (KEEPS) was designed. This trial is a randomized, controlled multicenter trial of HRT in recently menopausal women utilizing oral or transdermal estrogen with intermittent micronized progesterone. Women will be followed for a 5-year period, with common carotid intimal medial thickness (IMT) by B-mode ultrasound as its primary end point (20). Because HRT/ERT may convert from anti-atherogenic to proatherogenic in a diseased vessel, initiation of therapy at an earlier stage of atherosclerosis in women with shorter durations of estrogen deficiency should optimize the beneficial effects of ERT/HRT.

Although combined estrogen/progestin compounds are the most commonly prescribed hormone regimen in the United States, it is not known whether progestins interact with estrogen and diminish its neuroprotective effects. Experimental data suggest that progesterone increases subcortical damage after vascular occlusion in animals (27) and can reverse the beneficial effect seen on atherosclerotic plaque formation in nonhuman primates (21,22). However, clinical results argue against this hypothesis. The Estrogen Replacement and Atherosclerosis (ERA) trial utilized estrogen with or without a progestin and found no benefit in coronary disease progression as measured angiographically in either treatment group (28). Results from the Estrogen in the Prevention of Re-Infarction Trial (29) demonstrate that estradiol valerate did not reduce risk of recurrent myocardial infarction. Furthermore, the WEST did not demonstrate a beneficial effect of 17 beta-estradiol for secondary prevention of stroke and ischemic injury. The WHI convincingly shows that there is no benefit of HRT or ERT for primary stroke prevention. However, the women in these trials were estrogen deficient for prolonged periods prior to enrollment. Until the results of studies designed to mirror how HRT is used clinically and in previous observational studies (at the peri-menopause) are available, the debate of HRT and stroke risk continues.

Estrogen Receptors and Vascular Disease

One mechanism potentially attenuating the beneficial effects of estrogen is loss of arterial estrogen receptors (ER). Loss of the ER occurs with aging and is more prominent in atherosclerotic vessels (30-32). Population-based studies have shown an increased risk of myocardial infarction (MI) in postmenopausal women who carry ESR1 haplotype 1 (c.454-397 T allele and c.454-351 A allele: T genotype). Heterozygous carriers had a 2.23 times increased risk compared with noncarriers, whereas homozygous carriers had a 2.48 times increased risk (33). In the presence of a decreased number of alpha estrogen receptors that occurs in aging and diseased vessels, estrogen signaling may be less effective and, therefore, estrogen actions decreased. Interestingly, in males, homozygosity for the ESR1 c.454-397C allele (CC genotype) was associated with a three-fold greater risk of MI compared with those with the CT or TT genotype (34). The T allele, which increased MI risk in women, prevented heart disease in men. These striking gender differences demonstrate a level of complexity in gene/drug interactions that was previously unrecognized. These genetic polymorphisms have clear significance for stroke researchers as well. Recently, males carrying the CC genotype were found to have a 1.9-fold increase in stroke risk compared with men with the CT or TT genotype, even after adjustment for age, serum cholesterol, hypertension, diabetes, body mass index, and smoking status (35).

The effect of the menopause and HRT on ESR1 gene polymorphisms and vascular risk is not yet known. It is likely that changes in estrogen levels that occur at menopause interact with ESR1 genotype. Significant interactions between ESR1 and environmental risk factors clearly contribute to vascular risk. Women who smoked and carried the TT genotype have a >1.7-fold higher level of atherogenic LDL particles than women with the alternative genotypes. A dose-dependent effect of smoking was evident in both pre-menopausal and postmenopausal women (35,36), but the presence of the TT genotype was associated with a much larger increase in LDL in post-menopausal women on HRT. The differential responsiveness of women with the T allele to additional environmental insults could help explain the increased risk of MI and stroke in HRT trials.

The discrepancy between observational studies, pre-clinical data, and large randomized clinical trials emphasizes the need for further study of the mechanisms leading to the increased stroke incidence observed in post-menopausal women. The widening gap between clinical trial results and experimental laboratory-based data would suggest that our understanding of the cerebral ischemic pathophysiology and of estrogen's role as a cere-broprotectant is incomplete. Previously unrecognized genetic polymor-phisms and interaction with other environmental factors such as smoking demonstrates the importance of understanding the basic mechanism of estrogen's actions in the brain and vasculature. Because the largest burden for stroke is in post-menopausal women, there is great and continued inter-est in HRT as a means of preventing or treating cerebrovascular disease.

Conclusion

The guidelines for treatment of women with post-menopausal hormone therapy have changed dramatically since the release of the HERS, WEST, and WHI trials. Data clearly demonstrate that estrogen replacement either with or without a progestin increases stroke risk. Although the absolute increase in risk from ERT/HRT is small, it is significant. There is no role for ERT/HRT in the primary or secondary prevention of cerebrovascular dis-ease as currently prescribed. However, it is important to recognize the lim-itations of these clinical trials. HRT/ERT administration was begun well after menopause, which is quite different from how these therapies are utilized in clinical practice. But until data are available that demonstrate a protec-tive effect of HRT/ERT on stroke, women treated with HRT for menopausal symptoms should use the lowest effective dose, for the shortest possible duration. Women currently on HRT/ERT should be cautioned of the increased risk of stroke. Therapy should be withdrawn, especially in women with known vascular disease or at high risk for stroke until data are available showing efficacy of treatment. Younger women (especially non-smokers under age 35) have no excess risk from low-dose oral contraceptives. Oral contraceptives are generally considered to be safe and effective. Oral con-traceptives should be used with caution in older women, especially if they are smokers or have a history of complex migraine, although the risk remains quite small. Increasing attention to gender differences in clinical medicine will enhance our ability to treat patients of both sexes.

REFERENCES

1. **Gillum LA, Mamidipudi SK, Johnston SC.** Ischemic stroke risk with oral contraceptives: a meta-analysis. JAMA. 2000;284:72-8.
2. **Schwartz SM, Petitti DB, Siscovick DS, et al.** Stroke and use of low-dose oral contraceptives in young women: a pooled analsis of two US studies. Stroke. 1998;29:2277-84.
3. **Rosendaal FR, Helmerhorst FM, Vandenbroucke JP.** Female hormones and thrombosis. Arterioscler Thromb Vasc Biol. 2001;22:201-10.
4. **Leys D, Deplanque D, Mounier-Vehier C, et al.** Stroke prevention: management of modifiable vascular risk factors. J Neurol. 2002;249:507-17.
5. **Bousser MG, Kittner SJ.** Oral contraceptives and stroke. Cephalalgia. 2000;20:183-9.
6. **Siritho S, Thrift AG, McNeil JJ, et al.** Risk of ischemic stroke among users of the oral contraceptive pill. The Melbourne Risk Factor Study (MERFS) Group. Stroke. 2003; 34:1575-80.
7. **Lidegaard O, Kreiner S.** Contraceptives and cerebral thrombosis: a five-year national case-control study. Contraception. 2002;65:197-205.
8. **Kemmeren JM, Tanin BC, van den Bosch MA, et al.** Risk of arterial thrombosis in relation to oral contraceptives (RATIO) study: oral contraceptives and the risk of ischemic stroke. Stroke. 2002;33:1202-8.
9. **Tietjen GE.** The relationship of migraine and stroke. Neuroepidemiology. 2000;19:13-9.
10. **Bousser MG, Conrad J, Kittner S, et al.** Recommendations on the risk of ischaemic stroke associated with use of combined oral contraceptives and hormone replacement therapy in women with migraine. Cephalalgia. 2000;20:155-6.
11. **Silberstein S.** Headache and female hormones: what you need to know. Curr Opin Neurol. 2001;14:323-33.
12. **Langer RD.** Hormone replacement and the prevention of cardiovascular disease. Am J Cardiol. 2002;89(Suppl):36E-46E.
13. **Paganini-Hill A.** Hormone replacement therapy and stroke: risk, protection or no effect? Maturitas. 2001;38:243-61.
14. **Hulley S, Grady D, Bush T, et al.** Randomized trial of estrogen plus progestin for secondary prevention of coronary heart disease in postmenopausal women. Heart and Estrogen/Progestin Replacement Study (HERS) Research Group. JAMA. 1998;280:605-13.
15. **Grady D, Herrington D, Bittner V, et al.** Cardiovascular disease outcomes during 6.8 years of hormone therapy: Heart and Estrogen/progestin Replacement Study follow-up (HERS II). JAMA. 2002;288:49-57.
16. **Viscoli CM, Brass LM, Kernan WN, et al.** A clinical trial of estrogen-replacement therapy after ischemic stroke. N Engl J Med. 2001;345:1243-9.
17. **Writing Group for the Women's Health Initiative Investigators.** Risks and benefits of estrogen plus progestin in healthy postmenopausal women: principal results from the Women's Health Initiative randomized controlled trial. JAMA. 2002;288:321-33.
18. **Wassertheil-Smoller S, Hendrix SL, Limacher M, et al.** Effect of estrogen plus progestin on stroke in postmenopausal women: the Women's Health Initiative: a randomized trial. JAMA. 2003;289:2673-84.
19. **Anderson GL, Limacher M, Assaf AR, et al.** Women's Health Initiative Steering Committee. Effects of conjugated equine estrogen in postmenopausal women with hysterectomy: the Women's Health Initiative randomized controlled trial. JAMA. 2004;291:1701-12.
20. **Harman SM, Brinton EA, Cedars M, et al.** KEEPS: The Kronos Early Estrogen Prevention Study. Climacteric. 2005;8:3-12.

21. **Adams MR**. Medroxyprogesterone acetate antagonizes inhibitory effects of conjugated equine estrogens on coronary artery atherosclerosis. Arterioscler Thromb Vasc Biol. 1997;17:217-21.

22. **Williams JK, Manson JE, Colditz GA, et al**. Effects of hormone replacement therapy on reactivity of atherosclerotic coronary arteries in cynomolgus monkeys. J Am Coll Cardiol. 1994;24:1757-61.

23. **Grodstein F, Manson JE, Colditz GA, et al**. A prospective, observational study of postmenopausal hormone therapy and primary prevention of cardiovascular disease. Ann Intern Med. 2000;133:933-41.

24. **Prestwood KM, Unson C, Kulldorff M, et al**. The effect of different doses of micronized 17-beta-estradiol on C-reactive protein, interleukin-6, and lipids in older women. J Gerontol A Biol Sci Med Sci. 2004;59:827-32.

25. **Scarabin PY, Alhenc-Gelas M, Plu-Bureau G, et al**. Effects of oral and transdermal estrogen/progesterone regimens on blood coagulation and fibrinolysis in postmenopausal women: a randomized controlled trial. Arterioscler Thromb Vasc Biol. 1997;17: 3071-8.

26. **Alkjaersig N, Fletcher PD, de Ziegler D, et al**. Blood coagulation in postmenopausal women given estrogen treatment: comparison of transdermal and oral administration. J Lab Clin Med. 1997;111:224-8.

27. **Murphy SJ, Traystman RJ, Hum PD, et al**. Progesterone exacerbates striatal stroke injury in progesterone-deficient female animals. Stroke. 2000;31:1173-8.

28. **Herrington DM**. Effects of estrogen replacement on the progression of coronary-artery atherosclerosis. N Engl J Med. 2000;343:522-9.

29. **Cherry N**. Oestrogen therapy for prevention of reinfarction in postmenopausal women: a randomised placebo controlled trial, The ESPRIT Team. Lancet. 2002;360:2001-8.

30. **Losordo DW**. Variable expression of the estrogen receptor in normal and atherosclerotic coronary arteries of premenopausal women. Circulation. 1994;89:1501-10

31. **Post WS, Goldschmidt-Clement PJ, Wilhide CC, et al**. Methylation of the estrogen receptor gene is associated with aging and atherosclerosis in the cardiovascular system. Cardiovasc Res. 1999;43:985-91.

32. **Koivu TA, Fan YM, Matillas KH, et al**. The effect of hormone replacement therapy on atherosclerotic severity in relation to ESR1 genotype in postmenopausal women. Maturitas. 2003;44:29-38.

33. **Schuit SC, Oei HH, Witteman JC, et al**. Estrogen receptor alpha gene polymorphisms and risk of myocardial infarction. JAMA. 2004;291:2969-77.

34. **Shearman AM, Cupples LA, Demissie S, et al**. Association between estrogen receptor alpha gene variation and cardiovascular disease. J Am Med Assoc. 2003;290:2263-70.

35. **Shearman AM, Cooper JA, Kotwinski PJ, et al**. Estrogen receptor alpha gene variation and the risk of stroke. Stroke. 2005;36:2281-2.

36. **Demissie S, Cupples LA, Shearman AM, et al**. Estrogen receptor-alpha variants are associated with lipoprotein size distribution and particle levels in women. The Framingham Heart Study. Atherosclerosis. 2006;185:210-8.

Index

W